MW00344549

Addicts Who Survived

Addicts Who Survived

An Oral History of Narcotic Use in America before 1965

David Courtwright
Herman Joseph
Don Des Jarlais

With a new Epilogue

The University of Tennessee Press/Knoxville

Copyright © 1989 under the title *Addicts Who Survived: An Oral History of Narcotic Use in America, 1923–1965,* by The University of Tennessee Press, Knoxville. All Rights Reserved. Manufactured in the United States of America.
Cloth: 1st printing, 1989.
Paper: 1st printing, 2012.

Courtwright, David.
    Addicts who survived : an oral history of narcotic use in America before 1965 / David Courtwright, Herman Joseph, and Don Des Jarlais ; with a foreword by Claude Brown.
    p. cm.
    Bibliography: p.
    Includes index.
    1. Narcotic addicts—United Sates—Biography.
    2. Drug abuse—United States—History—20th century.
    3. Narcotics, Control of—United States—History—20th century.
    4. Methadone maintenance—United States—History—20th century.
    5. Narcotic addicts—New York (N.Y.)—Biography.
    I. Joseph, Herma, 1931–   .
    II. Des Jarlais, Don, 1945–   .
    III. Title.
HV5825.C68 1989
362.2'93'0922—dc 19   88-20583
    CIP

To Betty and Bob Courtwright
and to Lottie and Max Joseph
and to Mary Ellen and Robert Des Jarlais
and to the memory of Marie Nyswander

Contents

Illustrations

Smuggling Techniques
Arnold Rothstein
Louis "Lepke" Buchalter
Lucky Luciano
Making a Buy
The Hard Line
Lexington
Dr. and Mrs. Willis P. Butler
Drs. Vincent Dole and Marie Nyswander

TABLES

FIGURES

Foreword to the 1989 Edition

Surprisingly, *Addicts Who Survived* is a tome to which the banal books' blurb writers' adjective "riveting" deservedly applies. In fact the book is fascinatingly informative from the first paragraph of the introduction, and becomes increasingly spellbinding as the reader progresses through the text, encountering one unique real-life character after another. These people were remarkable survivors and their narratives are a priceless legacy.

Addicts Who Survived focuses primarily on what its authors have labeled the "classic period" of narcotic control—1923–65. Never before has the drug subculture of this time been described in such intimate detail. Unusual insights into the economic survival measures and strategies (hustling techniques) of the addicts provide interesting reading for the general public and a bonanza of specialized information for researchers.

This book has been very sensitively edited; there are no negative characterizations of the narrators or implications of their belonging to a subculture of reprobates. Nor is there anything in these pages that will elicit pity for any of the narrators; compassion, perhaps, but there is certainly nothing pathetic about any of them. The raconteurs of these memoirs are a unique group of individuals. The mere fact that many of them lived to become septuagenarians and octogenarians attests to their exceptional survival skills, above-average intelligence and amazing self-discipline—very few opiate addicts live so long . . . especially in the United States.

These narrators were proud addicts, not junkies. They draw a lucid distinction between themselves and ordinary junkies or subordinary dope fiends. Respectable and self-respecting addicts sound like patently contradictory terms, but that is what they were. These addicts took pride in their appearances. They ate properly, maintained their physical health, worked regularly and dependably at legal employment (some of them) and were often responsible parents, spouses, and family providers. They would seldom use more drugs than was required for them to feel "good," which was usually synonymous with normal.

The survivors were the elite addicts; they knew how to be addicted with class. Many of the narrators were, at various stages of their lives, engaged in petty criminal activity to support their addictions, but not even those individuals can be perceived as criminals in any conventional sense of the term. They are presented, or construed by an objective reader, as an ordinary group of people endowed with extraordinary vitality and mental vigor for coping with an intensely demoralizing and physically corrosive socio-medical affliction. These memoirs will certainly be of instructive value to scholars, bureaucrats, law enforcement agents, lawyers, judges, and all persons whose professions necessitate a more-than-casual comprehension of apparently antisocial behavior in opiate addicts. Through these personal histories, the reader can understand why an addict who sells drugs to help support his habit is no more a drug dealer than an indigent diabetic who steals insulin to stay alive is a thief.

An enormous amount of meticulous work went into the compilation and editing of *Addicts Who Survived*. The gathering of material was astutely planned and fastidiously conducted; the editors also implemented precautions to minimize fabrications, deceptions, and inaccurate recollections. Consequently, this book is probably the most honest and authoritative account of its subject matter obtainable today.

The introduction to *Addicts Who Survived* is in itself a minor treasure of American social history. It clearly presents the social conditions and attitudes that produced the initial and subsequent antinarcotic legislation and provides an honest and accurate account of the social and political background of drug control. It also reveals as much about the moral corruption and hypocrisy of America's legislative and administrative policy makers as it does about the illegal narcotics community. These disclosures point to the conclusion that practically all of the antinarcotic legislation and administrative decrees were rooted in prejudice or were responses to an extremely successful campaign to create public hysteria. At the very least, the revelations contained in the introduction, accompanied by an awareness of continued persecution of contemporary narcotic addicts, demand an immediate reappraisal and revamping of our country's narcotic laws, to render them compatible with and remedial for the anguished human condition of late twentieth- and early twenty-first century America.

The introduction also emphasizes and validates the postulate that increased narcotics usage by ethnic or racial minorities, especially by blacks, is a social problem that accompanied urbanization. Widespread narcotic use and abuse was and is more of a slum phenomenon than an ethnic trait or indulgence. As the ethnicity of the American slum dweller changed over the past ninety years, so did the ethnicity of the vast majority of drug users. Of course, there are several other factors contributing to the devastating blight of illicit drug abuse, such as the absence of a strong family bond, a religious foundation, a sense of personal dignity, etc. These con-ditions, however, are of considerably less significance than those related to urban migration.

The postwar period saw the renaissance of the American Mafia as well as the proliferation of black heroin addicts. Paradoxically, this country inadvertently facilitated the expansion and prosperity of organized crime through the enactment of increasingly harsh antinarcotic laws. Although it is neither specifically stated nor implied by either the narrators or the editors, *Addicts Who Survived* makes it evident that antinarcotic legislation has been as beneficial to organized crime as was Prohibition.

Reading this book made me wish that the addicts I've seen during the past three decades agonizing through their torturous affliction had been fortunate enough (if opiate addiction was their inevitable destiny) to have lived in America prior to the "classic period." This was an era when narcotic regulation had not yet evolved into oppression. The sad irony of the history of narcotic control is that, as the laws become progressively more punitive, even Draconian, they were conspicuously less effective.

The current AIDS epidemic and its alarming mortality demand new legislation to cope with the modern complexities and social perils emanating from the illicit narcotics community. These laws will have to be promulgated, not by self-righteous zealots, but by knowledgable and sensitive legislators who thoroughly understand the gravity of the current American drug crisis and its horrendous ramifications.

There are a minimum of 500,000 heroin addicts in America today. By sharing hypodermic needles, these addicts spread AIDS. New York City statistics show that 53 percent of AIDS-related deaths occur among intravenous narcotics users, a higher percentage of AIDS-related deaths than those attributed to gay and bisexual activity. In November of 1987, one of every sixty-one mothers of infants born in the state of New York tested positive for AIDS antibodies. These appalling statistics support the implied thesis of *Addicts Who Survived*: America needs a sane, compassionate, and humane national narcotic policy as soon as possible.

CLAUDE BROWN

Acknowledgments

We are indebted, first, to the New York State Division of Substance Abuse Services, whose cooperation and sponsorship made this undertaking possible. A National Endowment for the Humanities fellowship greatly assisted the principal author in the initial stages of preparing this book. Further support in the form of travel assistance came from the Department of Community Medicine and Health Care of the University of Connecticut Health Center. At the University of Hartford Blaise Lamphier indexed many of the tapes, Paul Zocco assisted with the illustrations, and Carol Roark and Carolyn Moore did most of the typing. Ann Spitzer, Gertrude Litzsky, Barry Grant, and the late Klaus Fischer provided and helped maintain our recording equipment. Librarians Ann Maio, Jean Prescott, John Mittnacht, and Mary Ann Nesto assisted with many reference questions; Shelby Miller, Terry Parssinen, Tom Grant, and Bruce Stephenson helped in reading over the manuscript. John Boile, the Drug Enforcement Administration's staff photographer, provided invaluable assistance in locating photographs, the reproduction of which was subsidized by a Coffin Grant from the University of Hartford. We are grateful to Claude Brown for contributing his views and insights, and to Cynthia Maude-Gembler, Lee Campbell Sioles, Sheila Hart, and Scot Danforth at the University of Tennessee Press. We also wish to thank the directors and staff of the several New York methadone programs and therapeutic communities who participated in this project and, above all, the addicts, former addicts, physicians, and administrators who gave so generously of their time and memories.

Alphabetical Table of Narratives

Narrator	Chapter(s)	Year Recorded
Al	3, 6	1980
Amparo	9	1980
Ann	10	1981
Arthur	4, 6, 11	1980
Brenda	1, 5, 13	1980
Burroughs, William S.	10	1981
Butler, Willis	12	1978
Charlie	8, 13	1980
Curtis	8	1981
Dole, Vincent	14	1982
Dusty	4	1980
Eddie	5	1980
Emanon	9	1981
Emily	3, 6	1980
Frieda	3	1980
Hubbard, S. Dana	12	—
Ivory	2	1980
Jack	4	1980
Janet	9	1980
Jerry	14	1980
John	5, 6	1980
Lao Pai-hsing	3	1980
Li	9	1980
Lotty	3, 7	1980
Low	9	1981

May	7	1980
Mel	3, 6	1980
Mick	2, 11	1980
Mike	5	1980
Nyswander, Marie	13	1981
O'Brien, William B.	13	1981
Otha	10	1980
Red	10, 14	1980
Salerno, Ralph	8	1982
Sam	2, 14	1980
Sophia	7	1980
Stick	1, 11	1981
Street, Leroy	12	1981
Teddy	1, 11	1981
West Indian Tom	10	1981

Introduction:

The Classic Era of Narcotic Control

From the early 1920s until the middle 1960s American narcotic policy was unprecedentedly strict and punitive, in comparison both to other western countries and to what it has become in our own time. To use a short-hand phrase, this was the classic period of narcotic control—"classic" in the sense of simple, consistent, and rigid. The purpose of this book is to describe, through the medium of oral history, what it was like to be a narcotic addict during those years. The narratives we have assembled are drawn from the recorded testimony of classic-era addicts who started using drugs as long ago as 1910 and who, against long odds, lived to tell of their experiences. Such an approach is, to our knowledge, unique: although there have been other interview-based studies of American ad-dicts, none has focused exclusively on older addicts whose memories reach so far back into the twentieth century.[1] Who our interviewees were, how they survived, and how we located them will be explained in due course. We shall begin, however, with a historical sketch of the period in question, to provide a conceptual and chronological framework for the personal narratives that follow.

THE SOCIAL AND

LEGISLATIVE BACKGROUND

During the nineteenth century there was virtually no effective regulation of narcotics in the United States. Various preparations and derivatives of opium were freely available and widely used. Although several states had statutes governing the sale of narcotics, and many municipalities forbade opium smoking, these laws were only sporadically enforced. In practice just about anyone could secure pure drugs with little bother and at modest cost. Pharmacists even delivered, dispatching messenger boys with vials of morphine to houses of high and low repute. Some customers were actually unaware of what they were purchasing: proprietors of patent medicines were notorious for slipping narcotics into their products, which before 1906 bore no list of ingredients on their labels. Doctors, too, frequently overprescribed narcotics. Opiates were among the few effective drugs they possessed, and it was tempting to alleviate the symptoms (and thus continue the patronage) of their patients, especially those who were chronically ill.

The result of all this was a narcotic problem of considerable dimensions, with perhaps as many as 300,000 opiate addicts at the turn of the century, plus an unknown number of irregular users.[2] Today there are an estimated 500,000 narcotic (mainly heroin) addicts in the United States, but the population is also much larger. On a per capita basis, narcotic abuse was certainly as bad and probably worse in the late nineteenth century.

Victorian Americans were much less worried about drugs, however, than they were about drink. An influential reform coalition, consisting mainly of native-born, white, middle-class Protestants, attacked alcohol as the principal source of social problems. Drinking was wrong because it led to drunkenness, and drunkenness led to battered wives, abandoned children, sexual incontinence, venal voting, pauperism, insanity, early death, and eternal damnation. Drinking was also objectionable because it was associated with groups whose morality was highly suspect: Catholic immigrants, machine politicians, urban blacks, demimondaines, criminals, tramps, casual laborers, and others of the lower strata. Reformers sought to uplift and reform drunkards, but they were also frank in their desire to control their behavior and to minimize the social costs they generated. The more ardent among them fought for and achieved prohibition, first on a local and state level, and then, in January 1920, on a national basis.

Given the prevalence of narcotic use, why were Americans initially so much more agitated over the drink question? One answer lies in the comparative effects of opiates and alcohol. It was a commonplace that drink maddened while opium soothed. Alcoholics were notoriously obstreperous and often injured others as well as themselves. Their behavior was a public nuisance and a scandal. Addicts, by contrast, tended to be quiet and withdrawn. Though they might merit reprehension for their enslavement to a drug, theirs was a private vice, unlikely to affect anyone outside their immediate family—and in some cases even the family did not know. These distinctions were grounded in pharmacological reality, insofar as narcotics are potent tranquilizers, capable of producing a pacific and languid state. It is easier for an addict to remain inconspicuous than a drunkard.

Who the narcotic users were was as important as how they acted. There was what might be termed a "hard core" of opium smokers, mainly Chinese laborers and white criminals; they were contemptuously regarded and likely to run afoul of the law. Opium smokers, however, made up only a minority of regular users. Addicts were more often found among upper- and middle-class women, many of whom had begun using morphine to relieve the symptoms of various illnesses. Surveys taken in the late nine-teenth century consistently showed that two-thirds of those addicted to medicinal opiates, such as laudanum or morphine sulfate, were female. Given that so many addicts were respectable women of ailing body and docile comportment, it is understandable that they were viewed with less alarm than heavy drinkers.

Not everyone saw the matter in this light: a handful of medical special-ists argued that addiction and alcoholism were in fact related, that both were a manifestation of an underlying nervous disorder called inebriety, and that "inebriates" needed institutional care, against their wills if nec-essary. They failed, however, to carry this last point. Although thousands of American addicts sought treatment in private asylums in the nineteenth century, they did so voluntarily; relatively few were coerced. The public thought of addiction as neither a crime nor a fit object for mandatory treatment. Whatever resentment existed against addicts was diffuse and lacked institutional expression.

Within twenty-five years these attitudes had dramatically changed. Even as the country was having second thoughts about alcohol prohi-bition, there was virtual consensus on the need to suppress narcotic addiction. Fears about narcotics became so pronounced that otherwise well-informed people began making foolish proposals. One 1936 article, published in the authoritative *Public Health Reports*, recommended that opiates be used sparingly to alleviate the sufferings of cancer patients, if at all.[3] Such advice was not only illogical (why worry about drug dependence in the dying?), it contradicted a well-established humanitarian tradition in American medicine, practiced by physicians as eminent as William Osler. Some extremists in the 1920s and 1930s even proposed firing squads as a permanent solution for the drug problem, on the theory that the only abstinent addict was a dead one.

This pronounced attitudinal shift was related to changing perceptions of who drug addicts were, how they acquired their habits, and how they behaved under the influence of drugs. After the turn of the century there were fewer new cases of medical addiction, as physicians became more conservative in their use of narcotics and the public became more chary of self-medication, thanks to the Pure Food and Drug Act (1906) and the efforts of muckrakers like Samuel Hopkins Adams. Some existing medi-cal addicts detoxified and remained abstinent, but the majority probably continued using morphine. Since many of them were old and ailing, however, they soon disappeared from the scene. That left a residue of generally younger, less sympathetic users who had begun experimenting with drugs in such decidedly nonmedical establishments as brothels and saloons. Opium smoking remained popular in the white underworld and continued to attract recruits, even though the number of Chinese living in America had begun to decline. Two powerful new drugs, cocaine and heroin, quickly spread outside medical practice and became popular euphorigenic agents. Cocaine, although not pharmacologically a narcotic, was often described as such and became associated in the public mind with crime sprees, particularly by black men. In the 1910s and early 1920s heroin use became widespread in the immigrant slums, where young men took to snorting small packets of the white powder. For some it was a passing fancy, but for others it became a lifelong preoccupation. In 1924 New York City Corrections Commissioner Frederick A. Wallis described what he took to be a typical case:

> The young man, 16 to 20, leaves school because he won't study, he doesn't like discipline, and shows inclination toward truancy and dishonesty.
>
> Out of school, his bad habits increase. He visits pool-rooms and dance halls, and chop suey restaurants and becomes one of the neighborhood rowdies or corner loafers. He goes with a gang and becomes reckless and is soon participating with the gang in neighborhood thefts. If he has a job, it becomes burdensome, and offensive to him. He then neglects his work, loses his job, and all his ambitions are in sympathy with criminal tendencies.
>
> He is arrested first for a minor offense, spends five to ten days in prison, loses self-respect, is released and returns to society with less regard for law and constitutional authority....
>
> Having served a term in prison, he is now qualified by the gang for exploits in the underworld.... He soon learns ... the easiest and most profitable way to get money with less personal hazard to himself and a lighter prison sentence, [and he] becomes a drug peddler and distributor. Before he realizes the danger he has been taught to use the drug. Soon he must have the drug at any price.
>
> He resorts to shoplifting and indulges in other petty offenses to obtain the drug. The next step is prison again, and he returns to society again, and then is arrested for a more serious crime. The craving for drugs is growing all the time. He must have more drugs. The requirement of $2.00 a day has grown into $5.00 or $10.00 a day. In his intensified craving he becomes a bandit, a hold-up man, murder follows. A wreck, mentally, physically and morally, he is given a life sentence or the electric chair.[4]

What is particularly interesting about this account is its judgmental tone, its depiction of the heroin addict as a modern version of Hogarth's idle 'prentice. It was not just that the old-fashioned medical addicts were disappearing and being replaced by a new breed, it was how people felt about the change. As had been the case with alcohol, disdain for users, tinged by ethnic and class prejudice, was an impetus for restrictive legislation. Change a very few words in Wallis's description and one has the old stereotype of the drunkard as a menacing, irresponsible wretch. Admittedly not everyone shared this view, and there were important individual and regional differences in attitudes toward narcotic addiction. The country as a whole, however, seemed to reach a psychological tipping point in the early twentieth century, as addicts dropped below an imperceptible but crucial line in the national consciousness and ceased to be the objects of benevolent pity.

Put another way, addiction went from being a pathetic condition to being a stigmatized one. Like venereal disease, it came to be understood as a condition that was acquired through forbidden indulgence with evil associates. Also like venereal disease, it was a condition that could afflict, or destroy, the lives of innocent others—the spouse, the family, the fetus, or the newborn child. Both diseases were, in a broad sense, communicable: addicts (and venereal patients) were alarming, not only because they had gotten themselves in trouble, but because they might put others in the same fix. After inadvertent medical addiction ceased to be much of a factor, it was clear that the majority of new users were introduced to drugs by and often became part of a network of experienced users and dealers. A deviant subculture was in place and perpetuated itself through continuous recruiting.

Deviant groups in American history have sometimes been dealt with by informal, local means—harassment, exile, even lynching. But when such groups become large enough, or threatening enough, they often evoke a legislative response. The resultant laws serve a dual purpose. They are symbolic, in that they define and reiterate majority norms; they are also instrumental, to the extent that they employ the police power of the state to restrict or eliminate the objectionable behavior. There have been many instances of this, from the 1675 Massachusetts law attacking the "damnable haeresies" of the Quakers to the 1940 Smith Act, used to prosecute domestic communists and Nazi sympathizers. Narcotic control seems to fit neatly into this pattern. As the legal scholars Richard Bonnie and Charles Whitebread have put it, "Once opiate use became identified with otherwise immoral or unliked populations, prohibition was almost automatic." [5]

The word "almost" must be stressed, however. The negative social and behavioral connotations surrounding nonmedical narcotic use were not, in any meaningful historical sense, a sufficient cause of the ensuing prohibition and criminalization. There was still room for the play of expert judgment and legislative discretion, and we know that contemporaries in other developed countries, such as Britain, arrived at less draconian solutions. It is fair to say, however, that the sinister transmogrification of narcotic addiction was a critical precondition for the legal developments that followed. It would have made no sense—politically, culturally, morally, or in any other way—to repress addicts who were mainly sick old women. Even after the laws were changed, physicians and law enforcement officers often tacitly permitted the dwindling number of iatrogenic addicts to continue their "medication." These patients were sympathetic figures and, because they were isolated from the street drug subculture, posed no threat to anyone.[6]

The transformation of American narcotic laws, like the transformation of the addict population itself, evolved over a period of time. The catalytic event was America's growing involvement in Asia, a region long notorious for its opium trade. American military governors in the recently acquired Philippines, missionaries in China, and diplomats studied the problem and sought to coordinate international efforts to eliminate or reduce the traffic. As a result of their efforts an international opium commission met at Shanghai in February 1909. The American delegation, anxious to assume a leadership role but fearful lest the laissez-faire narcotic market at home open them to charges of hypocrisy, pressed for at least token congressional legislation. This they received in the form of a hastily enacted law forbidding the importation of opium "for other than medicinal purposes," i.e., opium for smoking. Banning this form of the drug cost the federal government over $800,000 in annual revenues, but it was politically feasible, since opium smoking had such low-life connotations and few American firms had a large stake in its continued importation.

Reformers were not satisfied with this one measure, however. They continued to work for a more comprehensive narcotic law, both to address the domestic problem and to bring the country into line with the provisions of an international treaty then being negotiated. Their most forceful advocate was Dr. Hamilton Wright, American delegate to the Shanghai Commission and later the Hague Opium Conference (1911–12). Wright compiled an official report for Congress, complete with authoritative references to drug-inspired rape and miscegenation, as well as statistics that seemed to show that narcotic use was outstripping population growth. (In fact it was not; per capita consumption was down after 1900, due largely to increased therapeutic conservatism.)

Wright also played up the prevalence of lower-class and criminal use, as may be seen from his specific addiction estimates in Table 1. The percentages reproduced here are as unfounded as they are pretentious: Wright's research was highly unsystematic, and hardly merited numerical expression, let alone two- and three-decimal-point precision.[7] He was, however, magnifying an epidemiologic reality: by 1910 criminals and prostitutes did have much higher rates of use than the general adult population, and possibly (although this is not certain) higher rates than medical personnel, who historically had a serious addiction problem. Wright was, moreover, believed. His statements and statistics were given wide circulation in the popular press, medical journals, congressional committee reports, and other official documents.

Despite his skills as a propagandist, Wright got a bill neither as soon as nor as stringent as he wanted. He ran into opposition, especially from

TABLE 1: Opiate Addiction Estimates for Various Groups in the
United States Made by Hamilton Wright in 1910

Group	Percentage Addicted
General Criminal Population	45.48
Chinese	25.0[a]
Prostitutes and Their Companions	21.6
Prisoners in Large Jails and State Prisons[b]	6.0
Medical Profession	2.06
Trained Nurses	1.32
Other Professional Classes	0.684
General Adult Population[c]	0.18
College and University Students	"Practically Unknown"

Source: U.S. Senate, *Report on the International Opium Commission and on the Opium Problem as Seen Within the United States and Its Possessions* (Washington, D.C.: G.P.O., 1910), 42, 47.
[a] Percentage estimate includes those who smoked a pound and a half or more per annum, but excludes "social smokers."
[b] As distinct from the "general criminal population," which committed lesser crimes and hence ended up in local jails rather than large jails or state institutions.
[c] Exclusive of the groups enumerated above.

drug companies that did a large wholesale business in narcotics. He also encountered philosophical and constitutional difficulties, since the limits or even the existence of a federal police power were not then generally agreed upon. (Indeed, in 1918 and again in 1922 the Supreme Court would strike down something as seemingly proper and desirable as federal child labor laws.) The regulation of medical practice was a matter traditionally left to the states, and narcotics were still very much a part of medical practice.

The measure that finally passed, the Harrison Narcotic Act of 1914, was a complex compromise. It required anyone who sold or distributed narcotics—importers, manufacturers, wholesale and retail druggists, and physicians—to register with the government and to pay a small tax.[8] When they sold or otherwise distributed narcotics, they had to make a detailed record of the transaction, open to government inspection. Unregistered persons caught with narcotics in their possession were presumptively guilty of violating the law, unless they had been "prescribed in good faith by a physician, dentist, or veterinary surgeon registered under this Act." If convicted, they could be fined and imprisoned for up to five years. It was anticipated that such sanctions would make the narcotic traffic transparent and confine it to legitimate medical channels.

Two features of the Harrison Act are of particular interest. One is the definition of narcotics as opium- and coca-based drugs. As previously noted, opium and coca are medicinally distinct. One is a central nervous system depressant, the other a stimulant. They were combined legislatively, however, because of the assumption that both were euphorigenic, potentially habit-forming, and associated with crime. It was for similar reasons that marijuana would also later be described as a narcotic.[9]

(2)   The second point is the law's failure to address the question of whether an addict could receive, on an indefinite basis, a prescribed supply of narcotics. In retrospect, this was one of the most crucial lacunae in any federal statute enacted in the twentieth century. The Treasury Department officials who administered the law assumed a negative stance and initiated several prosecutions against addicts, physicians, and pharmacists for conspiracy to violate the Harrison Act. At first the Supreme Court rebuked the Treasury Department for attempting to stop physicians from prescribing for addicts; ultimately, however, it reversed itself and narrowly ruled in favor of the antimaintenance position. In two cases decided March 3, 1919, the Court sustained the constitutionality of the Harrison Act and ruled that a physician might not write prescriptions for an addict "to keep him comfortable by maintaining his customary use."

The circumstances of these cases, *United States* v. *Doremus* and *Webb et al.* v. *United States*, are revealing. Doremus was a physician who prescribed, for a price, large quantities of heroin to one Alexander Ameris, alias Myers, who was "addicted to the use of the drug as a habit, being a person popularly known as a 'dope fiend.' "[10] Ameris's ethnic surname, use of heroin, and large habit were all negatives, summed up in the epithet "dope fiend." Dr. Webb was similarly accused of gross overprescription; before he was arrested he averaged more than eighty morphine prescriptions a week, at fifty cents apiece. This may seem modest in comparison to today's inflated medical prices, but it was a lucrative sideline in an era when practitioners earned only a few thousand dollars a year and milk retailed for eleven cents a quart. Government attorneys decried such unprofessional behavior, likening it to a barkeeper dispensing whiskey to a drunkard.[11] Five members of the Court agreed, and Webb's original conviction was upheld. Had either case involved only small amounts of narcotics prescribed by a reputable physician, it is highly likely that the decision would have gone the other way. Six years later, in *Linder* v. *United States*, the Court unanimously reversed the conviction of a respected Oregon practitioner who had prescribed one tablet of morphine and three tablets of cocaine for a stool-pigeon addict.[12]

The Prohibition Unit of the Treasury Department nevertheless treated *Webb* as the governing decision and pursued an aggressive antimaintenance policy. By threats and actual prosecutions they were able to drive a wedge of fear between the legal providers (physicians, pharmacists) and the addicts. Prosecutions of those who supplied addicts might fail, as they had with Dr. Linder—but they might also succeed, as they had with Dr.

Webb and numerous others. Even if a defense were successful, the potential legal fees and loss of reputation made a physician think twice before reaching for his prescription pad. Doctors, moreover, were less and less favorably disposed toward nonmedical addicts, whom they perceived as devious, troublesome, and notoriously resistant to cure.

There were, however, some physicians who continued to write for addicts, if only on an occasional basis. They were motivated by pity, or greed, or simply by a desire to get the users off their backs and out of town. This book has a good deal of information about such doctors, from the point of view of the users who "made" them. It is interesting that, even at the height of its powers, the Bureau of Narcotics never completely succeeded in closing off all medical supplies to addicts. A small but significant gray market of pure drugs persisted as an alternative to the black market of adulterated heroin. Some users managed to develop extensive connections in the former and stay out of the latter altogether. Still, medical sources were chancy and could not be counted on indefinitely; doctors who wrote prescriptions too often or too openly were sure to be visited by a federal agaent. That, as far as addicts were concerned, was the chief legacy of the Harrison Act and the 1919 Court decisions.

There was one other alternative to the black market, but it was short-lived. Following the *Webb* ruling, a number of cities and towns set up facilities to dispense narcotics to addicts. If private maintenance were disallowed, then organized, public maintenance, either with or without gradual detoxification, might yet take its place. Two of the more famous of these "clinics," in Shreveport, Louisiana, and New York City, are described in chapter 12. It is enough to say here that the Treasury Department objected and, by one means or another, managed to force closure of the clinics within a few years. February 10, 1923, when the hold-out Shreveport clinic finally broke off maintenance operations, is as appropriate a date as any to mark the beginning of the classic period of narcotic control, since it represented the end of legal access to organized maintenance treatment.[13]

The unprecedented nature of federal narcotic policy is underscored by the fact that alcoholic beverage prohibition applied only to manufacture and sale. Neither the Eighteenth Amendment nor the Volstead Act barred personal use and consumption by alcoholics or, for that matter, anyone else. National prohibition, moreover, was controversial from the start and lasted only fourteen years. Large numbers of apparently normal people continued to drink; they resented both the prices they had to pay for bootlegged alcohol and the prohibitionists who meddled with their customary freedoms. The laws proved virtually unenforceable, as criminals manufactured or diverted alcohol and speakeasies spread across the land. The byproducts of Prohibition—gangsterism, corruption, and methanol poisoning—filled the front pages. Ardent supporters grew disenchanted.

Powerful business and opinion leaders such as Pierre du Pont and William Randolph Hearst campaigned for repeal. A well-funded national organization, the Association Against the Prohibition Amendment, maintained a drumfire of criticism and propaganda. The public was told that the noble experiment had backfired and was creating a nation of drunkards. The war against narcotics, by contrast, was thought to be successful in reducing nonmedical addiction, and was so portrayed by government officials.[14]

The onset of depression in 1929 handed the antiprohibitionists a new and decisive argument: money. "If the liquor now sold by bootleggers was legally sold, regulated, and taxed," one writer observed, "the excise income would pay the interest on the entire local and national bonded indebtedness and leave more than $200,000,000 for other urgently needed purposes."[15] The Democrats adopted a repeal plank in 1932, and nominee Franklin Roosevelt pledged to the convention that "the 18th Amendment is doomed."[16] True to his word, he announced on December 5, 1933, that three-quarters of the states had ratified the Twenty-first Amendment, thereby ending national prohibition.

Virtually no one spoke up for the narcotic user, however; there was no Association Against the Harrison Act. On the contrary, the national champions of repeal, including Hearst and Roosevelt, persisted in seeing drug use as a criminal menace and condoned restrictive measures. One "wet" argument, dating back to the early state prohibition battles, had been that frustrated drinkers would turn to narcotic drugs, which would madden and enslave them.[17] Drink was the lesser evil. Hostile toward addicts anyway, it suited the purposes of the antiprohibitionists to maintain them as a negative reference point, the dead end of their *ad horrendum* stories.

As for the addicts themselves, they were too few and too marginal to carry much political weight. Many of them were convicted felons and thus could not even vote. There was little that they could do about the refusal to allow maintenance, a policy that lasted more than forty years. When the antimaintenance regime was finally challenged, it was not by the narcotic users but by an elite group of professionals—mainly lawyers, physicians, and social scientists—who had become convinced that it was unjust and unworkable. In attacking the Bureau of Narcotics, they too invoked the alleged failures of Prohibition, arguing that it was useless and counterproductive to outlaw addictive substances. It also seemed a double standard to permit pathogens like alcohol and tobacco, while proscribing "narcotics" of lesser or unproven danger, and without which regular users would become violently ill. This was a fair point but, like all rational arguments, it had its limits. There was still a powerful, visceral fear of narcotic addicts and all that they stood for. It was the social and moral connotations of narcotic addiction that mattered, not just the mental and physical effects of the drugs themselves.

LIFE UNDER ANSLINGER

The personification of the antinarcotic regime was Harry Jacob Anslinger, head (or, to his critics, "czar") of the Bureau of Narcotics. Anslinger was a minor diplomat who in the 1920s became involved with efforts to prevent liquor from being smuggled into the country. He was a competent and honest functionary in a field not known for either trait, and in 1929 he was made Assistant Commissioner of Prohibition. After Levi Nutt, boss of the Prohibition Unit's Narcotic Division was tainted with scandal and demoted, Anslinger took his place. When the Bureau of Narcotics was spun off as a distinct organization in 1930—partly to distance it from the furor over alcohol prohibition—Anslinger was named its first commissioner, a post he retained until 1962.

There was a peculiar, almost Jekyll-and-Hyde aspect to Anslinger's personality. The private man was humorous, cosmopolitan, fluent in several languages, musically accomplished, devoted to his wife, and loyal to his hometown friends. Anslinger also possessed a keen political intelligence. Like his contemporary Lyndon Johnson, he knew exactly whom to cultivate to advance his interests. His most powerful weapon was undoubtedly his telephone. Anslinger is remembered, however, not as man of exceptional gifts, nor as a deft bureaucrat, but as the ultimate tough cop. His appearance—bald, barrel-chested, square-jawed, and unsmiling, a sort of beefy Mussolini—had much to do with this. By all accounts Anslinger was intimidating; one visitor described him as "a man whose eyes seem to be cataloguing you—your features, build, clothes." "He had a disposition about him that used to scare the shit out of people . . . ," recalled Howard Diller, a former Bureau agent. "He was like a Napoleonic guy."

Anslinger enjoyed power and relished its trappings. Once he was met at the airport by some agents who had improvidently brought along a medium-sized car. Anslinger demanded to know where his Cadillac was and, when told that it was at the office, reportedly said, "Well, go get the damn thing. I'll wait. It performs much better for a large man." They went. Wherever Anslinger traveled, he was accompanied by an entourage; he was also fond of carrying about a small, leather-bound book, listing names of known or suspected traffickers. Even in retirement, he would walk up to an agent, punch him in the chest, and exclaim, "Young man, you got a goddam tough job ahead of you." When explaining or defending his policies, he was given to curt aphorisms: "Wherever you find severe penalties, addiction disappears," or "The best cure for addiction? Never let it happen." [18]

Anslinger summed up his basic approach in similarly brief manner. "We intend to get the killer-pushers and their willing customers out of selling and buying drugs," he said. "The answer to the problem is simple —get rid of drugs, pushers and users. Period." Interdicting smuggling and jailing dealers made narcotics scarce and expensive; confining addicts made it impossible for them to spread the vice. It was, moreover, their only hope of cure. Unless addicts were confined where there was no possibility of obtaining drugs, Anslinger believed, withdrawal treatment was bound to fail. He strongly favored compulsory commitment and fretted that most states lacked statutes permitting them to pick up addicts and force them into institutions. [19]

Yet even this was not enough. Anslinger understood that narcotic trafficking was international in scope and required diplomatic efforts as well as strict domestic enforcement. He tirelessly attended meetings sponsored by the League of Nations, seeking agreements that would make it more difficult to smuggle drugs. In 1931, for example, he took an active role in negotiating an international pact to limit the manufacture of narcotics. Nations ratifying the treaty, of which there were twenty-five by 1933, were to make or import no more narcotics than necessary for estimated annual medical use, thereby reducing the surplus available for diversion into the illicit traffic.

Like many American diplomats of his generation, Anslinger saw the world in black and white terms. Most nations were good, in that they were willing to assist others in the international campaign against the drug evil. There were also bad states that not only refused to cooperate but actually used narcotics as an instrument of subversion and conquest. At the head of Anslinger's renegade list were Imperial Japan and Communist China. "Wherever the Japanese Army goes," he charged, "the drug traffic follows. In every territory conquered by the Japanese, a large part of the people become enslaved with drugs." In the 1950s and early 1960s he attacked the leaders of the People's Republic of China, accusing them of narcotic sales to the West to support their invasion of Korea and later of joining with Castro's Cuba to create an illicit drug network. It is not coincidental that all of the bad nations were, at the time Anslinger assailed them, military and ideological rivals of the United States. Narcotic policy dovetailed with foreign policy, a fact that enhanced Anslinger's prestige as well as his bureau's budget. [20]

The one eventuality that Anslinger had to guard against was the return of legal maintenance. This, he felt, would utterly defeat his plans to keep drugs out of the hands of addicts and their associates. The potential danger was great. The medical profession was enormously powerful and prestigious, having achieved what sociologist Paul Starr has called "sovereign" status by the 1930s.[21] If physicians took seriously the idea that addiction was a disease and that, lacking a sure cure, the most favorable course of treatment was maintenance,[22] then they might challenge, and ultimately defeat, the tenuous legal basis for narcotic prohibition.

Fortunately for Anslinger, most practitioners were disinclined to rock the boat. Like the public at large, physicians tended to see drug users, especially heroin addicts and opium smokers, as vicious and declassé. They were in any case oriented toward treating somatic disorders, and the dominant medical opinion of the day declared narcotic addiction to be a manifestation of psychopathology, that is, not a physical disease at all. The psychopathy thesis was popularized by Dr. Lawrence Kolb and his coworkers at the United States Public Health Service, who also oversaw the two federal narcotic farms at Lexington, Kentucky, and Fort Worth, Texas. These facilities, described in chapter 13, were quasi-penal in nature, and were strictly geared toward detoxification, rehabilitation, and abstinence. As such, they were perfectly acceptable to Anslinger. Kolb challenged Anslinger from time to time, complaining that too-zealous enforcement was causing problems, but on the whole the approaches of the two men were compatible.[23]

Anslinger never let down his guard, however. He not only monitored and occasionally prosecuted individual physicians whom he suspected of writing too many prescriptions, he fulminated against organized maintenance at every opportunity. He blamed the rudimentary clinic system of the early 1920s for "a tremendous rise in teen-age drug addiction" and predicted that a return to such folly would increase the narcotic problem nearly tenfold. Maintenance was also deeply repugnant: "the idea of giving a teenager heroin for the rest of his life is unthinkable. . . . Why not set up bars for alcoholics or department stores for kleptomaniacs or brothels for homosexuals." Or research projects for professors. "You know, there are so many experts in drug addiction," he complained in 1957, "that I think if we made a survey we would find more experts than addicts."[24] Anslinger appealed to the conservatism and anti-intellectualism of ordinary Americans, and also to their nativist and racial fears. He relied on the antinarcotic consensus to help him in his long, preemptive battle against maintenance; he was abetted by reporters, editorialists, political cartoonists, and filmmakers, who consistently portrayed narcotic traffickers as murderous villains. Again and again, Americans were told that the role of the government was to eliminate peddlers, not to assume their role.[25]

MINORITIES AND NARCOTIC USE:
THE SECOND TRANSFORMATION

Anslinger may have exploited public antipathy toward narcotic dealers and users, but he did not invent it. The antinarcotic consensus had arisen from the earlier transformation of the addict population, a real demographic event helped along by imaginative statisticians and propagandists. During Anslinger's long tenure the addict population continued to evolve, and in a way that further strengthened his hand. The key change was the growing use of heroin by black men.

Blacks were not considered heavy drug users early in the century. They lived mainly in the rural South, were poor, and had less access to opiates than whites, who could afford doctors and patent medicines. Black workers occasionally used cocaine as a pick-me-up, a few field hands smoked marijuana, and some unemployed men drank excessively, but, with these exceptions, blacks had neither a disproportionate nor a very serious drug problem. On the contrary, the prevailing racial stereotype of the narcotic addict was white or Oriental.

After World War II the situation changed completely. Middle-class whites came to "imagine that ghettos [were] filled with black men mugging whites for money to pay for heroin and then injecting this evil drug so that they can spend the rest of the day nodding away in a blissful vacuum."[26] Figure 1 displays the statistical basis for these fears. Not only were black addicts turning up more often in federal treatment centers, they were being booked more frequently by the police, to the point that, by the 1950s, half or more of all narcotic arrests involved blacks. Something similar was happening in the Hispanic communities. In 1936 only about 1 percent of the addicts treated at Lexington were Hispanic; by 1966 over a quarter were—13.9 percent Puerto Rican and 12.2 percent Mexican.[27]

Data of this sort have been criticized as misleading, since minorities are treated prejudicially and are hence more likely to end up in institutions or jails. They are particularly vulnerable during periods of racial or nativist tension, economic dislocation, or politically motivated crackdowns.[28] Even in normal times it is tempting for the police to fill their quotas in the ghetto; it is easier to ticket, arrest, or prosecute those who are relatively powerless.

These biases are real but in one sense irrelevant. Statistics such as these, amplified and personalized by news stories and photographs, shape public opinion, regardless of their factual basis. Rightly or wrongly, the black junkie became a stereotype, and that made a difference. Moreover, even though these percentages may overstate the degree of involvement, there is no reason to doubt that minorities were using drugs in the 1940s and 1950s in a way they had not before. Black narcotic arrests, for exam-

FIGURE 1   Indices of Black Narcotic Use

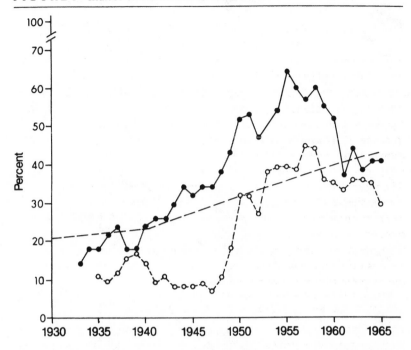

●—●—● Percentage of Those Arrested for Narcotic Law Violations in U.S. Cities of Population Greater than 2500 Who Were Black

o-o-o Percentage of Those Admitted to Lexington and Fort Worth Hospitals Who Were Black

— — — Percentage of U.S. Blacks Living Outside the South

Sources: Patti Iiyama et al., *Drug Use and Abuse among U.S. Minorities: An Annotated Bibliography* (New York: Praeger, 1976), 5; John C. Ball and Carl D. Chambers, eds., *The Epidemiology of Opiate Addiction in the United States* (Springfield, Ill.: Charles C. Thomas, 1970), 180; Bureau of the Census, *Historical Statistics of the United States: Colonial Times to 1970*, Part 1 (Washington, D.C.: G.P.O., 1975), 22.

ple, were increasing absolutely as well as relatively, rising from a mere 362 nationally in 1933 to 4,262 in 1950 to 11,816 in 1965. An increase of that magnitude, sustained over a long period of time, is due to something more than prejudice. Black writers and intellectuals were also sounding the alarm. Claude Brown's *Manchild in the Promised Land* (1965) contains a bitter account of the "shit plague" that befell New York City's neighborhoods in the early 1950s. Not only Harlem, "but in Brooklyn, the Bronx, and everyplace I went, uptown and downtown. It was like horse had just taken over."[29] This impression is confirmed by the people we questioned.

TABLE 2: Onset of Addiction by Race and Sex for Forty-one
Interviewees Addicted before 1965[a]

Decade	White	Chinese	Hispanic	Black	Totals
1916–25	M M M F F F[a]	M			7
1926–35	M M F F F F F F	M[b]		M	10
1936–45	M M M M F		M[c]	M M M F	10
1946–55	M M M F	M	F	M M M M M M	12
1956–65				M F[d]	2
Totals	23	3	2	13	41

[a] M = Male Subject; F = Female Subject
[b] Date of addiction approximate, due to the subject's difficulty with chronology.
[c] Mixed ancestry: father from Virgin Islands, mother Puerto Rican.
[d] Mixed ancestry: father Chinese, mother black.

Individually, they commented on this change; collectively, their histories
attest to it. Table 2 shows the onset of addiction by race and sex for the
first forty-one subjects interviewed, all of whom were addicted prior to
1965. It is apparent that there was a shift away from the white and Chinese
addicts who predominated before 1935, to more Hispanic and especially
black addicts after that date.

It is not hard to understand why this happened. Black narcotic use
was a concomitant of urbanization. During 1915 to 1930, and again during 1940 to 1960, millions of blacks left the countryside for larger towns
and cities. Jim Crow, disfranchisement, poverty, boll weevils, and agricultural mechanization made it difficult to stay; higher-paying industrial
jobs, especially during the war years, made it tempting to leave. Some migrants settled in southern cities; most eventually moved on to the North
or West. Three major routes developed: from the South Atlantic seaboard
toward the northeast urban corridor; from Mississippi toward Chicago;
and from Texas and Louisiana toward California. In 1910 not a single city
in the country contained 100,000 blacks; by 1960 New York City alone
had more than a million. In 1910 73 percent of the black population was
rural; in 1960 73 percent was urban.[30]

The blacks who fled the South were mainly young, unattached adults
whose futures lay before them. They left with high hopes, singing hymns

like "Jesus, Take My Hand" and "I'm on the Way." What actually awaited them, the ghetto slum, has been likened to the frying pan instead of the fire. Not only did they have to face the classic dilemma of an uprooted peasantry—how to adjust to the city when what they knew was the land—but to do so under the worst possible circumstances, crowded into stinking, overpriced tenements.[31] They also had to cope with the usual array of urban vice figures: pimps, prostitutes, thieves, con men, numbers runners, and all manner of drug retailers, from marijuana distributors like the legendary white hipster Milton Mezzrow to black opiate users and dealers like Malcolm Little, later Malcolm X. Disoriented and demoralized, the newcomers were exposed to narcotics in a way they had never been before. So were their children, particularly those who had left school, were out of work, could scrounge a buck, and spent their time on the street. The result could easily have been predicted: a growing incidence of black heroin addiction, particularly among the traditional high-risk group of single males in their late teens or early twenties.

To say that such an event was predictable is not to indulge in historical hindsight. There was ample precedent for what happened to the black urban community. It had happened before to other immigrants living in the same or similar neighborhoods. The white ethnic addicts we interviewed, who started using narcotics in the 1920s and 1930s, told substantially the same story as the blacks who began in the 1940s and 1950s. They grew up in or moved to neighborhoods where drugs could be procured; they were on their own or unsupervised; they had friends who were users; they yielded to curiosity or peer pressure and tried it for themselves. Thus the ethnic slum, matrix of heroin use from about 1910 on, continued to spawn illicit narcotic use throughout the classic period.[32] When the color of the faces in the tenement windows changed, so did the color of the addicts on the street.

Several factors, however, made the immigration-slums-narcotics tangle worse for blacks than for previous groups. First, because of their color, blacks had been and continued to be the objects of especially virulent racism. To the extent that this racism translated into educational and occupational handicaps, and to the extent that unemployment and poverty were conducive to drug and alcohol abuse, urban blacks were especially vulnerable; living for what Norman Mailer called "the enormous present" made more sense for those who felt excluded from the future.[33] Partly because of this legacy of racism, blacks had fewer political and organizational resources than other groups. There was, for example, no black counterpart to the New York Kehillah's Bureau of Social Morals, which monitored drug dealers in the Jewish immigrant community. Even the Mafia, the country's leading narcotic importer and wholesaler, kept the peddlers off its home turf.[34] Ghetto blacks also had fewer familial resources. Why this was so has become a political and intellectual *cause célèbre;* the fact remains that minority family dislocation did occur and it did contribute to addiction. *The Road to H*, a major study of young heroin users in New York City in the 1950s, found that 97 percent of addicts' families were characterized by "a disturbed relationship between the parents, as evidenced by separation, divorce, open hostility, or lack of warmth and mutual interest." The mother was the most important parent; about half the fathers often presented "immoral models through their own deviant activity with respect to criminality, infidelity, alcoholism, and the like." [35] Keeping teenagers away from drugs in an environment where they are plentiful requires especially active, watchful parenting. It is not likely to be done very well if parents are distracted, absent—or busy shooting up in the bathroom. Finally, there was the permanence of the black ghetto. Many of the white urban immigrants and their descendants were able to distance themselves from the tenements, moving to better quarters in safer neighborhoods and eventually to the suburbs. New York City's Jews, for example, went from Manhattan's chaotic Lower East Side, to Brooklyn and the Bronx, to Long Island, Westchester County, and New Jersey. Each step took them further away from the primary illicit narcotic markets; indeed, to distance themselves from drugs and crime was one of the reasons suburbanites moved in the first place. Low-income blacks were not as fortunate. Even as the Civil Rights movement achieved its judicial and legislative triumphs, a collective decision was made to abandon blacks in the inner city, to leave them behind with inferior schools and inadequate services in an environment virtually assured to perpetuate poverty. This was the result, not of a single grand conspiracy, but of a thousand private, uncoordinated ones: restrictive covenants, realtors' whispered advice, bankers' lending practices. The federal government generously subsidized the fleeing whites, via its tax, transportation, and mortgage policies. Urban abandonment soon developed its own momentum; as inner-city conditions progressively worsened, pressure grew on the remaining whites to escape beyond municipal lines, taking their tax dollars with them. Educated and upwardly mobile blacks were able to follow them to the suburbs, but those who were unemployed or underemployed had to stay behind. The decaying neighborhoods in which they lived were areas of heavy drug trafficking and use. Heroin became a staple in the ghetto economy, and black children grew up around older users who were both role models and potential initiators. Continued exposure, persistent discrimination, and progressive familial breakdown assured that subsequent generations of urban blacks would also suffer high rates of addiction. What began as an epidemic among black youth in the late 1940s and 1950s has long since become endemic to the urban underclass.

The growing involvement of blacks and Hispanics with narcotics, and the consequent racial transformation of the addict population, did not go unnoticed in high places. Anslinger himself emphasized this development. "Fifteen years ago, the Lexington and Forth Worth Hospitals had mostly white patients," he pointed out in 1957. "Today, they are filled with Negro addicts. What happened to the white addicts? You don't see them." Asked about the postwar rise in youthful addiction, Anslinger responded, "The increase is practically 100% among Negro people in police precincts with the lowest economic and social standards. . . . There is no drug addiction if the child comes from a good family, with the church, the home, and the school all integrated." [36]

There was truth in what Anslinger said, however bluntly he expressed it. Historically, children who were not poor, who were raised in intact families and socialized by middle-class institutions, were impervious to heroin. He did not, however, advance to the conclusion implied by his analysis: doing something about black addiction meant doing something about black economic and social conditions. Instead, Anslinger fell back upon what he knew best, enforcement. During the 1950s he pushed for ever tougher sanctions against traffickers, believing that the ultimate solution lay in choking off the illicit supply. Congress, alarmed by stories of teenage users, the darkening racial cast of institutionalized addicts, the postwar renaissance of the Mafia, and the alleged trafficking of nonwhite communist countries like China, was in a mood to agree. In 1951 it passed the Boggs Act and in 1956 the Narcotic Control Act, providing progressively stiffer, mandatory sentences for possession and sale. The inflexible provisions of these laws sometimes resulted in pathetic miscarriages of justice. In one instance a Chicano epileptic with an IQ of 69 was given two life terms for selling heroin to a seventeen-year-old provocateur; in another a black veteran with no previous record was sentenced to fifty years without parole for selling marijuana. Many states, nevertheless, followed suit, passing "Little Boggs Laws" that pegged minimum prison terms at or beyond the federal levels. A 1956 Louisiana statute provided mandatory sentences ranging from five to ninety-nine years for persons who sold, possessed, or administered narcotics; in Texas, possession of marijuana was punishable by two years to life. One celebrated Texas case was that of CandyBarr, a Dallas stripper who was given fifteen years after police found marijuana in her room. (It was her first offense and not even her own marijuana.) These were not isolated events; across the country nonfederal narcotic prosecutions were up sharply during the 1950s. [37] As the narratives in this book attest, many addicts were forced to endure long stretches in prison. A few who were well connected were able to avoid the law altogether, but they were the clear exceptions.

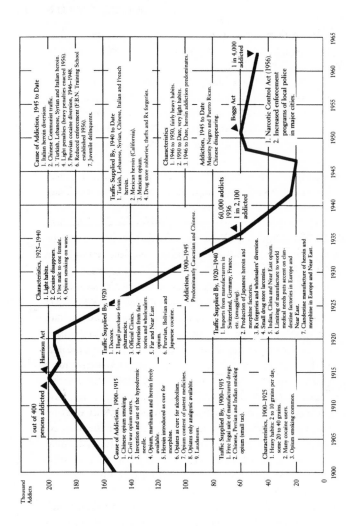

FIGURE 2

History of Narcotic Addiction in the United States

This chart represents the Bureau of Narcotics' version of classic-era history and epidemiology. Every time a federal law was passed, the prevalence of addiction allegedly diminished. Note also the comment on "Majority Negro and Puerto Rican" after 1945. Not all of the information presented above is erroneous; nevertheless, the slope, coordinates, and assumptions of the "ski-jump curve" have been repeatedly questioned. Anslinger was notorious for his willingness to manipulate prevalence data to achieve legislative ends.

Source: U.S. Senate, *Organized Crime and Illicit Traffic in Narcotics: Hearings before the Permanent Subcommittee on Investigations of the Committee on Government Operations*, Part 3 (Washington, DC: G.P.O., 1964), 771.

THE END OF THE CLASSIC PERIOD, 1960–1965

Historians who have studied American narcotic policy are agreed that the 1950s marked the zenith of the punitive approach. The "new spasm of concern" felt during this decade translated into "increased regulation in familiar patterns," comments H. Wayne Morgan. "On the surface, the consensus against drug use and for enforcement seemed stronger than ever."[38] Yet by 1965 the consensus had eroded and the old order, especially the categorical denial of maintenance, had been successfully challenged. Why did this happen?

The question must be answered on several levels. In the broadest terms, the Bureau of Narcotics and allied organizations were unable to bring about a lasting solution, as urban narcotic addiction remained a serious, widely publicized problem in the early 1960s. A Vietnam-like disillusionment began to set in: despite decades of escalating sanctions, narcotics were still finding their way onto the streets of America's cities. It was not for want of trying that the Bureau failed to stop the traffic permanently; under Anslinger it was one of the country's more efficient police organizations and the one most feared by organized crime. The problem lay in the nature of the case. Narcotics are highly compact, easily hidden substances. Two kilos in a false-bottomed suitcase are worth a small fortune. They are also reasonably easy to acquire, since opium is a major cash crop and only a fraction of the world's harvest is sufficient to supply American addicts' needs.[39] From the smugglers' vantage the United States is ideal: it is an open society with excellent transportation facilities, 88,633 miles of tidal shoreline, and two long boundaries with Mexico and Canada. Traffickers would forego these geographical advantages if deterred by threat of punishment, but here the Bureau encountered a paradox. Successful prosecutions take suppliers out of circulation and heighten the level of risk. Given what economists call an inflexible demand curve (addicts are generally steady customers), restrictions on supply and increased risk quickly translate into higher prices. The profits to be made from selling adulterated heroin to addicts tempt other criminals to jump into the market—criminals who are generally more ruthless and better organized than those previously arrested or deterred.[40] Narcotics enforcement is like antibiotics: it wipes out disease-producing organisms, but over time it also produces more resistant strains.

Anslinger realized that the way out of this paradox was to simultaneously reduce demand by isolating and then curing addicts. Fewer customers would mean smaller profits for dealers, and at some point the illicit trade would cease to be worth the risk. The catch was that Lexington-style institutions failed to effect many permanent cures: classic-period addicts like Brenda (see chapter 13) often went through several times, relapsing after every treatment. Narcotic wards were not without value: detoxification brought respite from the street grind and helped addicts to keep their habits within manageable bounds. But the generally high relapse rates provoked skepticism and lent credence to the cliché "once a junkie, always a junkie."

There were some alternatives to the big, revolving-door institutions: the 1960s saw a revival of the group approach to addiction treatment. Inspired by Synanon, therapeutic communities like Daytop Village, established in 1963, sought to rehabilitate addicts through structured, communal living. Addicts were reprogrammed in artificial, authoritarian families. They had to accept restrictions, work at tasks, stay clean. Peer pressure, sometimes of a brutal sort, was used to keep them in line. Group encounters, usually under the direction of an experienced former addict, probed the feelings of the participants; they aimed to produce an emotional catharsis and an atmosphere of truth-seeking. The ultimate goal was to learn to confront challenges openly and honestly, rather than to escape them by using drugs. Once addicts could do that, they could theoretically return to the straight world. In practice, however, many patients (called "splittees") left before completing the treatment; even full-fledged graduates often relapsed.[41] Therapeutic communities were in any case small and experimental—in the 1960s they had nothing like the scale or financial resources they enjoy today—and were not widely seen as the solution to the demand side of the narcotic control equation.

It is one thing to question whether a given institutional arrangement is working; it is another thing altogether to question its very moral and political basis. Increasingly in the 1960s liberal commentators asked why the country had a narcotic problem. Were drugs evil because they were physical and social pathogens? Or were they pathogens because illegal, hence adulterated and exorbitantly priced? Would addicts behave differently if the maintenance taboo were broken and they could receive cheap, pure medication? Specifically, would maintenance reduce the number of crimes addicts committed? Would it provide a way out of a destructive subculture, back into the productive world of family and work?

These were not new questions: they had been pointedly asked by the pioneers of organized maintenance, physicians like Charles Terry and Willis Butler. But now, after forty years of apparently self-defeating police solutions, they were being raised again by critics such as the sociologist Alfred Lindesmith. Like most twentieth-century liberals, Lindesmith was a negative utilitarian. He believed that if a law produced many costs and few benefits, then it was irrational and should be modified or abolished. This was the premise of his influential 1965 study, *The Addict and the Law*, in which he argued that American addicts were both more numerous and more "impoverished, degraded, and demoralized" than elsewhere in the western world. He cited police estimates that up to 50 percent of big-city crime was due to addicts hustling to support their habits.[42] Someone like John (chapter 6), who stole an estimated seven million dollars worth of merchandise and money during his addiction career, would be Exhibit A in Lindesmith's case; Exhibit B was the British system of medical maintenance, which to that point had resulted in neither serious crime nor an inordinate amount of addiction. Lindesmith and others essentially charged the Bureau with benighted prohibitionism, resulting in huge costs to both users and society. "The American narcotics problem," summed up Marie Nyswander in 1965, "is an artificial tragedy with real victims."[43]

If the crime issue was one fault line along which the narcotic consensus fractured, then marijuana was another. Marijuana had come under the Bureau of Narcotics' jurisdiction as a result of the 1937 Marijuana Tax Act, passed by Congress at Anslinger's urging. Like cocaine, marijuana was identified with an internal minority (Mexicans) and alleged to produce insanity and violent, unpredictable behavior. Later, its prohibition was rationalized by what came to be known as the stepping-stone hypothesis: marijuana was not in itself habit-forming but its use led to drugs like heroin that were. "The danger is this," testified Anslinger in 1951. "Over 50 percent of those young addicts started on marijuana smoking. They started there and graduated to heroin; they took to the needle when the thrill of marijuana was gone."[44]

Again Anslinger had appropriated a partial truth. Minority addicts treated at the federal narcotic hospitals typically smoked marijuana a year or two before using heroin. It did not follow, however, that marijuana led ineluctably to heroin. Many adolescents from the same milieu, including delinquents and gang members, smoked marijuana but refrained from trying opiates.[45] Nor was there any scientific evidence to substantiate the horror stories Anslinger was fond of circulating. Growing numbers of college-age marijuana smokers discovered this for themselves in the 1960s. Marijuana might not be good for their lungs, or their memories, or their waistlines, but neither did it lead to rape, madness, or axe murder. Moreover, if the authorities had misrepresented the dangers posed by marijuana, what of the other drugs they controlled? Just what was wrong with "narcotics"?[46]

What, in fact, was wrong with all the great American taboos? The ultimate basis for the suppression of nonmedical drug use lay in the realm of moral assumptions. Americans of the classic period were, to a degree unknown today, governed by a popular moral code, postulated on the self-evident correctness of patriotism, self-discipline, hard work, self-reliance, family stability, personal honesty, and self-restraint.[47] However dishonored in practice, these virtues were consistently affirmed by religious and civil institutions, and served to justify the proscription of drugs, just as they had earlier served to rationalize the prohibition of drink. During the 1960s, however, these traditional values—Harry Anslinger's values —were increasingly questioned. The principal challenges came from the mass media, the youthful counterculture, and skeptical "new class" intellectuals disenchanted by the status quo and optimistic that they could replace it with something better. Whatever the merits of their critique, American society did change, becoming noticeably more permissive and secular. Although this social revolution did not peak until the 1970s, it was well underway by the mid-1960s, and it did not augur well for strict narcotic control.[48] Recall Anslinger's remark that maintaining addicts with drugs was like pandering to homosexuals. That analogy would be effective with a traditionalist, one who was instinctively homophobic. But for someone beginning to doubt the received wisdom, wondering if the suppression of homosexuality might not itself be unfair and counterproductive, the argument would not carry much weight. It might even backfire, lending credence to the belief that America (or Amerika, as it was soon to be called) was blindly opposed to all forms of social and political liberation, of which drug use was but one instance.[49]

As for narcotic officials, they had more on their minds than the unfavorable turn of the *Zeitgeist*. A more immediate problem, which Anslinger concealed but never resolved, was their shaky legal foundation. The denial of maintenance was predicated on distant and narrowly decided Supreme Court cases; there were also contrary precedents, like the *Linder* ruling. These weaknesses were not apparent to the general public, but they were known and discussed within the legal and medical communities, together with the more general question of the propriety of maintenance. The eventual outcome of this discussion was *Narcotic Drugs: Interim Report of the Joint Committee of the American Bar Association and the American Medical Association on Narcotic Drugs* (1958). Authored by a panel of physicians, lawyers, and judges, and based upon three years of research in the United States and Britain, the *Interim Report* was a temperate critique of the police approach with suggestions for further research and trial programs. Doubting "whether drug addicts can be deterred from using drugs by threats of jail or prison sentences," it recommended the establishment of an experimental outpatient clinic that might, under certain circumstances, supply addicts so they would not have to patronize illicit dealers.[50]

Anslinger, who saw this guarded proposal as the hole that would sunder the dike, immediately plugged it with his fist. Denouncing the committee's plan as "so simple that only a simpleton could think it up," he launched a campaign of villification against his opponents. The *pièce de résistance* was *Comments on Narcotic Drugs* (1959), a rebuttal by the "Advisory Committee to the Federal Bureau of Narcotics" which Anslinger quickly assembled. Clinics were portrayed as proven failures, liable to spread addiction and to provide comfort to the nation's communist enemies. The solution was not less punishment, but more: "Only under the impact of heavy prison sentences can we hope to rout the scum of the criminal world." And routing they deserved, since what they were really peddling was "murder on the installment plan." Experts who disputed this approach were feckless dreamers, or worse. As far as Anslinger was concerned they ought to join the addicts in jail. "He had no tolerance for disagreement," Howard Diller explained. "He completely disagreed with the free exchange of ideas on the subject." His Bureau spokesmen openly accused the critics of Hitlerian "Big Lie" tactics and of endangering the health and morals of the nation.[51]

It did not work. Anslinger not only failed to discredit or suppress the report—it was published in 1961 as *Drug Addiction: Crime or Disease?* and went through seven printings by 1969—his tactics backfired and brought unfavorable publicity to the Bureau. "The whole tenor of the [rebuttal] document," wrote Stanley Meisler in *The Nation*, "indicates Anslinger does not want to win the discussion as much as he wants to eliminate it."[52] Historian David Musto has commented, "the bureau's vituperative attack . . . can be seen as a desperate response to the belief that, regardless of congressional support and official bureau statements, its control of narcotic enforcement in America was beginning to slip."[53]

The year 1962 brought further slippage. On June 25 the Supreme Court decided, in *Robinson* v. *California*, to strike down a California statute making addiction to the use of narcotics a misdemeanor, punishable by ninety days to a year in the county jail. The Court, recalling the language of *Linder* that addicts "are diseased and proper subjects for [medical] treatment," condemned prison as a cruel and unusual punishment for the sick. "It is unlikely that any State at this moment in history," Justice Potter Stewart wrote, "would attempt to make it a criminal offense for a person to be mentally ill, or a leper, or to be afflicted with a venereal disease."[54] The decision did not do the appellant, Lawrence Robinson, much good—he had died in 1961—but it did scotch Anslinger's long-standing ambition to take addicts out of circulation to prevent crime and the further spread of addiction.

The addiction-as-disease theme was being sounded elsewhere as well. In 1962 Lawrence Kolb published *Drug Addiction*, a collection of articles and essays pointedly subtitled *A Medical Problem*. Kolb, once Anslinger's wary collaborator, had grown increasingly disenchanted with punitive tactics. He now called openly for Americans to rid themselves "of the fury that propagandists have injected into our laws, administrative practices, and attitudes concerning addiction."[55] Even as Kolb was airing his doubts, the chief perpetrator of the narcotic fury was being quietly eased from power; in 1962 Anslinger was forced to retire, having reached the age of seventy. He was succeeded by the Bureau's Deputy Commissioner, Henry L. Giordano. Anslinger did not disappear from the scene altogether; he put in an appearance at a large White House Conference on Narcotic Drug Abuse in September 1962 but seemed uncharacteristically subdued.[56] This same conference recommended the establishment of a presidential commission, which met and issued its report the following year. Among its recommendations were more flexible sentencing, wider latitude in medical treatment, and more emphasis on rehabilitation and research.[57]

Heresies were spreading about the land now, and they even bore the imprimatur of a presidential commission. The time was ripe for someone to heed the many calls for research and actually put together an experimental maintenance program. That task was accomplished in 1963–64 by Marie Nyswander, a psychiatrically trained clinician who had experience treating addicts, and Vincent Dole, a metabolic disease specialist who had no such experience but who brought a fresh approach to the problem. The story of the development of methadone maintenance is narrated by Dr. Dole himself later in this book; here the important thing to note is that the Bureau failed utterly to stop his and Nyswander's experimental work. He defied the agents sent to harass him, at one point suggesting that they take him to court "so we can have a determination on this point." The Bureau demurred. It might well have prevailed against an unscrupulous doctor writing prescriptions for cash, but its chance of winning against a distinguished scientist, backed by a major research institution, with a liberal majority on the Supreme Court, and in a climate increasingly hostile to the police approach, was effectively nil. The Bureau also failed to prevent the program from expanding. In 1965 a ward in the Manhattan General Hospital was given over to methadone maintenance, as Dole and Nyswander came under the sponsorship of the New York City health department. Although miniscule in comparison to what it would become in the early 1970s, methadone maintenance was by 1965 officially and permanently established. It was also beginning to attract widespread and favorable attention, both in medical journals and in popular periodicals such as *Look*, *Time*, *Newsweek*, and *Science Digest*. (Marie Nyswander was accorded the ultimate symbol of arrival, a profile in *The New Yorker*.) The antimaintenance regime was over.

There are other reasons for designating 1965 as the terminal date of the classic period. During that year new forces and personalities were emerging. The escalation of the war in Vietnam, sharply increased marijuana use by students, and the participatory "acid tests" staged by Ken Kesey and his Merry Pranksters were among the most notable developments, or at least the best publicized. Worries about opiates were compounded by new concerns over hallucinogens and the spread of drugs outside the ghetto. Popular music, which had steered clear of drug lyrics since Cab Calloway's heyday in the 1930s, became increasingly explicit about drug use. Three songs from 1965–66, The Association's "Along

Comes Mary," Bob Dylan's "Just Like Tom Thumb Blues," and Richard and Mimi Fariña's "Mainline Prosperity Blues," made reference to marijuana or narcotic use. Such allusions would become commonplace in the following decade.[58] After 1965 drug use also began to take on radical overtones; to light up a joint was to oppose the war, to question the system, to reject the square virtues. (Whatever else veteran narcotic addicts may have been, they were not social revolutionaries. They were too preoccupied with survival.)

The designation of a year or a decade as the end of an era is not likely to mean much unless it somehow affected the lives of those who passed through it. It seems, however, to have made a difference for many of the people we interviewed. We asked one woman, a methadone patient, whether she would stay away from drugs if she had her life to live over again. "Oh, definitely, brother!" she replied. "See, in my times, they didn't have the programs that you've got today. Today a kid can go *anywhere* for help, pick up the telephone and call for help with alcohol and narcotics and all that stuff. In my day you couldn't do that, they didn't have no place. A drug addict? 'Get out of here! We can't do nothin' for no dope fiend.'"

Others remarked that the zeal had gone out of narcotic enforcement. "The difference between now and the fifties is incredible," commented one man, who had used narcotics on and off for forty years. "Then you could get arrested for talking about it on the subway." Since then, however, "there's been very little attempt on the part of the police to make arrests for possession. . . . Now [in 1981] they're lined up over there on the East Side to buy drugs, and the police are making no attempt to arrest dealers—but they sure did under Anslinger." Although there are many continuities between American narcotic use today and during the classic period, not the least of which is the heavy minority involvement, there is still an important sense in which the years between 1923 and 1965 were unique. Never before and never since has there been such a vigorous attempt to suppress narcotics, such a determination to narrow the choices of addicts to two stark alternatives: jail or abstinence.

THE ORAL TESTIMONY

The primary purpose of this book is to offer multiple, first-person accounts of what it was like to be an addict during this unprecedentedly harsh period of narcotic control. Although there are articulate exceptions, such as William S. Burroughs, most addicts of this era did not leave written accounts of their experiences. Even if they possessed the talent and motivation to write, it was inexpedient to do so, given that the police might suddenly kick in the door and start seizing evidence. Any social historical account, emphasizing the experiences of the addicts themselves, must therefore rely heavily on oral history.

The gathering of such oral testimony was made possible by a chance discovery. In 1979 researchers at the New York State Division of Substance Abuse Services began noticing a growing number of older methadone patients—persons in their sixties, seventies, and even eighties— enrolled in New York City methadone maintenance programs. Almost all of them had lengthy addiction histories, in some cases more than fifty years. It seemed likely that they possessed valuable, unrecorded information about the history of narcotic addiction, that they could offer insiders' accounts of how American drug use and trafficking had evolved since federal controls were first imposed. It was also apparent that these men and women could not go on defying the actuarial tables much longer. So the agency decided to sponsor an oral history project. In May 1980 a team of interviewers, consisting of a historian (David Courtwright) and a sociologist (Herman Joseph), began arranging and taping interviews. A social psychologist (Don Des Jarlais) took part in a number of interviews and helped to coordinate the project.

Our research strategy was straightforward. Using computer printouts, we identified those clinics serving patients over the age of sixty. With the permission and assistance of the clinical staff, we approached patients and asked if we could tape anonymous interviews with them. At first we concentrated on the oldest individuals, for the simple reason that they might soon be dead. (In fact, several did die within weeks or months of our interviewing them.) Later, after we had accumulated a number of interviews with subjects over sixty, we began taping individuals in their fifties, provided that they had lengthy addiction histories. With the assistance of therapeutic community staff, we also located and interviewed three veteran addicts who had managed to quit using illicit narcotics through means other than methadone. We did not, however, interview young or middle-aged addicts, partly because this had already been done, but mainly because we were interested in probing as far back into history as possible.

Most of the interviews were conducted in familiar surroundings: the subjects' homes, or the clinics where they regularly received their medication. All were strictly voluntary, the only incentive to participate being a small honorarium. As it turned out, a large majority of those we contacted participated willingly, even enthusiastically. They had time on their hands, and were pleased (or perhaps amused) that someone should think their lives of historical interest. The fact that we were not addicts, or former addicts, was not held against us. Indeed, it often worked to our advantage. Precisely because we were nonaddicts, we had a license to ask questions that would otherwise be inappropriate or unproductive. For example, one addict would be unlikely to ask another what it was like to experience withdrawal symptoms, because they both already knew the answer, and in a visceral way. Should the question be raised, the answer would likely be a terse "Well, man, you know how it is." Empathy abbreviates. But when the same question is put by a nonaddict, subjects are forced to articulate their feelings, to explain themselves for the benefit of someone who cannot intuit the answer. They are, therefore, more likely to produce a detailed description of events.[59] Sometimes also a revelatory one: the insider-outsider dynamic can make things clearer to the subject, as well as to the interviewer, since it may be the first occasion when the former has been asked to enlarge upon some aspect of a personal experience. It is a sudden imagining of the forest for one who has spent a life among the trees.

Interviews of this sort, however informative, are of still greater value if they are structured and comparable. It was for this reason that we devised a list of core questions, reproduced in the Appendix. These questions were designed to elicit the life histories of the interviewees, with special reference to their use of narcotics and other drugs. They were asked about their childhood, their family and neighborhood, their schooling, their first use of drugs, why they used narcotics, the prices and sources of various drugs at different points in time, how they supported themselves, their prison histories, how they got into a methadone or other treatment program, what they thought of it, and so forth. When a person showed himself or herself to be especially knowledgeable on some point, we naturally departed from the prepared agenda and began asking other questions. Several subjects were so articulate and possessed such good recall that their interviews ran to several sessions. By 1981 we had recorded sixty-five life histories, amounting to more than two hundred hours of oral testimony.

It soon became apparent that we had more than enough material for a book conceived as a collection of first-person narratives. That is to say, our model was the edited anthology rather than the work of formal ethnography or statistical analysis. We have consciously adopted the format of such oral history classics as Ronald Blythe's *Akenfield: Portrait of an English Village* (1969), Studs Terkel's *Hard Times: An Oral History of the Great Depression* (1970), and Tamara Hareven and Randolph Langenbach's *Amoskeag: Life and Work in an American Factory-City* (1978). The virtues of these books are several: they are readable, they are concrete, and they are empathic. Although it is by no means the only way to describe the history of narcotic addiction, the oral tableau nevertheless appealed to us as a fresh and personal way of approaching the topic.

The oral history model is not without risks and limitations, however, and these should be considered as well. One problem with any finite collection of narratives has to do with their representativeness. How typical are the remembered experiences and feelings of a given group of interviewees? This question is raised in a particularly interesting way by our study. As mentioned earlier, the people we interviewed were mainly in their sixties or seventies and enrolled in methadone programs in the New York City area.[60] Did the fact that they were old, using methadone, and living in New York make them unrepresentative of narcotic users in the classic era?

The answer is yes and no. Begin with the problem of location. Although several of the interviewees had traveled extensively, most had lived in New York City for many years; some had lived there all their lives and had the accents to prove it. This distribution, however, was typical of the national pattern. Throughout the classic period, New York City was a mecca for narcotic users, home to an estimated half of the country's active addicts.[61] (Once, in 1938, Bureau of Narcotics officials needed a survey showing that the number of nonmedical addicts had declined since the 1920s, proving that the police approach had worked. They therefore sampled areas outside of New York City and any large northeastern states. They got their decline.[62]) Although our sample was geographically concentrated, so was the population of illicit narcotic users during the decades in question.

The problem posed by age and survival is more subtle. Why did these people live when so many of their compatriots died? One answer is that they were more cautious and disciplined than the average narcotic user. They kept up their appearances and hygiene, were careful about using clean needles, and were more scrupulous about the quality and amount of drugs they consumed. "I wasn't greedy," was a remark we heard repeatedly. "I can always be very realistic," explained one long-time user. "I've got so much, and it's got to last me, and not get myself in a position of being sick, because I couldn't control myself." Control and discipline were recurring themes—ironically so, in view of the stereotype of the dope fiend. "I think for about twenty years I shot one bag or two bags of dope a day," commented another user,

I've always had my own needle, and I never let anybody use it. I don't have any abscesses or nothing. Using that way, it was very easy for me to see how other people abused drugs. I felt, and I still feel that, if a person can afford it, and use drugs moderately, it wouldn't be detrimental to them in any way. But, it's like everything else: it ain't what you do, it's the way you do it.

The desire to avoid "drug abuse" extended to other substances as well. With one or two exceptions they shunned barbiturates and amphetamines, and drank heavily only when they were off narcotics, never concurrently. H.G., who worked as a railroad coach attendant during the 1940s, told a typical story:

I never did take pills, but I drank quite a bit of whiskey when I was on the railroad. I'd drink and smoke marijuana at the same time. But that was before I started using heroin. After I started using heroin I slackened up off the drinking. I never stopped—during the winter when it's cold I always take a shot of bourbon as a tonic to stimulate my body. But not just for pleasure or for kicks—mostly as a tonic.

One woman, who worked as a call girl, was addicted to heroin but detoxified in 1935 and remained abstinent for five years. She began frequenting nightclubs, however, and "got addicted to alcohol by drinking more than what I should have drunk." She went back to heroin as the lesser of two evils. "Heroin stopped the shakes and everything. I think drinking is the worst thing that could happen to a person." Arguably, she and the others we interviewed were better off with narcotics than with alcohol. Better off, that is, if they were mindful about dosage and needle hygiene. While these scruples did not eliminate the possibility of overdose or disease, they at least reduced the risk. ⟵

One significant detail that fits the pattern of restrained use is that many of our older subjects were, or aspired to be, opium smokers. Before World War II white opium smokers were a breed apart, a self-consciously elite group. Show-business personalities, underworld notables, musicians, confidence men, chorus girls, politicians, and assorted high rollers would gather in posh apartments or hotels, recline on mattresses, and take turns passing the communal pipe. These were people who possessed money and style, and they in no way identified with or shared the lifestyles of heroin addicts. "We never bothered with the needle users," recalled one smoker, a prostitute who earned up to $900 a week. "We looked down on them as something very scummy, very low." As it happened, most of the addicted opium smokers were eventually forced to inject street narcotics, as illicit supplies of prepared opium were drastically reduced during and after the 1930s. But many former smokers retained the habits and attitudes of this "better" class of narcotic users; to the extent that this made them more careful and discriminating, it helped to preserve their lives.

The same point can be made linguistically. All of our interviewees conceded that they were or are "addicts," but they often balked at the word "junkie." A junkie was a no-account, a slovenly type who could neither keep up his habit nor keep it within reasonable bounds. Junkies gave narcotic addicts a bad name. To become a junkie was to become a failure, to lose one's identity and self-respect. Janet, whose narrative is among those included in this volume, summed up the matter thus:

When I was using drugs, I enjoyed it. There's no use in me lying. It was good back in those years. I had plenty. I didn't have no sick days. I didn't have nobody running off with my money or giving me no bad stuff. . . . Drugs never killed nobody. All you've got to do is to get plenty of them. Drugs preserve you. But when you've got to be sick, and dissipating, and don't eat, and you're cattin' in them abandoned houses, winter and summer, you're *calling* for death. But I had a pretty good life; drugs and everything else I needed, I always had. I have never begged for cotton in my life, and everybody who knows me knows it.

To beg for cotton is to be so hard up as to crave the residue from the wisps of cotton used to filter impurities out of liquified heroin; it is to addicts roughly what drinking cheap wine is to alcoholics. "I certainly wouldn't have led the life that some lived," commented another addict. "I would have quit." Most of them did quit, insofar as they entered methadone programs in the late 1960s or early 1970s. Methadone maintenance came along at a time when they were reaching late middle age, and thus finding it harder to keep up a heroin habit. The programs gave them a graceful way out. They also helped to keep them alive, in that they provided controlled dosages of an unadulterated drug, as well as ancillary social and medical services.[63]

In short, the people we interviewed behaved in a businesslike way during their active careers as narcotic users. To cope with decades of ever-tightening legal and economic strictures they had to be organized and tenacious, or exceptionally well connected. They were a select group; they were the survivors. Their addiction was of a paradoxical sort. They were physically and psychologically dependent on narcotics, yet relatively cautious about the amount and circumstances of their use.[64] These addicts were "in the life," but not entirely of it.

Considered as subcultural history, there is thus a measure of bias in this collection of narratives. Three groups are missing or underrepresented: the "chippy users," or dilettantes; regular users who became addicted but then kicked and remained abstinent; and the dope fiends who shot up everything they could lay their hands on. The absence of these types is an unavoidable problem in an interview-based study with this time frame. It is nearly impossible to locate people who dabbled in narcotics a half century ago, quit, and then disappeared back into the general population. It is also extremely difficult to identify abstinent former addicts who were active prior to the 1950s.[65] As for the greedy or incautious users (or users who gave up narcotics for drink), they met with premature deaths and thus escaped interview. "I knew a lot of people who used drugs," remarked Teddy, "but most of them is dead, ain't around. If I go uptown, I see a few, and they look fucked up. Some of them are still using drugs, but most of them can't afford it, they can't get out and hustle. So what they do is go and get on the methadone." It happened that Teddy was one of the veteran addicts we interviewed who had never participated in a methadone maintenance program, but he conceded that his situation was unusual, that his generation of addicts had largely died, disappeared, or gone onto methadone. This is why any oral history of the classic era is likely to gravitate toward one part of the narcotic-using spectrum, that of controlled long-term addiction transmuted to methadone maintenance. There are, needless to say, plenty of other, current users to be interviewed—but their memories do not embrace fifty or sixty years of street experience.

Our method, then, has led us to focus on a subculture-within-a-subculture. It would be wrong, however, to suppose that the testimony of survivors is completely unrepresentative of the experiences of ordinary narcotic users during the mid-twentieth century. Much of what the survivors observed and commented on would have been described in the same terms by other types of users in the subculture: trends in the price and quality of drugs, for example, or the rituals associated with smoking opium or injecting heroin. Their attitudes toward the police, constant need for cash, reactions to imprisonment and withdrawal, techniques for inveigling physicians, all would have been much the same. The addicts may not have been like the junkies, but they all had to swim in the same sea.

An analogy may be useful. Much of what we know about life in concentration or labor camps comes from the testimony of survivors. These survivors were not a random group. The concentration camp inmates were spared immediate death only because their age and health made them suitable for slave labor, or because they had certain skills useful to their masters. They also presumably had unusual physical and psychological resources to get through the ordeal, as did their counterparts in forced labor camps. Despite the fact that they were in some ways atypical, we do not doubt (although we may occasionally wish to qualify) their collective description of camp life and routine. The same applies to those who managed to beat the odds and to survive as addicts: there is no reason to dismiss their collective account of the subculture and its history, even if we must bear in mind that their circumstances and talents were not always of the usual sort.

The question of representativeness is not the only possible evidential problem to arise from the oral history approach to narcotic addiction. There is also the more general issue of truthfulness. Addicts are popularly believed to be notorious liars. They also have shameful or illegal deeds in their past which they might wish to hide. How do we know that they were not deceiving us? How do we know that they were forthcoming?

The answer is that addicts do lie, but usually only when their freedom or their supply of drugs is at stake. Since most of our subjects were already in a methadone program and were receiving a legal supply of medication, this was not a factor; the interviews placed them in no jeopardy. To make doubly sure, we instructed them to avoid using surnames, either their own or those of living persons who may have been involved in various crimes. The given names used were, for the most part, aliases. This anonymity, together with our complete disassociation from any law enforcement agency, made for more relaxed and truthful interviews. As a rule people will tell the truth if they have nothing to fear.[66]

But what if, even with the best of intentions, the addicts suffered lapses of memory, or misremembered key events? This is a more difficult question to answer. Our subjects were old; many were ailing; and most had been using memory-impairing drugs (notably marijuana and alcohol) intermittently over the years. Consequently there were gaps and vagaries in some of their recollections, and we would not want to vouch for either the literal truth or the strict order of every single episode recounted to us. But this is once again a largely unavoidable problem: the limits of your memory are the limits of my interview.

Countermeasures are possible, however. We have weeded out the vaguest and most contradictory interviews; excerpts from them do not appear in this book.[67] We have also sought to corroborate individual stories by checking them against other sources, especially written ones. When a particular event or individual was mentioned on tape, we would examine newspapers, periodicals, government documents, memoirs, biographies, and histories, seeking to fix a precise date or to glean additional testimony. This was doubly useful, in that it permitted us to elaborate, as well as corroborate, a given story. Often we discovered material in written sources that made an oral episode more resonant and comprehensible, or vice versa. We could not intrude this information directly into the narratives—that would literally have been putting words into someone's mouth —but we did preserve part of it in the form of footnotes. We have also included a glossary for the convenience of readers who may be unfamiliar with twentieth-century criminal argot and drug terminology.

Research in traditional printed sources, although crucial, is not the only way of enriching oral narratives. Visual material, especially photographs, can be extremely valuable. But here we faced a dilemma. We could not use photographs, past or present, of interviewees whose identities we had agreed to conceal. The problem was solved by a discovery, of the sort that historians dream about, of three boxes of photographs from the 1920s through the 1960s in the photo archive of the Drug Enforcement Administration, the present-day successor of the Bureau of Narcotics. Many of the more interesting and unusual of these photographs are reproduced in this book, together with illustrations from several other sources.

Another challenge posed by an oral history of narcotic addiction—in many ways the most interesting and difficult challenge—is the transition from tape to printed narrative. Unless the subject is a natural storyteller, a polished speaker, or experienced in fielding questions, a literal transcript is liable to contain a certain amount of backtracking and repetition, as well as corrections, clarifications, lost threads, solecisms, spoonerisms, "uhs" and "you knows," and other locutions of twentieth-century speech. Transcripts, in other words, do not make for easy reading. In their own way they can be as frustrating and exhausting as a barrage of statistics or the arcana of scholarly discourse. They are also unmanageably long; word-for-word, these interviews would run to several thousand typed pages. We therefore found it necessary to cut and reshape this raw material into concise and readable accounts. In practice this meant deleting or summarizing certain sections, inserting occasional transitional words and phrases, translating gestures, making some grammatical changes, conflating scattered remarks, and altering dates or descriptions about which the speakers later changed their minds. A common occurrence in an oral history interview is for the subject to return to a particular episode, expanding, embellishing, and correcting it as the conversation gains momentum and the memories come flooding back. We sought to combine these verbal accretions into more complete and topically unified paragraphs. In order to enhance the narrative flow, we also elided or incorporated our own questions, except in instances where they were unusually long or otherwise would have been awkward to remove. These editing procedures are illustrated in the Appendix. Only when we, for reasons of confidentiality, changed the names of persons unduly or unnecessarily compromised by the interview, was meaning deliberately altered. And this happened rarely, since the subjects (who were themselves anonymous) were cautioned beforehand. When they did name names, it was usually of individuals like Billie Holiday or Arnold Rothstein, whose involvement with narcotics was so much a matter of public record as to make concealment unnecessary.

We realize, however, that there are those who prefer their oral history verbatim, who trust only untouched primary sources. In consideration of their needs, and to provide an eventual check upon our selection and editing, the tapes will be housed at the Columbia University Oral History Center, where they will be open to researchers beginning in the year 2000. The tapes are being restricted until then to help protect the interviewees, most of whom will have passed from the scene by the end of the century.

If the evaluation and editing of oral histories are challenging, so too is their arrangement into a book. The scheme we have used is one of topical chapters with brief introductions, followed by several related narratives. This form of organization is based on the assumption that the book will be of interest to both specialist and nonspecialist readers. Those who are seeking a systematic overview of American narcotic addiction during the classic era should read the book straight through. The chapters have been placed in a logical order, from the first use of narcotics through the onset of addiction, through the behavioral changes associated with addiction, to various forms of punishment and treatment. Readers who are not seeking a step-by-step account, however, and who have more precisely defined interests, can use the topical arrangement to pinpoint the narratives that are most likely to be of value to them. Someone who is researching historical patterns of addict crime, for example, may wish to begin *in medias res* with the chapters on "Hustling," "Hooking," and "Dealing." Because the book is an anthology, it can be read either sequentially or nonsequentially. It can also be read as a collection of memoirs; those who wish to proceed one-narrator-at-a-time, bypassing the chapter divisions, should use the alphabetical table of narratives at the beginning of the book.

In assembling the narratives for a given chapter, we adopted the same strategy that an addict might use in instructing a neophyte. We included prototypical examples, but with significant variations. If an interview contained good, detailed illustrations of common experiences, expressed in a clear and interesting way, then it was a prime candidate for inclusion; however, we also consciously incorporated special viewpoints—someone who was a medical addict, for example, or someone who had pursued an unusual criminal career. Unfortunately, we did have to leave out some excellent passages and even entire interviews, largely for considerations of length. But at least these will remain as a part of the archival collection.

Although this book is about narcotic addicts, it does not consist of their testimony alone. One attraction of an oral anthology is that it can provide, as in a novel or a film, several different and conflicting perspectives on the same events. A conventional scholarly work embodies the author's interpretation; it keeps the argument up front. A collection of narratives, on the other hand, is more inclusive, more diverse, and therefore potentially better suited to describe a complex and controversial phenomenon like narcotic addiction. This virtue did not occur to us at once, however. Our original intention was to confine ourselves to older addicts. But, as we progressed, we decided to interview some of the pioneers of methadone maintenance, such as Drs. Vincent Dole and Marie Nyswander, who could offer a medical interpretation of the problem and who, because of their own historical significance, were obvious candidates for interviews. For the sake of balance we taped sessions with leaders of various therapeutic communities, whose methods and philosophies stressed the drug-free approach. Finally, we considered the enforcement problem, conducting interviews with police officers who had first-hand knowledge of the narcotics field and who could comment on historical patterns of trafficking from their special vantage. We have included one former policeman's and several physicians' narratives; the testimony of the latter is especially valuable, insofar as it details the revolution in maintenance treatment. The aftermath of that revolution is, finally, the subject of an epilogue. What are the similarities and differences between classic-era narcotic addiction and the situation today, and what policy implications can be drawn from the contrast? It is a natural question to ask, and an important one to try to answer, since drug use has reemerged as a priority item on the national political agenda.

NOTES

1. Studies based mainly on interviews with younger addicts include Jeremy Larner and Ralph Tefferteller, *The Addict in the Street* (New York: Grove Press, 1964); Seymour Fiddle, *Portraits from a Shooting Gallery: Life Styles from the Drug Addict World* (New York: Harper and Row, 1967); and Michael Agar, *Ripping and Running: A Formal Ethnography of Urban Heroin Addicts* (New York: Seminar Press, 1973). Bruce Jackson, *In the Life: Versions of the Criminal Experience* (New York: Holt, Reinhart and Winston, 1972), is not devoted to addiction per se, but nevertheless contains reminiscences of several narcotic users. Bill Hanson et al., *Life with Heroin: Voices from the Inner City* (Lexington, Mass.: Lexington Books, 1985), focuses on black male heroin users and contains useful bibliographical material on the ethnography of drug use.
2. For a review of the statistical evidence on late nineteenth- and early twentieth-century addiction, see ch. 1 of David T. Courtwright, *Dark Paradise: Opiate Addiction in America before 1940* (Cambridge, Mass.: Harvard University Press, 1982). The argument that follows in the first section of this introduction is in part a recapitualtion and elaboration of the thesis of *Dark Paradise*.
3. Ernest M. Daland, "The Relief of Pain in Cancer Patients," *Public Health Reports*, Suppl. no. 121 (Washington, D.C.: G.P.O., 1936).
4. Address delivered at Syracuse, New York; copy forwarded to Katharine Bement Davis, November 22, 1924, Papers of the Bureau of Social Hygiene, Series 3, Box 3, Folder 126, Rockefeller Archive Center, North Tarrytown, N.Y.
5. Richard J. Bonnie and Charles H. Whitebread II, *The Marijuana Conviction: A History of Marijuana Prohibition in the United States* (Charlottesville: University Press of Virginia, 1974), 26–27.
6. As will be seen in ch. 5, nonmedical addicts sometimes exploited this double standard by feigning illness in order to receive narcotic prescriptions.
7. The correspondence and questionnaires that Wright assembled before making these estimates may be found in the Records of the United States Delegation to the International Opium Commission and Conference, 1909–1913, Record Group 43, National Archives, Washington, D.C.
8. The purpose of the tax was less to raise revenue than to justify the constitutionality of the bill, by making it seem an expression of the congressional taxing power in Article I, Section 8 of the Constitution. This was one of two standard gambits, the other being an evocation of the commerce clause. Those who drafted major social and economic reform legislation could be almost certain of constitutional challenges, and the Supreme Court had a reputation for frequently voiding such laws, at least prior to the "constitutional revolution" of 1937.
9. Bonnie and Whitebread, 28. "A Chemist" published the following letter in the *St. Louis Star-Times* of February 4, 1935: ". . . Marijuana, cocaine, morphine, heroin, opium, all alcoholic beverages and five other drugs are habit forming and known by all expert chemists. I think the best cure is to let dopers have all they want and get rid of them."

10. 249 U.S. 90; *Transcript of Record . . . The United States of America . . . v. C.T. Doremus* (filed 1918), 2.

11. 249 U.S. 98; *W.S. Webb and Jacob Goldbaum v. The United States of America . . . Brief on Behalf of the United States*, 34–35. The choice of metaphor is interesting, and reveals the extent to which the stereotypes of the addict and the alcoholic had become intertwined by 1918.

12. 268 U.S. 5. For a discussion of *Doremus, Webb, Linder,* and related cases, see Rufus King, *The Drug Hang-Up: America's Fifty-Year Folly* (Springfield, Ill.: Charles C. Thomas, 1972), 40–46. King argues that the government deliberately selected the most blatant and unsavory cases of "scrip doctors," thereby enhancing its chances of securing antimaintenance precedents. A reading of the government briefs in *Doremus* and *Webb* reveals a complementary strategy: statistical manipulation. Both documents assert that Congress was wrestling with a massive social problem, involving as many as 1.5 million addicts, concentrated in urban and industrial areas. These figures were frightening; they were also fabricated. One is struck by the fact that, at virtually every crucial juncture in the evolution of narcotic policy between 1909 and 1919, the key legislative and judicial decision makers had to rely on distorted and exaggerated figures. Addiction was understood as not merely bad but malignant, threatening to engulf the entire nation. This belief made restrictive measures seem necessary, despite doubts about their constitutionality. Finally, there was at the time of these rulings still widespread optimism that addicts could be cured and remain abstinent, especially if their supplies of drugs were cut off and they were left without an alternative. These assumptions were subsequently proved to be naive, but in historical terms they were nevertheless important to the passage and interpretation of the Harrison Act. See ch. 4 of David F. Musto, *The American Disease: Origins of Narcotic Control* (New Haven: Yale University Press, 1973).

13. The Shreveport closure was bracketed by two other noteworthy legal developments. In 1922 Congress passed the Narcotic Drugs Import and Export Act, placing further restrictions on the international narcotic trade and strengthening provisions against unauthorized possession; in 1924 it outlawed heroin altogether. In both practical and symbolic terms, however, it was the elimination of organized maintenance in 1923 that most clearly demarcated the classic period of narcotic control. The 1922 and 1924 statutes were essentially refinements or expansions of the established policy of forbidding certain drugs to nonmedical users.

14. It is now clear that Prohibition actually reduced the per capita consumption of alcohol, perhaps by as much as 50 percent. See Paul Aaron and David Musto, "Temperance and Prohibition in America: A Historical Overview," in Mark H. Moore and Dean R. Gerstein, eds., *Alcohol and Public Policy: Beyond the Shadow of Prohibition* (Washington, D.C.: National Academy Press, 1981), 164–66. However, as Aaron and Musto point out, this was not necessarily the perception of contemporaries. Repeal advocates conducted a skillful campaign of mystification; in 1932 no less a public figure than Franklin Roosevelt declared that "instead of restricting, we have extended the spread of intemperance." (*The Public Papers and Addresses of Franklin D.*

Roosevelt, Samuel I. Rosenman, comp., vol. 1 [New York: Random House, 1938], 685.) This myth is still widely entertained by Americans. On the official line that strict enforcement reduced nonmedical addiction after 1921 and the problems with this claim, see ch. 5 of Courtwright, *Dark Paradise.*

15. Quoted in Larry Engelmann, *Intemperance: The Lost War Against Liquor* (New York: Free Press, 1979), 199.

16. *The Public Papers and Addresses of Franklin D. Roosevelt*, vol. 1, 653.

17. E.g., Bonnie and Whitebread, *The Marijuana Conviction*, 19; Edward H. Williams, "The Drug-Habit Menace in the South," *Medical Record* 85 (1914), 247–49. Musto, in *The American Disease*, 61, 65–68, makes the interesting point that most of the key sponsors of the Harrison Act were drinkers and/ or opposed to alcohol prohibition. Some public figures, however, remained consistent in their opposition to both drink and drugs, e.g., Richmond P. Hobson and William Jennings Bryan. Generally speaking, only evangelical Protestants opposed both after the 1920s; most other Americans accepted moderate drinking (and tobacco smoking) but were vehemently opposed to narcotic use.

18. "Anslinger, H(arry) J(acob)," *Current Biography, Ninth Annual Compilation—1948* (New York: H.H. Wilson, 1949), 20–22; John Finlator, *The Drugged Nation: A "Narc's" Story* (New York: Simon and Schuster, 1973), 69–73; interview with Howard Diller in Larry Sloman, *Reefer Madness: The History of Marijuana in America* (Indianapolis: Bobbs-Merrill, 1979), 194–98; Harry Anslinger and Kenneth W. Chapman, "Narcotic Addiction," *Modern Medicine* 25 (1957), 182; H.J. Anslinger and William F. Tompkins, *The Traffic in Narcotics* (New York: Funk and Wagnalls, 1953), 241. The fullest and most balanced biographical treatment is John Caldwell McWilliams, "The Protectors: Harry J. Anslinger and the Federal Bureau of Narcotics, 1930–1962" (Ph.D. diss., Pennsylvania State University, 1986).

19. "Harry J. Anslinger Dies at 83; Hard-Hitting Foe of Narcotics," *New York Times*, November 18, 1975, p. 40; Anslinger and Chapman, 183, 189.

20. "Anslinger, H(arry) J(acob)," 21; Douglas Clark Kinder, "Bureaucratic Cold Warrior: Harry J. Anslinger and Illicit Narcotics Traffic," *Pacific Historical Review* 50 (1981), 169–91; and Douglas Clark Kinder and William O. Walker, "Stable Force in a Storm: Harry J. Anslinger and United States Narcotic Foreign Policy, 1930–1962," *Journal of American History* 72 (1986), 908–27.

21. Paul Starr, *The Social Transformation of American Medicine* (New York: Basic Books, 1982), 3–144.

22. One physician who took this stance was Charles Terry. His story is told in David T. Courtwright, "Charles Terry, *The Opium Problem*, and American Narcotic Policy," *Journal of Drug Issues* 16 (1984), 421–34.

23. Anslinger himself accepted Kolb's view on the psychopathic makeup of nonmedical addicts and made use of his findings that users were generally criminals before becoming addicted. Anslinger's predecessor, Levi Nutt, also declared that addicts were "mentally deficient or psychopathic characters" who needed to be taken off the streets and placed in institutions, thereby destroying the demand for smuggled drugs. Thus there was theoretical and practical continuity at the highest levels from the 1920s through the 1930s

and beyond. Or, as H. Wayne Morgan puts it, "by the time Anslinger headed the federal antinarcotic effort in 1930, the patterns of law enforcement were well set. He merely made them more efficient." Morgan, *Drugs in America, 1800–1980: A Social History* (Syracuse, N.Y.: Syracuse University Press, 1981), 124. See also Anslinger and Tompkins, 223, 268, and Courtwright, *Dark Paradise*, 141–45.

24. Anslinger and Chapman, "Narcotic Addiction," 175, 187, 191. See also Stanley Meisler, "Federal Narcotic Czar," *The Nation* 190 (February 20, 1960), 159; Morgan, *Drugs in America*, 134–35.

25. Gary Silver and Michael Aldrich have assembled a large number of sensational feature stories, editorial cartoons, and the like in *The Dope Chronicles: 1850–1950* (San Francisco: Harper and Row, 1979). Many of these come from the Hearst papers. The Hearst cartoons are of particular interest, not only as vivid illustrations of how the hard-line narcotic policy was reinforced by mass media, but because they sharply differentiated between drug and alcohol prohibition, upholding the former and condemning the latter. The comic strips of the Prohibition era also generally portrayed alcohol in a neutral or slightly favorable way. See Sylvia Lambert, "The Social History of Alcohol as Portrayed in the Comics up to the End of the Prohibition Era," *Journal of Drug Issues* 16 (1986), 585–608.

26. Patti Iiyama, Setsuko Matsunaga Nishi, and Bruce D. Johnson, *Drug Use and Abuse among U.S. Minorities: An Annotated Bibliography* (New York: Praeger, 1976), 16–17.

27. John C. Ball and Carl D. Chambers, eds., *The Epidemiology of Opiate Addiction in the United States* (Springfield, Ill.: Charles C. Thomas, 1970), 312–15. Note that the 1966 percentages include addicts in both the Lexington and Fort Worth hospitals.

28. Iiyama et al., *Drug Use and Abuse among U.S. Minorities*, 6.

29. *Manchild in the Promised Land* (New York: Macmillan, 1965), 99. See also pp. 179–91.

30. Richard B. Sherman, ed., *The Negro and the City* (Englewood Cliffs, N.J.: Prentice-Hall, 1970), 14; Mabel M. Smythe, ed., *The Black American Reference Book* (Englewood Cliffs, N.J.: Prentice-Hall, 1976), 178–79; Bureau of the Census, *State and Metropolitan Area Data Book, 1982: A Statistical Abstract Supplement* (Washington, D.C.: G.P.O., 1982), 201; Karl E. and Alma F. Taeubur, *Negroes in Cities: Residential Segregation and Neighborhood Change* (Chicago: Aldine, 1965), 1.

31. Thomas C. Holt, "Afro-Americans," in Stephan Thernstrom et al., eds., *The Harvard Encyclopedia of American Ethnic Groups* (Cambridge, Mass.: Belknap Press of Harvard University Press, 1980), 15; Brown, *Manchild*, 7–8.

32. See Sylvester Leahy, "Some Observations on Heroin Habitués," *Psychiatric Bulletin of the New York State Hospitals*, n.s. 8 (1915), 260, on the propensity of white immigrant children to become involved with narcotics.

33. "The cameos of security for the average white . . . ," Mailer wrote, "are not even a mockery to millions of Negroes; they are impossible." Trapped in a violent, fear-filled existence, the black man "could rarely afford the sophisticated inhibitions of civilization, and so he kept for his survival the

art of the primitive, he lived in the enormous present, he subsisted for his Saturday night kicks, relinquishing the pleasures of the mind for the more obligatory pleasures of the body. . . ." From the 1957 essay, "The White Negro," reprinted in *Advertisements for Myself* (New York: Perigee Books, 1981), 302–303.

34. Alan A. Block, "The Snowman Cometh: Coke in Progressive New York," *Criminology* 17 (1979), 75–79, describes the Bureau of Social Morals. Ralph Salerno comments on the Mafia in ch. 8 of the present study. The most important black organization to campaign against narcotics was the Nation of Islam, but whatever success it may have had was on the level of individual conversions. They were unable to keep the dealers off the streets for any sustained period of time.

35. Isidor Chein et al., *The Road to H: Narcotics, Delinquency, and Social Policy* (New York: Basic Books, 1964), 271–75. Familial disorganization was also common among blacks who migrated to southern cities. See Joel Williamson, *The Crucible of Race: Black-White Relations in the American South Since Emancipation* (New York: Oxford University Press, 1984), 59.

36. Anslinger and Chapman, "Narcotic Addiction," 182, 189–90.

37. Musto, *American Disease*, 230–32; Bonnie and Whitebread, *Marijuana Conviction*, 215; Edward M. Brecher et al., *Licit and Illicit Drugs* (Boston: Little, Brown, 1972), 419–20; Alfred R. Lindesmith, *The Addict and the Law* (Bloomington: Indiana University Press, 1965), 25–28, 33–34, 108; Lawrence Kolb, *Drug Addiction: A Medical Problem* (Springfield, Ill.: Charles C. Thomas, 1962), 157–59. There is an extensive file on the CandyBarrcase in the Kolb Papers, History of Medicine Division, National Library of Medicine, Bethesda, Maryland. See also John Bainbridge, "The Super-American State," *New Yorker* 37 (April 22, 1961), 100–10.

38. Morgan, *Drugs in America*, 147. See also McWilliams, "The Protectors," 193.

39. John Kaplan, *The Hardest Drug: Heroin and Public Policy* (Chicago: University of Chicago Press, 1983), 70–72.

40. Chein et al., *The Road to H*, 370–71. "The dope trade is by its very nature an extremely ruthless industry," Claude Brown has written. "Indeed, it attracts and is controlled by the most vicious, predacious, esurient and desperate elements of this society, who become negative idols for youth." ("Manchild in Harlem," *New York Times Magazine*, September 16, 1984, p. 54.)

41. Lewis Yablonsky, *Synanon: The Tunnel Back* (Baltimore: Penguin Books, 1967), especially 56–59; Morgan, *Drugs in America*, 151–52. Morgan also shows that group therapy in narcotic treatment was not an entirely new idea. See his description of the late nineteenth-century Keeley Institute, 78–89.

42. Lindesmith, *The Addict and the Law*, 124–28. For a more recent and balanced discussion of the heroin-crime connection, see Kaplan, *The Hardest Drug*, 51–58.

43. Nat Hentoff, "The Treatment of Patients" [Profile of Dr. Marie Nyswander], *New Yorker* 41 (June 26, 1965), 45. More recently Louis Nizer, in "How About Low-Cost Drugs for Addicts?" *New York Times*, June 6, 1986, p. E23, has complained that the illegality of cocaine, as well as heroin, has been responsible for a huge wave of street crime.

44. Bonnie and Whitebread, *Marijuana Conviction*, 213 et passim; Howard S. Becker, *Outsiders: Studies in the Sociology of Deviance* (London: Free Press of Glencoe, 1963), ch. 7; Lindesmith, *The Addict and the Law*, ch. 8; H.J. Anslinger with Courtney Ryley Cooper, "Marijuana: Assassin of Youth," *American Magazine* (July 1937), 18–19, 150–53.

45. Ball and Chambers, eds., *The Epidemiology of Opiate Addiction*, 167–77, 194–96, 229–30, 312.

46. Brecher et al., *Licit and Illicit Drugs*, 422, report that marijuana arrests in California rose from 1,156 in 1954 to 7,560 in 1964; two years later, in 1966, the total stood at 18,243. The growing skepticism over the harmfulness of marijuana during the 1960s is discussed in ch. 6 of Jerome L. Himmelstein, *The Strange Career of Marijuana: Politics and Ideology of Drug Control in America* (Westport, Conn.: Greenwood Press, 1983).

47. James Hitchcock, *Years of Crisis: Collected Essays, 1970–1983* (San Francisco: Ignatius Press, 1985), 57.

48. The head of New York's Phoenix House drug-treatment program, Dr. Mitchell S. Rosenthal, makes a similar point in "Time for a Real War on Drugs," *Newsweek* 106 (September 2, 1985), 12–13. Conventional prosecute-the-dealer tactics, he concludes, are ineffective "unless we reach a consensus on the strict enforcement of drug laws. . . . What is needed is broad societal *disapproval* of illicit drug use" (his emphasis). Rosenthal is correct. Informal social controls such as the disapproval of parents or peers are undoubtedly more effective than formal controls; moreover, drug laws are better enforced when an antinarcotic consensus exists. The problem is that there has been no such consensus since the middle-1960s; nor can it simply be willed back into existence, since the moral and social climate is so profoundly different from that of the classic era.

49. Morgan, *Drugs in America*, 159–61.

50. *Drug Addiction: Crime or Disease? Interim and Final Reports of the Joint Committee of the American Bar Association and the American Medical Association on Narcotic Drugs* (Bloomington: Indiana University Press, 1961; seventh printing in 1969), 19, 104–105.

51. *Comments on Narcotic Drugs* (Washington, D.C.: Bureau of Narcotics, 1959), 1, 51, 81, 95, 119, 135, et passim; Diller in Sloman, *Reefer Madness*, 199–200. Anslinger had reacted in a similarly violent fashion to the so-called LaGuardia Report of 1944, which deemphasized the dangers of marijuana smoking. McWilliams, "The Protectors," 189–90.

52. "Federal Narcotics Czar," 162.

53. *American Disease*, 234. The ABA-AMA report controversy is discussed further in King, *Drug Hang-Up*, ch. 18; Lindesmith, *The Addict and the Law*, 247–48; and William Butler Eldridge, *Narcotics and the Law: A Critique of the American Experiment in Narcotic Control*, 2nd ed. (Chicago: University of Chicago Press, 1967), ch. 3.

54. 370 U.S. 660; quotation at 666. Stewart's language reminds us again of addiction's status as a stigmatized disease. By the early 1960s, however, the Court, as well as the medical research establishment, was placing more emphasis on the disease aspect and less on the stigma.

55. *Narcotic Addiction*, 169. Eldridge's *Narcotics and the Law*, cited above and first published in 1962, carried a similar message: "the treatment of addiction and research into possible preventative medicine are medical problems and should be dealt with as such." Eldridge accorded a role to law enforcement, but argued that physicians should be free to individualize treatment, just as judges should be free to individualize sentences (118–25). *Narcotics and the Law* was published under the auspices of the American Bar Foundation.

56. King, *Drug Hang-Up*, 235.

57. President's Advisory Commission on Narcotic Drug Abuse, *Final Report* (Washington, D.C.: G.P.O., 1963), 6–9.

58. John P. Morgan, " 'Golden-Leaf Rag' to 'Angel-Dust': A 55-Year History of American Drug-Related Music" (typescript). We are grateful to Dr. Morgan for sharing his research with us.

59. This point is borne out by the experience of the authors of *Life with Heroin*, a 1985 ethnographic study of black, male, inner-city heroin users. Black ex-addicts were trained to act as interviewers. Although they gathered much valuable information, there were also lapses. The principal author, Bill Hanson, comments:

> In some ways, the indigenous interviewers were too familiar with many aspects of the users' surroundings and lifestyles which the project was designed to investigate in more depth. As a result, despite the precautions given during the training and subsequent supervision sessions, interviewers sometimes neglected to probe more deeply or ask the meaning of some comments, events, or phraseology. This problem was not related to the amount of time allowed for the interview or to interviewers' probing skills, but rather stemmed from interviewers' assumptions that the project directors knew more than they did or, more likely, that they simply would not be interested in much of what the interviewers considered the trivia of everyday life. (195)

60. It should be noted, however, that two of the methadone patients had recently detoxified completely and that several others were in the process of detoxification, or stated their intention of doing so.

61. Granville W. Larimore and Henry Brill, "Epidemiologic Factors in Drug Addiction in England and the United States," *Public Health Reports* 77 (1962), 558–59. See also U.S. Senate, *Organized Crime and Illicit Traffic in Narcotics: Hearings before the Permanent Subcommittee on Investigations of the Committee on Government Operations*, Part 3 (Washington, D.C.: G.P.O., 1964), 764.

62. Courtwright, *Dark Paradise*, 121.

63. The longevity issue is considered at greater length in Don C. Des Jarlais, Herman Joseph, and David T. Courtwright, "Old Age and Addiction: A Study of Elderly Patients in Methadone Maintenance Treatment," in Edward Gottheil et al., eds., *The Combined Problems of Alcoholism, Drug Addiction, and Aging* (Springfield, Ill.: Charles C. Thomas, 1985), 201–209. See also John C. Ball and John C. Urbaitis, "Absence of Major Medical Complications Among Chronic Opiate Addicts," *British Journal of Addiction* 65 (1970), 109–12. Ball and Urbaitis point out that it is the "hectic way of life" pursued

by most addicts that has such serious consequences, not the effects of opiates *per se.*

64. Strong support for the continued existence of a controlled addict subculture may be found in Hanson et al., *Life with Heroin.*

65. This problem is well illustrated by Patrick Biernacki's pioneering study, *Pathways from Heroin Addiction: Recovery Without Treatment* (Philadelphia, 1986). Using chain-referral sampling, Biernacki located and interviewed 101 former users who were in many respects the opposite of our group: heroin addicts who had managed to quit and remain abstinent without benefit of medical treatment. But not one of his subjects became addicted before World War II, and only a handful did so during the 1950s. The large majority dated their addiction to the 1960s or 1970s (xiii, 226–29). This is in no way to fault Biernacki's method, only to point out the difficulty of locating very old, abstinent addicts with extensive knowledge of the classic era, particularly of the years from 1923 to 1950.

66. See John Paul McKinsey, "Transient Men in Missouri: A Descriptive Analysis of Transient Men and of Agencies Dealing with Them" (Ph.D. diss., University of Missouri, 1940), 64–66, and John C. Ball, "The Reliability and Validity of Interview Data Obtained from 59 Narcotic Drug Addicts," *American Journal of Sociology* 72 (1967), 650–54. Ball's subjects were asked about their addiction history, employment, criminal record, and current drug use. Their answers were checked against hospital files, FBI arrest records, and fresh urine samples. "The research results indicate a rather surprising veracity on the part of former addicts," Ball concluded. On the question of first arrest, for example, 80.7 percent of the sample either reported the first arrest correctly or even admitted an earlier offense than those listed in the FBI files. Disassociation with the police was essential to obtaining such results.

The only conspicuous episode of lying we encountered, where the details of the story simply did not make sense, involved two female patients attending the same methadone clinic. It turned out that they had had a lesbian relationship over many years and had agreed upon a cover story to conceal that fact. It is interesting that they attempted to disguise their homosexuality, yet spoke freely of their experiences with drugs.

67. As a double check, we asked a researcher who had himself been an addict to read the manuscript and identify any episodes or narratives that seemed suspicious or contradictory to him.

PART ONE:
BECOMING AN ADDICT

1.

Turned On

Almost all of the persons we interviewed had a vivid memory of their first use of a narcotic, as well as the circumstances leading up to it. Like most twentieth-century addicts, they were introduced to opiates by acquaintances, rather than by pharmacists or physicians. Coming into contact with someone who sold or gave them narcotics was not just a matter of bad luck. As members of lower-class or deviant subcultures, they traveled in circles in which opiate use was commonplace and exposure therefore likely to occur. Because they were jazz musicians, or ghetto dwellers, or marijuana smokers they stood a much better chance of discovering the joys and sorrows of heroin than people whose activities were confined to the straight world. This was a fact of political as well as epidemiological significance, since the pattern of low-life narcotic use reinforced the consensus behind the police approach. The relationship was circular, insofar as criminalizing drug use kept it pretty much confined to criminal circles. Heroin belonged to the night, and Anslinger meant to keep it there.

We asked our subjects how they felt when they first used narcotics. The reactions varied. Some individuals, like the late saxophonist Art Pepper, claimed to experience a pure and powerful euphoria. In his autobiography, Straight Life, *Pepper recalled that his first sniff of heroin gave him a sense of warmth and peace he had never known; for the first time in his life he was free from the demons of guilt and self-hatred. "I looked in the mirror," he wrote, "and I looked like an angel."*[1]

For the majority, however, the high was accompanied by an intense nausea. Like the novice drinker who has had one too many, they became miserably sick. This was partly a matter of natural aversion, the body's response when first challenged by a dose of an external opiate. It may also reflect the somewhat higher

1. Art and Laurie Pepper, *Straight Life: The Story of Art Pepper* (New York: Schirmer Books, 1979), 85.

purity of street heroin during the classic era, something that the addicts themselves remarked upon.

TEDDY

Teddy was born of black parents in Savannah, Georgia, in 1927. His family life was extremely unstable. His absentee father drank himself to death, and his mother tried repeatedly to foist Teddy on other relatives: "I was like a burden to her." Eventually she ran away to New York City, but he found her and joined her in the mid-1930s.

When I was a youngster Harlem was alive. You could hear laughter. The streets would be full of people. Lenox Avenue, Seventh Avenue, all had businesses: there wasn't an empty store front along there. Seventh Avenue was like Broadway downtown. There was dope in Harlem, and crime, but it wasn't like it is now: people weren't getting mugged. Sure, there were fights, but it was basically just fights.

The section I lived in was integrated. There were white people living right down the block on 132nd Street, and on 134th. I went to school with white kids. We even had gangs or clubs with the white kids in them. The people who owned the stores, most of them were Jews or Italians; they used to bring their kids there in the morning, and the kids would go to school with us to grammar school. When they'd complete grammar school, they'd go someplace else. I went to P.S. 89: it was the first school I'd gone to. I didn't go all that much down South—there wasn't nobody to make you go down there; it was left to your family. It wasn't compulsory to go to school the way it was here in New York. So my mother had to take me to school. I went as far as the eighth grade. I started ninth grade but I was just *going*, if you know what I mean: I went when I wanted. There was no one there to guide me; there was never no one home. My mother worked as a maid on Long Island. She would leave in the morning to go to work, or whatever, and she might come home two days later. So I'd be runnin' around on the streets and stealing. At that time you could go to all the five-and-ten-cent stores, where they'd have cookies and candies just laying on the shelves. I'd go and pick them up and eat them. It was like a picnic. Everything was in the open—it wasn't like it is now, where everything is in cases.

I had run-ins with the police, like for stealing cases of soda off of trucks. See, back then the police had a different system. The police knew just about everybody on their beat: all the kids, where they lived, who their mothers were, and their fathers. This way, if something happened in the neighborhood—if someone said, "Why, them kids stole so-and-so"

—he'd round up all the kids in the block and find out who it was. Most of the time they'd take you home. But if your mother wasn't home, they'd take you to the precinct, slap you around, beat you up, and send you on home. Then they'd notify your parents and say, "Listen, Teddy did this, this, and this." That's when I was getting to be about thirteen, fourteen years old.

The first time that I actually got arrested was for cuttin' a guy. I was in a teenager's gang; maybe I was about fifteen. It was a territory thing: we've got this block, this is our block, and you can't come in this block unless you've got permission from us. We were fighting, but we weren't fighting really to *kill* one another, even though we had sticks and knives. You had to carry this stuff. If you stuck somebody, it made you a big guy. If you stuck so-and-so, they'd give you a name like "Ice Pick Slim" or "Killer Ray." You'd try to get a nickname for yourself. The police would take us in, and line up all the clubs, and ask, "Who did this?" So you'd say, "I stuck the guy," right? It was a thing where, if you did it, you told them. You did it because it looked good—you'd get a name for yourself, you know. People would say, "Teddy sticked that guy, yeah," or "Teddy'll kill ya," or "Don't mess with Teddy, 'cause he's a bad guy." This is how you started to get that rep, or that bad-guy image.

I started with dope around fourteen, but I wasn't actually using it. I was handling it. First, I have to tell you that dope back then was handled entirely differently from what it is now. People that were dope fiends, you'd never know that they were dope fiends, for the simple reason that they didn't nod on no corners, they weren't greasy, and if they stole anything, you would never know. They were clean, their clothes looked good, and they only stole the best. They kept money in their pockets, and nobody talked, nobody said, "Oh, listen, there's Teddy who's a dope fiend." It was a quietly kept thing.

How did we find out about it? Well, by being kids in the block, we knew everything: we knew who took numbers, where the whiskey was. I was making whiskey in a bathtub. The person that started me handling dope was the same person with the whiskey. They used us kids because we were better to use than an adult: they could give us twenty-five or thirty cents, or a dollar, and that seemed like big money. They'd let us run the stuff, and the police would be less suspicious of the kids, you know.

I was working in this house that dealt in sex, alcohol, and drugs. There were girls there, and whiskey for sale, and narcotics. The police knew this was going on, but they didn't arrest anybody because they'd come buy and pick up their payoff. My position was more or less a hanger-on-er or a flunkie. I used to put the liquor in the bottles. I'd add one shot of brown sugar that I cooked up on the stove to make it look just like whiskey. I would sit on the stoop, where I had a string with a bell. When somebody *surprising.*

wanted some whiskey, they would come up in their car; I'd go up and get it, bring it out. I was a lookout man. If the cop came, I'd ring the bell and start running.

The johns who came to this house were mostly white people. It was downtown trade, not uptown. In fact, we didn't want to deal with the blacks at all because you'd have to hassle with them. They'd want to come in and try to make love to the girls, stay all night, make a home. With a white person, they'd come in and do what they gotta do and leave. No problems. Get in their car and—phewww!—they're gone. There was no argument about, "I paid this amount of money and I don't think she did it right." And most of the time the blacks who would come for the girls would be drunk on alcohol, and that would be a problem. You can't just tell them, "No," so you have to deal with them some way. If possible, we'd try to steer them away: "Hey, man, why don't you go across there to so-and-so."

These white johns were mostly in business or, if they weren't business-men, they were well dressed when they came up. Usually they'd come in twos, sometimes even in threes. I guess this was a safety thing, although we had a policy not to beat nobody—nobody'd come in there and get robbed, because if they got robbed or something, the business is gone. So as long as they were in the house with us, they were protected. The block was the same way: once they left the house, nobody'd do nothing in the block. They were protected, and that kept our business going. This was a thing also with the people who were using dope. They didn't tell who they copped from. If they got busted, they didn't say, "Well, I went over to Teddy and got it." You got busted, and that was it. The police used to deal different with people who used dope, because their addiction wasn't a known thing. The only time a guy would get found out was when he got sick.

Protection

The only narcotics they sold in this house were heroin and cocaine. Marijuana was never big, it wasn't a good seller, business-wise. There was nothing in it. But heroin and coke just turns over—on Fridays, Saturdays, you had people who were like regular customers going in a store. They had their hours; they'd call up and say, "Listen, I'll be there," or, "Could you get Teddy to drop this off at this place for me."

The people who bought the drugs were mostly black men and women: waiters, musicians, showgirls. Some of them were hustlers. They would go downtown and shoplift or pickpocket. This is what you call *slickness;* very few would rob somebody, or actually cause bodily harm. 'Cause, like I said before, every store in New York was opened up, things weren't chained down. Shoplifting was the big thing—you didn't have no muggings.

When I first started working there, I didn't know what dope was. I'd go into the house and see people shooting it in their arm, and I thought it was medicine. It wasn't until I was sixteen that I used my first dope. I'd run errands for the prostitutes upstairs, if they wanted something from the store. Every time I'd do this they'd give me a tip. So one day I went up to the third floor, and the girl had this white powder on her table. She was doing it in her nose. I said, "What you doing?" She said, "You want some?" And I said, "Yeah!" and I snorted some heroin. The first reaction is hard to explain. I got a big itch in my groin; I started scratchin' and scratchin'. I don't know if I got high, or what, but I had to scratch. The girl said, "What's wrong with you, boy? What you got, the crabs? You been fuckin' around, or something?" I said, "No man, but my mother-fuckin' thing's itching down there!" Then I got sick. Your stomach feels upset. I felt like I was going to bring it all up, like my stomach was floating in shit. And when I did bring it up, it was all green, if you know what I mean. After I got over the scratchin', and the first sickness, I was fucked up one way or the other for damn near all day. See, the grade of heroin they sold back then would probably O.D. a couple of people out here now.

A couple of days later I tried it again. Why? Curiosity. It was *there*, you know. And within these crowds, you don't want to say no. You want to be known, you want to be down, you want to be hip, to know everything that's going on. Say, if you drank and it's all right for you, then, why not, I'm going to try it too. If it made you feel good, it'll make me feel good. Then it'll give me something to talk to you about on your level; I'm coming up. I'll say, "Well, shit, we had that same stuff, and it was good, man," and you'll say, "Yeah." I can't relate it to you if I never tried it. To talk about it, I have to know what I'm talking about. This way, if people said, "We have something here that we want to get tested," somebody would say, "Well, we can go get Teddy. He'll test it. He's all right. He knows what's happening."

It was like coming up through the ranks. That's what they did for the black kids coming up back in them days. The majority of us, we didn't have no plans or no future. We never planned anything. We never expected no more than what we were. The only thing, if you were lucky, you would say, "Wow, if I finish high school, I might be able to get me a department of sanitation job." That was about the biggest: there were very few black conductors. In fact, on 125th Street, there were very few black salesmen in the stores. All the stores in Harlem had white clerks. There was no future to look for, like there is today. They're *paying* kids to go to school now; all the colleges and everything have opened up. Your parents now could send you to college and it doesn't cost them anything. But when I was coming up, it was a scuffle just to try to get through high school. So the kids were running in the street like I was. It was a relief for the parents to get rid of us: this was a responsibility they didn't have to worry about. And we'd do whatever the people in the block were doing—

if they were writing numbers, or selling dope, or whatever. It was a part of the neighborhood. You either did it, or you got out of the neighborhood. A person who worked, or went straight—what we'd call a "square"—would go his own way. Most of them were better off than we were in the long run. Look at what happened to me. I wish I was a square—I wish I was a square now, but not before. Back then I thought it was the hippest thing in the world to be with somebody that shot dope, or drank whiskey, or smoked reefer, rather than to be with somebody who had a job.

STICK

I was born in 1922 in a house on Fifty-ninth Street and Tenth Avenue. That part of New York was called Hell's Kitchen. There were real tenement houses; we called them "cold-water flats." That meant you ain't got no hot water, unless you heat it. And when you stood at the door, you could look straight through the apartment, because there were no rooms off by themselves. Some called them "railroad apartments." The bathtub was in the kitchen, because that was the warmest part of the house. We had five rooms, and plenty of closet space, because we always used one room for all the excess junk like winter clothing in the summertime.

My family moved to 103rd Street between Second and Third avenues before I started school. It was pretty much the same thing: cold-water flats, railroad flats, naked light bulbs burning, no heat, no hot water. We had to stuff the windows with rags in the wintertime to keep the heat in and the cold air out. To save money you put your food on the windowsill —everybody had a window box in them days. Instead of buying ice, they'd nail a box to the window that faces the back yard and put a piece of linoleum over it so the rain wouldn't get in. In the wintertime you could put all your meats and stuff in there. That's the kind of winters we used to have, man. It used to be real cold.

I had twelve brothers and sisters: six girls and six boys. I was the last one on the vine. I had a twin brother, but he died. My father had been a farmer before I was born, but when he came up to New York, he had only one job that I knew of, working for the WPA. But he raised thirteen children. He was like a witch doctor. He sold roots and home remedies for all kinds of different ailments that people would tell him about. He had cures for them; the house stayed full of people all the time. And he never even had a social security card. My mom used to do housework. Long ago they used to have certain areas of the Bronx, white neighborhoods, where the black ladies would go and stand on various corners. The white ladies would come out, you understand, and hire them for a day's work to clean their houses, cook, whatever. That's what my mother used to do, every morning, five days a week. Sometimes she'd work three days a week for this lady, or two days a week for that lady. A houseworker, that's what she was. Neither my mother nor father could read nor write.

It was a struggle during my childhood, but that wasn't unusual, because everybody was struggling. There wasn't nobody who could point me out and say, "There goes Stick, man," because we *all* had patches in our pants and we *all* had holes in our shoes with cardboard stuffed down in them. There wasn't no exception; it was like a regular, real thing. That's the way it was.

I left school in the ninth grade, after my father died. Although my mother didn't want me to stop school, I could see that we didn't have no money, no regular money like when my father was alive. I didn't quit school right away; I tried to go to school and work for Loew's movie at Seventy-second Street. I worked at night cleaning the movie theater from twelve o'clock to eight o'clock. Then I'd get on the Lexington Avenue bus and shoot to school. I went to P.S. 171, then to the machine and medal trades school on Ninety-sixth Street between First and Second avenues. But after awhile I started sleeping in the classroom, because I'd been up all night cleaning the movie. I'd sit in the classroom, trying to do the schoolwork, and I'd be sleeping like I was on dope or something. [Laughs.] I smoked a little reefer in school, but it wasn't a big thing. If somebody came up and said, "Look, man, I got some pot, man. Y'all want to get down?" we'd say, "Yeah, man." But nobody didn't look for no pot. Maybe we'd drink us a little wine; you could get wine twenty-five cents for a milk bottle full. The pot was twenty-five cents a stick. That's not the reason I was sleeping in class, though. I was just tired.

I was seventeen when I stopped school. I was working for the next two years, or running the streets. I was hanging out, you know, going to dances, planning parties, gang-fighting. We always had plenty of that. They called the gangs "social clubs." [Laughs.] We'd all chip in with the money and we'd give dances and stuff, or buy jackets, or maybe all get together and buy a raggedy car for the gang. East Harlem is Spanish today, but it wasn't when I lived there. We had everybody: we had Gypsies, we had Spanish people, we had Irish people, we had Italian people. Everybody was down there. There was no prejudice as far as I could see: I used to go to their houses; they used to come to my house. Their mothers used to beat me up if they catched me doing something wrong; my mother used to beat them up . . . It was a real community. There wasn't no "Hey, we hate the white guy," or "Hey, we hate the nigger," or "Hey, we hate the spic." There wasn't no shit like that.

But it wasn't that way in the army. I was drafted and went into the army in January of 1943. When they called me I was glad, because there would be more money for the family. I would be able to send them a check every month. I was sent to Camp Upton. I think it was out there on Long Island or some damn place—I don't even know where it was at.[2] Joe Louis was inducted at Camp Upton; now they send everyone to Fort Dix.

After six weeks of basic training I went to Camp Butner in North Carolina, then to South Carolina, then to Boston, then to Le Havre, in France. The camps were segregated—segregated to the core. Whites went one way, blacks went the other. This was the first time that I was segregated because I was black. I can't lie and say that I never encountered racial discrimination until I went into the service. But it was an underlying thing that wasn't really mentioned. We all knew that there was something wrong, something different between the white people and the black people, but it wasn't no *confrontation* thing, you know. We'd only whisper about it, not holler out like they do now.

There was no patriotism amongst the blacks that I knew. The army wasn't about fighting for your country. It was something that we had to do or suffer consequences we didn't want to pay. If you said, "Look, man, I'm not going in the army," then you were going to jail. If you didn't want to go to jail, you went into the army. And, after you went into the army and you got up tight in a position where it was either your life or your death, either kill or be killed, you're going to kill if you can. It was about fighting for your life, not no country. There was very, very, very little patriotism that I have ever felt or witnessed. I have never felt patriotic toward this country, or met anyone who has, in the service or out.

I'll tell you an interesting thing, though. Later on, when I was driving with a convoy of four ammunition trucks in Liège, Belgium, there was a Frenchman standing in the road, waving us off. He was telling us, "*Roosevelt kaput, Roosevelt kaput.*" We said, "Man, what are you talkin' about, '*Roosevelt kaput?*' What are you crazy, or something? What does that mean? Is he dead?" That's the first time I ever felt anything about this country, that I ever had any real feelings about America. The second time was when they killed Kennedy.

I was in several battles in Europe. I was in the Ardennes, I was in the breakthrough to Belgium, and I was on the Red Ball Highway. Shit, that damn thing was a battlefield in itself. The Germans kept hitting it anytime they felt like it during the early part of the war. There were some guys in my trucking outfit who were killed or injured.

I got a punctured lung myself, but I didn't get that in Germany. I went to the Philippines after the war was over in Europe. We thought we were going home, but they changed our uniforms, gave us new weapons and khaki outfits and mosquito netting. We drove all night and all day leaving

2. It was on Long Island, in Suffolk County, and was used during both world wars.

Germany. We went from Marseilles, past Gibraltar, through the Panama Canal, straight to Luzon. We were two months and a week on that ship. It was horrible.

The first night we got to Luzon we found that the harbor was all choked up with sunken ships. Our ship couldn't navigate, so it moored outside the port, and they had to come all the way out and get us on them damn amphibious ducks—do you remember them?[3] To get to them we had to climb off the boats on rope ladders. Naturally, some guys got drowned. They'd fall into the water with all that gear and shit on and go straight to the bottom.

Well, anyhow, we went to the area that we were supposed to be in. We chopped down all this foliage and made us a camp site. Everything was cool now; the mess sergeant fixed us up some jive meal—you know how it is in the service, a bullshit meal—but it was something to eat anyway. Then we went out to see what the joint looked like. We didn't have our vehicles, but we all had weapons; man, we were armed to the teeth. We were bunched up in little groups—you know how two or three guys will hang out together. We went out and drank this new whiskey called *sake*. Then we came back and we were sitting around and rapping about what the girls were like, and how the whiskey was, and the food, and all that stuff, when a bunch of guys came back all beat-up. We said, "Hey, what happened to you guys? Goddam!" They ran it down to us how they went to this whorehouse, and the white guys beat them up because they weren't supposed to go in there. Everybody got their weapons and said, "C'mon, man, show us where it's at." So we went down to this place and tore the town up. The whorehouse was sitting on bamboo sticks, up above the ground. [Laughs.] We snatched the sticks out from under the house and destroyed it.

It happened that a couple of guys got killed. So the white MPs came and surrounded our outfit with half-tracks. Their lieutenant said, "All right, y'all gotta give up your weapons." Our first sergeant rapped with the lieutenant, then he came and rapped with us. The sergeant said he wanted to talk to us in private, because at first we weren't going to give up the guns. He said, "Look, everybody in this outfit's got a private weapon. I know goddam well you got your own guns, so give them their guns. And if you ain't got a weapon, see me. If you ain't got no ammunition, see me." So we gave the MPs all the regulation weapons, the rifles and the forty-fives. They even took the fifty-caliber machine guns. If we had had to face an attack by the Japanese, we would have been in trouble, because

3. These were two-and-a-half-ton, six-wheel-drive trucks equipped with a propeller and watertight hull. They were called ducks because of their code designation, DUKW.

all we had was pistols. We'd have been up shit creek. But the only time we faced the Japanese was on skirmishes. It was snipers and like that; we never faced a whole Japanese unit.

I got the punctured lung from a bayonet. There was this young Japanese prisoner—I don't know where he got the bayonet from. He caught me off guard, even though I was looking right at him. He ran up to me and plunged the bayonet down into my shoulder. I was so shocked I didn't even move; that's the only thing that saved my life. The doctor later said he didn't know why it didn't cut a nerve. It just went straight down and pierced my lung. Then he snatched it out of my shoulder.

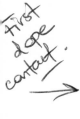

I stayed out in the field for three days; there wasn't no pain or nothing. *Three days,* and I still performed my duties. But on the fourth day I began having difficulties breathing. [Mimics rapid panting.] Blood was filling up my lung, and it got infected. My whole side was in pain. They took me to the hospital. They gave me a shot of morphine. It took the pain away, and I went on to sleep. That was my first shot of dope. While I was in the hospital I only got three shots, and that wasn't daily either. That was "as needed," or as they thought I needed it.

After that, I was seeking it on my own. I was asking guys in the hospital how you would go about getting it. I was seeking this information because I enjoyed the morphine. I felt nauseous after the first shot, but there was something that overrode the nauseousness, and the pins-and-needles feeling. There was something that was greater than the discomfort.

What was it about the morphine that you liked so much?

Peace. Peace. An inner peace. Yes, an inner peace. Relaxed. Yeah, relaxed. Away from all the goddam tension and anxieties and dissatisfaction and all that stuff that "reality" is about. Everybody says that when you use dope you're escaping from reality. You're goddam right—what do you think reality is, something funny? Or something pleasant? Shit. Damn right: who the hell wants to look at reality?

From the Philippines we went to Japan. My outfit was one of the first outfits over there; we started moving in right after the atomic bomb. We were all packed up because, if they didn't drop the bomb, they were getting ready to invade Japan. They had turned us from a trucking outfit to an amphibious outfit. They took away our trucks and gave us ducks: we were a land-and-sea force. [Laughs.]

There were black-market drugs in Japan: heroin, opium, and hashish. That was the first time I came into contact with pure, raw opium. It was like a plug of chewing tobacco. You took a little pinch and chewed it. It was a downer—a relaxer, I guess you'd call it. Peace and tranquility. I preferred the opium to morphine, although I didn't use it no more than four or five times while I was in Japan. I didn't get a nauseous feeling from the opium, although I probably didn't take that much.

I received an honorable discharge. I came out of the army in April. I had terminal leave; I was still getting paid by the army even though my discharge date didn't come up until the fourth of June. I had a little money, and one of my brothers got me a job on the waterfront on the North River here in Manhattan. Then I tried to get a truck driver's job. That didn't pan out at all. I tried to get a job with Jack Frost sugar refineries, and plenty of other companies that had tractor-trailers on the road, but I could never land one. You couldn't get a job driving in New York State if you were black back in '47. Some companies would let me go as far as filling out an application, but they'd never call me. So I couldn't get a job doing what I wanted to do.

Then I got married. My woman was a dress designer for Bergdorf Goodman. She was making nice money. She wanted to get ahead, you know. So I got a job in the post office, and she was as pleased as punch. "My old man works in the post office," she said—that fucking bourgeoisie shit, right. [Laughs.] But, hey, I only worked there for three or four nights. I didn't want the job. I only filled out the application and took the test just to please her. They gave me ten points on the test because I was a veteran. They called me one day to go get the job. I said, "Damn," but I went on down to the general post office on 33rd Street, that big joint down there. Three nights and I quit. It wasn't the hard work; it was that I was cooped up. I had just gotten out of the service and I wasn't settled. I didn't have any intelligence at all—I just walked away from the damn job and they mailed me my check.

After that I went back on the waterfront for a while. But my wife was becoming more and more "dissatisfied" with my fucking "actions," 'cause I'm spending up her money, and my money. She was making some nice money, and I was fucking it up. Then one day a guy came around the house. We were talking and he told me about selling dope. He needed a runner—this was when the East Side was the dope center for the city. The guy who owned the dope was Italian, but everyone who worked for him was either Spanish, or Italian, or black—it was a whole conglomeration of people. So I started working for this Italian dude, carrying dope from the East Side down to the Penthouse Ballroom on Union Square. There was a nightclub on top of this office building. All I had to do was drop the dope off and get the hell on out of there. I got a hundred and a half a trip.

I wasn't using then. I mean I was using, but I wasn't hooked. I started using heroin the same year I started running dope. Here's what happened. I was sitting out there and bullshitting with this guy. He tells me, "Hey, man, this other guy is sick." I said, "What are you talkin' about, he's 'sick'?" He said, "He needs some dope, man." I said, "What? Damn, he got a Jones?" He said, "Yeah, he got a Jones, man." I had some money, so I went and got some dope, and the two of us took it down. We gave it to this dude, and he snorted it. Then my friend snorted it, and I snorted it. That's the first time I got high in America.

I got sick. I threw up. But, as I said before, there's an overriding feeling of peace that erased the memory of all that other bullshit, the nausea and the discomfort. It reminded me of the opium in Japan. That night I just sat out on the stoop. The doors were open because it was in the summertime. I was sitting on the stoop by myself; nobody was in the street. I could see the light coming from the bar and, hey, I was listening to Billy Eckstine singing. I was at peace with myself and everything around me.

That was the beginning, or another beginning. I snorted again about a week later. Each time I said, "Man, I'll never use none of that shit no more." But then it came around, and I couldn't resist it, and I went on along. Same thing: I said, "I'll never use it no more." Then again and again, though I kept saying it. [Laughs.] I went down fightin', but I wound up getting hooked.

BRENDA

Ever since the 1930s, when Prohibition was repealed, Americans have tended, both attitudinally and behaviorally, to separate alcohol from drugs. Franklin Roosevelt, the chain-smoking president who signed the 1937 Marijuana Tax Act into law and who once conveyed to Harry Anslinger the threat that "should he ever forward to the White House a recommendation for clemency for a drug pusher, he could attach his resignation to it," liked to unwind in the afternoon over cocktails. Anslinger himself kept a bar in his home and was fond of Jack Daniels.[4] Neither man felt the least embarrassment over drinking, or saw it as contradictory behavior. They, like the vast majority of Americans—evangelicals excepted—were adhering to the dominant post-Prohibition code: moderate drinking is acceptable, but narcotics are taboo.

Despite the legal and cultural divorce of drinking from drug use, alcoholism historically has been an important antecedent of narcotic addiction in this country, both during the classic period and in the decades preceding it. This arose from the fact that heavy drinkers often discovered that they could use opiates as a sure cure for their hangovers, as well as for other pleasurable effects. As late as 1940 Garland Williams, the Bureau of Narcotics' District Supervisor for New York, remarked how frequently he was told by an addict "that he became addicted when

4. David F. Musto, *The American Disease: Origins of Narcotic Control* (New Haven: Yale University Press, 1973), 212; Frank Freidel, *Franklin D. Roosevelt: The Triumph* (Boston: Little, Brown, 1956), 142; James Sterba, "The Politics of Pot," *Esquire* 70 (August 1968), 58, 118.

*an associate induced him to take 'shots' of heroin in order to ease the pains of a
'hang-over' from a long drinking spell."*[5]

*Brenda is a case in point. Born of white parents in Brooklyn in 1923, she was
raised in her grandparents' home, following her mother's death and her father's
confinement in a Veterans' Hospital. A gifted student, she won a scholarship to a
Catholic high school, where she received a liberal education. Then, shortly after
graduation, her life fell apart.*

I was introduced to liquor by a young man I had met in the neighborhood.
I was seventeen, just in the last six months of high school. It wasn't that
I'd drink heavy in the beginning. It was, you'd say, social drinking. But I
could never control social drinking. Two or three drinks or highballs and
I was out of control.

I was never allowed at a young age, in the early teens—thirteen, fourteen—to even associate with a boy. I was told that, if boys were at a
party, I couldn't go. In other words, the upbringing was strict. Too strict.
Too cautious, as I see it today. But I was the one sister, of the two of
us, that wanted the freedom of going out and having friends. I was more
aggressive, and she was very passive.

After I finished high school, I went to work for a short while as an
assistant bookkeeper for a company. I left there and went to work for the
Insurance Company of North America. I wanted to be an underwriter.
But, in the process of this, I became very infatuated with the young man
I told you about. I was a romantic young girl, I'd never been with another
boy. And, under the influence of alcohol, I conceived a child.

This brought a terrible disgrace to the family. I was ostracized, I guess
you'd call it. I was constantly being called names by grandmother, like
"the whore" or "nasty, filthy, dirty girl." While I was going through the
pregnancy, she'd look at me with such disgust. I think you know in them
times what people were like. My grandmother and grandfather were naturally very moral people and very religious people. You didn't have sex with
a young man unless you were married. You were in no way promiscuous—
that was a horror to them. Abortion? Oh, forget it. That was unheard of.

This made me feel terribly dejected for a young girl, terribly hurt, even
though I felt an enormous amount of guilt. I knew, the way I was raised,
that I wasn't supposed to have gotten involved in a situation like this. The
two together—my own religious upbringing in Catholic school and their
constant downgrading of me—kept me filled with enormous guilt.

I married in January of 1942, and I had the child in August. My

5. Letter to Harry Anslinger, February 9, 1940, Treasury Department file 0120-9,
accessed through the Freedom of Information Division of the Drug Enforcement Administration, Washington, D.C. See also ch. 9 of John A. O'Donnell, *Narcotic Addicts in Kentucky*
(Washington, D.C.: G.P.O., 1969).

grandmother would accept me back home, but she didn't want any part of the father, even though I married him. He didn't have anything, so he couldn't provide a home. But his mother agreed to have us and, right after the child was born, I went to live with his parents.

They were altogether different from my grandparents. They were alcoholics, the mother and the father. The father passed away shortly after that. The mother was from the old country, Ireland. She was very abusive, physically abusive to her four children. It was a frightening home for me, very uncomfortable. I disliked the woman intensely. Years later, when I looked back on it, I was able to understand her behavior. At the time, of course, I didn't.

My husband went into the service when the baby was three months old. He went into the army. I stayed with the mother for five months, then he came home on a leave. He was stationed in the States still. I left New York with him and went to Orlando, Florida, where there was an air base. My mother-in-law took care of the baby. He insisted that I go. I didn't want to go; I wanted to stay with the baby. But it was a short stay, and he was sent overseas. When I came back to New York, I was pregnant again. Still no home, and another child.

After I had the baby, that was it. I couldn't live there with my mother-in-law any longer. I tried to find an apartment, with the fifty or sixty dollar allotment you got from the government. I found a small apartment in a horrible tenement in Brooklyn, in Greenpoint. I don't know today if I could even describe it, with the cockroaches—which I was scared to death of. It was just a fearful place. No bath, just a toilet. Twenty or twenty-five dollars a month. There were two rooms, a kitchen and a bedroom.

I didn't even know public assistance existed. All I knew was the check from the government. But then my husband overextended his last leave in New York. After he caught up with his outfit and got to London he was court-martialed. The court-martial gave him a dishonorable discharge and so much time in prison. But all of that, once the war was progressing, was changed from a general court-martial to a summary court-martial, and he was later reinstated in the service because he was called to active duty. Now, this stopped the allotment check for me altogether at the time I was pregnant with the second child. Three or four months before I was ready to give birth to her I had no allotment; everything stopped because he had gone through that general court-martial. When he was reinstated I didn't receive any back pay; I didn't receive *anything* until the baby was four and a half months old. In the meantime it was a process of running to my grandmother for food, to his mother for food, of learning how to go to the grocery store on the corner before they opened up in the morning. They used to have milk cases outside that the milkman would deliver, and all the bread and rolls would sit outside the grocery store. I began to get up early in the morning and help myself to the rolls and two or

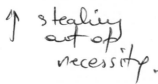
stealing
out of
necessity.

three bottles of milk. I saw this as a necessity; I knew no other way to get it. While I was waiting for the baby, my grandmother helped me with the rent. The gas and the electricity were turned off. In other words, I was solely dependent on the grandmother, and whatever I could get from the mother-in-law. But neither one of them would agree to mind the two children and let me go to work.

My husband came home in the early part of '46. No doubt he could have got out sooner, because married men with families were the first ones to leave. He was working as a bartender in an officers' club in London. He made money on the side doing that, of course, but never sent me anything for the care of the children. When he came home, much as I thought of him when I first married him, this was a very crude, really cruel man. He drank twice as much as he had when we first got married. He was really, by this time, a heavy alcoholic. I lived with him for a short time after he came home in this small apartment. He made no attempt to find a home for me and the children. It was the responsibility he didn't want, as I see it today. He was young. It was too much for him. He wanted out in any way, shape, or form. His only way of resolving the whole thing was to go out and get drunk and come home and beat me up, until my grandmother pleaded with me. "You'll have ulcers on your eyes," she'd tell me, "by the time you're twenty-five years old. The man'll blind you." Every week I had a black eye.

It finally came to a head when he came in one evening and broke my leg. He kicked me from the ankle to up above the knee and gashed it in so many places that when the police came they wanted to know who had done this. I was so fearful of him—which is hard to explain today, but people don't really know what it's like—I told them I fell down the stairs. Much as they tried to tell me they knew that that was impossible, that whoever did this should be put away, I was still too fearful to say anything. That was when my grandmother agreed that, if I would get away from New York and get away from him, she would take care of one of the children, if his mother would agree to take care of the other one. She said, "You'll have to get away from here. The man is going to kill you." I said, "But how can I leave? I have nothing to leave on. Where could I go?" I didn't know any place to go, and I didn't want to leave the children. You know, you love your children no matter how bad things are. But she kept after me, and she was a very strong lady. "I'll give you the money. Take a bus, go anywhere, and get a job. Once you're straightened out with a job you can get your children."

Well, it doesn't always work out the way things are planned for you. I left. I went to Chicago. My grandmother took the youngest child, and his mother took the older one. I went back to school. I took a job at night, and I went into nurse's training. The job at night was so different from what I was trying to go for in the daytime. I was going to school to be a nurse

Drinker's outlet.

in the daytime and looking for the money at night, in a nightclub, where I could make the most of it. At that time they had a dice game going in most nightclubs in Chicago; I was a dealer at one of the tables.

During the period when my husband was away in the service I stopped drinking. But the minute he came back I started to drink, the very second he came back. After that I couldn't get away from the drinking, even when I left and was going to school. The nightclub provided the drinks. It was an outlet for me, being lonesome for the children and wanting to go home, and still wanting to make some money. Twenty-three was very young, immature, to go off by yourself to a strange city, where you knew no one, with a few dollars in your pocket, which wasn't very much, and have to go to work. And, of course, a girl alone always meets the wrong people.

I continued with the school, but the nighttime drinking was my problem. At school I ended up meeting a young nurse; we roomed together to save expenses. She was older than I was by ten years. She had been taking Demerol for quite some time. She didn't have any pains or sickness that I knew of. I came in one night: I was drinking quite heavy. I got up the next morning sick—really, terribly, sick. I thought, "Oh, how am I going to make it today?" She told me, "Well, why don't you take a shot of Demerol? I have some." It was a 30 cc bottle. She withdrew some with a syringe, and I took it intramuscular. In a short time—say twenty minutes, thirty minutes—no hangover. I was fine, ready to start all over again. This, little by little, became the habit of pulling away from alcohol. I was advised by her, "You can't function, and hold your school together, and have a hangover all the time. You can't be intoxicated when you go to school. If you want to finish up, you're going to have to straighten yourself out some way." Well, my "straightening out" became the Demerol.

I didn't take the Demerol to get high. I took the Demerol because it relaxed me—no problems. The feeling of having to get home passed away. All the pressures were taken away with the Demerol. It also gave me energy. Not only energy, but a very relaxed, confident . . . sense of well-being.

2.

Hooked

Classic-era political cartoons often portrayed drug dealers as vampires or snakes —creatures who, once they plunged their fangs into a victim, produced ineluctable death. Any contact with drugs posed mortal danger. Hence, the cliché "it's so good don't even try it once."

Recent research, however, has downplayed the necessary link between narcotics and addiction. Researchers such as Norman Zinberg have shown that many people can use heroin once, twice, or even semi-regularly without becoming full-blown addicts.[1] *This does not mean that heroin is safe, only that some individuals manage to use it occasionally and recreationally in such a way that it does not take over their lives. Narcotic users themselves have long recognized this pattern, and have a host of names for it: "weekend habit," "chicken-shit habit," "ice cream habit," "Saturday-night habit," "chippy habit."*

The problem is that, while some persons can continue to use occasionally, others cannot. Our subjects all began as chippy users. Not one of them started with the intention of becoming an addict. If they were aware of addiction at all, it was something that they feared. What happened was that they drifted into regular use over a period of several weeks or months. By gradually increasing the size and frequency of their doses they became, without knowing it, physically dependent. When a chance event interrupted their use of narcotics, they experienced withdrawal symptoms. These included yawning, chills, running nose, watering eyes, goose flesh, sweating, cramps, tremors, vomiting, and severe diarrhea:

When you're kicking, your bowels bust, you get nauseous. You're puking, you're sick. You lay there like a dog. You don't care what goes on; people could step all over you. You lay in your own dirt and everything else, and you don't think

---

1. Norman E. Zinberg, "Nonaddictive Opiate Use," in James C. Weissman and Robert L. DuPont, eds., *Criminal Justice and Drugs: The Unresolved Connection* (Port Washington, N.Y.: Kennikat, 1982), 5–23.

nothing of it. It takes about seventy-two hours or so to get it out of your system—that's if you've been any kind of a user at all.

But physical dependence and withdrawal symptoms, however unpleasant, are not quite the same thing as addiction. To become fully addicted, or "hooked," users had to understand why they were sick, that their sudden, confusing illness was caused by the absence of narcotics. Once they made the connection and understood that they could solve (or "fix") the problem with another injection, then a powerful association was established between the continued use of opiates and the prevention or relief of pain. To the original motive of pleasure was added a second, even more compelling incentive: keep using or get sick. They were now addicts. They had to have narcotics, and they knew it.[2]

One theme that ran through the interviews was the important role played by veteran users in the addiction process. Not only did they provide the subjects with opiates, they also acted as interpreters of the experience. They explained, for example, that the nausea they suffered as novices would pass after the second or third trial. The experienced users were also often the ones to provide the crucial information that the way to alleviate withdrawal distress was simply another fix, setting the stage for the dramatic recognition of addiction. Conversely, addicts who were loners, who were afraid or ashamed to associate with other users, took longer to realize what had happened. They had to puzzle out the facts of addiction for themselves.

IVORY

Ivory was born to poor black parents in Port Arthur, Texas, in 1920. His father, "a street guy who did nothing," left when he was six years old: "I don't know whether he's dead or living." Ivory was arrested for stealing when he was eleven years old, and was in and out of reformatories and prisons for the rest of his life. Between terms he married, conceived a child, and divorced. He also supported himself as a pickpocket and as a "mechanic," or card shark, first in Houston and later in Los Angeles. It was in Los Angeles that he first used heroin, in 1952.

I had been in jail. I had gotten into a couple of fights in jail, and they moved me out of the tank I was staying in. A tank was where a lot of people stayed—they tried to have you segregated, they tried to have all the robbers together, all the burglars together, all the junkies together.

---

2. For an extended discussion of the addiction process, see Alfred R. Lindesmith's classic study, *Addiction and Opiates*, rev. ed. (Chicago: Aldine, 1968).

They moved me into the tank where the junkies were. They said, "If he wants to fight, we'll put him where he'll get a lot of fighting." But I knew all those guys from the street, and I was glad to get in there, because a lot of them were my friends.

I would sit down at night and hear all these stories they'd tell about dope. The first time I used some dope was there in jail. A guy got his wife to bring some heroin in a dollar bill. See, they used to let us have cash money. She took the dollar bill and saturated it with heroin, and then she took her iron and smoothed it out. Then she wrinkled it all up. The bill was encrusted with dope. We'd have to go up to the screen to get money; he would take it, and put it on the table, and take a razor blade and cut little pieces off. He would take those little pieces and put them in a spoon, put some water on it, put a match to it, and stir it, and the dope would come right out. Then they would fix up. They asked me, "Do you want some? Ohhh, this is good." They asked about three times.[3] I said no, I don't want none of that. I was scared. Actually I was really scared to death. I always was scared of the needle. I'm still scared of the needle now, if it isn't in my own hand.

But they just kept on. A guy I knew he just kept on. He said, "Come on, take a little bit. Come on, Ivory, take a little." I said, "OK, fix me up some." So he fixed me up a little bit in a dropper. I held my head back, and he shot it, and it made me sick. I throwed up all over the place—I didn't even feel good. I told him I didn't want no more of that. So I didn't fool with it no more in jail.

I got out, and I went to another friend of mine. He and his old lady were in the bed. She had just gone out and got some stuff. He fixed up and said, "You want to try a little bit?" I said, "No, man, the last time I tried that, it made me sick." He said, "Whoever gave it to you, gave you too much. We'll give you some that will make you feel good." So I said OK. He fixed me up, gave me a little taste. After awhile I had a feeling coming over me that I'd never felt before. It was strange, and then it felt so good. I started laughing and getting happy and going on with myself.

When I left, me and some guys went riding in the car. I puked all over the car and everything. After I got through puking I went into a washroom and washed up. But I felt so good, you know.

Now, I didn't just go straight into using it. I don't think I used no more for maybe a long time, seven or eight months. What I did, I started to selling dope. A guy told me how I could make some money—see, I had

3. This detail of the story is highly unusual and should be taken with a grain of salt. Drugs are scarce in jail, and addicted inmates are not known for their generosity in sharing them.

two girls on the street hustling, so I had money in the bank. He talked me into buying some dope to sell, so I went and drew some money out of the bank. I bought an eighth of an ounce, and I gave it to him to sell for me and him. But he was a junkie, so he beat me out of the money.

I started talking to another boy I knew in jail. He said, "Ivory, I've got some dope I'll sell you cheap." So, I said, "What about four hundred dollars' worth?" He said, "I'll give you a good deal." During that time they were selling dope in caps. I bought it, and I got someone to show me how to cap it up.

In the olden days, heroin was heroin. L.A. was noted for good dope. Some dope came directly into L.A., but it didn't come in like it did to New York. New York is the seaport of the world for dope. See, we used to pool our money and send a guy to New York every month to pick up the dope, until the dope there went to getting bad in the fifties. Then we had it the other way: we used to have more people coming from New York to Los Angeles and picking up dope. That's one thing I was always scared of, when they'd send a guy to pick up dope to make a drop.[4] I didn't like that. You could get busted that way, or robbed.

Dope is maybe 97 or 98 percent pure—they say it will never be 100 percent. The big boys, they'll sell it to somebody who's damn near as big, somebody who'll buy a quarter of a million dollars' worth of dope. They'll take the dope—they call the places where they cut up the dope "mills"—they'll take it and put twice as much cut on it as there is dope, so they've made their money back two times. If they paid a quarter of a million dollars for it, they'll get three-quarters of a million back.

The next guy comes to buy, say, he wants two, three hundred thousand dollars' worth of stuff. Then he takes it home, whacks it up, puts the same cut on it: two-on-one, or three-on-one, or four-on-one. All right, then he sells it to someone else—now we're getting down to the riff-raff. He puts his cut on and sells it to another guy, maybe the type of dealer I was. I get it, put the whack on it, put three spoons to every one. I'll sell it to the next guy—now we're getting around to the ordinary dealer. He'll ask you, "Man, how many cuts can I put on it?" You tell him, "Man, you can put four." That means he'll put one good spoon with four spoons of cut. Then he's going to sell it to the ordinary guy who don't do nothing but sell stuff on the street out of caps and bags. *He's* going to get a whack out of it. And you know what the dope is when you get it on the street? Something like one and a half, two percent.

That's why the L.A. dope was better: there were more cuts in New York. Big as New York was, it had the sorriest dope in the country. New York City is more crooked than L.A. New York City's got twice as much

4. I.e., to pick up drugs for delivery to a third party.

of everything. Anything Los Angeles will do, New York will do it bigger. You can believe that.

Anyway, I was making a good living off of selling heroin. Every day I was putting five, six hundred dollars in the bank. I wasn't addicted. I wasn't even using—I told you about the first two times.

A very good friend of mine used to come to the house. He used to buy dope from me and shoot it at my house. My old lady, she laughed at him, but she'd let him get off because she liked him. He was a pretty good guy. Another friend worked in Lionel Hampton's band. He was addicted. Every time he would come to town, he would come by the house. He'd buy seventy, eighty dollars' worth of dope, and he'd always bring show people with him. Entertainment people, a lot of guys in Count Basie's band. I used to meet some interesting people, especially women. Like the girl that died, Billie Holiday. So I got curious. This is how I got hooked— I got curious. I said to myself, "Good God, look at all these people. They aren't like the average addict I see on the street, dirty and nasty. These people are clean, they've got a pocketful of money, a profession, they sing in big bands, travel all over the country. They're using that stuff? Then, sure, I'm going to try it again." I told this guy I knew, "Man, I want to try it." He said, "OK, I'll fix you up." He fixed me up some and I shot it in my leg. See, in Los Angeles, they've got a law there, if they see tracks on your arm, they would put you in jail—they call it "vag-addict." So I shot in my leg. It began to get so good, every day I'd want some. That must have went on for about six months.

One day this other guy—not the one who played in the band, but the one who came to my house all the time—he came around with some show girls. They were burlesque dancers, and they would fix 'n' go. I was in the bed this particular day. He said, "Man, get up." It was about three o'clock. I said, "I feel bad. I'm sick. My stomach's hurting. I must have a bad cold, my nose is running. Man, I don't know what's the matter with me." I'm hooked, but I don't know it. So he started laughing. He said, "Oh, Goddam! Whoa!" He's laughing at me. He said, "You've got a habit." I said, "Oh, bull." You see, I'd never been to the point where I had to hustle for no dope, or to where I knew how it felt to be sick, because I'd always had all the dope I wanted. He said, "Boy, you're sick, and you're getting sicker and sicker." So I said, "What happens now?" He said, "You got to get out of that bed and fix you some stuff. Let me show you." He made my old lady get the works, and he fixed me up some and shot it in. In about three or four minutes, I'm feeling just marvelin' good. He said, "Boy, I told you, you're hooked." That's the way I got hooked. From then on, it was an everyday thing.

MICK

Mick was born into a large white family in Brooklyn in 1909. There were nine sons and one daughter; he was the youngest of the boys. His father, who ran a livery stable and fruit stand, died suddenly when Mick was six years old. But the older brothers took over the business, and his mother, a multilingual native of Alsace-Lorraine, earned fees by acting as advisor and translator for newly arrived immigrants.

I used to go out fooling around with a wild bunch of kids. They were mainly the sons of immigrants: Irish, Italian, German, Polish, Jewish. In them days we used to run up after the wagons—you know, they used to deliver the groceries and stuff in wagons. We'd get on the back of the wagon and get a couple of cases of tomatoes or whatever the hell was on there, then we'd go out and sell it. We used to go over to the railroad and get coal, "heave coal" we used to call it. Then we'd sell it. That's how we made our money to go to the movies and buy cocaine. You could buy it in a drug store then. We could buy a half-ounce for fifty cents over the counter.

The other fellas in the gang introduced me to cocaine. I was around thirteen, fourteen. But it was only snorting in those days; there wasn't no shooting or anything. Just put a little cocaine on the back of your hand and sniff it. That was it. It'd get you a little high. It was all good cocaine, pure cocaine. It gave you a lightheaded feeling, you got little hallucinations, fantasies—you went off into fantasies, like.

After we sniffed cocaine we'd just hang around and maybe go to a movie or sit around the parks. And vaudeville, they had vaudeville in them days. We'd go to the RKO—at that time it was Keith's Orpheum, Keith's Theater. And we'd go to burlesques. They had Gaiety Burlesques, forty cents, fifty cents. We went in to see a show, and we'd have cocaine. But there was no robbing or none of that. It's just that we raised a little hell amongst ourselves. We'd get high, sit around and talk, and that's it. You could buy beer then, you could buy all the beer you wanted. It was only a nickel a glass. [Laughs.] But I didn't drink that much. I never was much of a drinker.

See, it was no disgrace to be a cokie—they used to call them "cokies." People who passed by never made no remarks or said "look at that cokie" or anything like that. Your eyes got glassy, and that was it, and that was the only way they could tell. You'd stare, but you wouldn't actually be seeing anything, you know what I mean? Everything you'd see would be in your own imagination.

It wasn't a steady diet. Don't get me wrong—it wasn't that you had to have it. It was something that you could take, or something that you could leave alone. That's the way it was. If we thought that going to the show was more important than buying the cocaine, why we'd go to the show. It wasn't real habit-forming unless you dipped in every day. But none of us did that, none of the fellas I knew. One of them went off to be a policeman; he retired, he died. The other fella, he turned out to be a tug boat captain. This cocaine use was just a passing fancy, being with the crowd, like. Going to the beach, or something like that. We used to go to North Beach out here in Queens and have a couple of sniffs of coke.[5] Same as these kids today: they smoke this pot and they get high. But it's a different feeling to them—half of them go nuts. Cocaine didn't make you feel like that.

My mother and my older brothers didn't worry about my being in this gang—everybody ran around in them days. It was no big thing to be in; it was no *gang* like a mischievous gang or anything. No, whatever you did, you did. It was just what you'd call "pranks" today. Wildness. You'd do a little nod; you'd steal a little here; or you'd go heaving coal; go pick junk; miss school. Truancy was the biggest thing in them days. They had a truant officer, and they'd pick you up. Your parents had to go down to Jeralemon Street, Schermerhorn Street, and explain why you didn't go to school if you was staying out too much. I went as far as the ninth grade. I used to play hookey a lot. Then I beat it when I was fourteen. I got out of school; I quit altogether.

After I dropped out of ninth grade, I went aboard a ship. I was out at sea most of the time then. I got away from the gang. I got away from all that. I got on as an apprentice oiler on the United States Line. I went on from there to be a fireman, and so forth. I worked for American Exports; they covered every port in the United States, in Europe, and all over the world. American Exports—it was one of the very biggest.

There wasn't much money in it, but it was a good life. It kept you good and healthy. Of course, you had your freedom when you went ashore in different countries—and they weren't as strict, like the customs and all. You'd go ashore, and you could drink or fool around with women or do whatever you wanted. You could buy cocaine or morphine or opium when you hit certain ports, like in Africa.

Sometimes I used drugs on liberty; most of the time I just got drunk. I didn't bother with drugs until I went into the service. I went in in '41 and I came out in '45. I was in the navy, I was a Second-Class Petty Officer in the fireroom. The only time I used drugs then was when we took the medical kits out of the lifeboats. We used to take the morphine

5. North Beach, the site of present-day LaGuardia Airport, was a small-scale Coney Island used mainly by local German and Irish immigrant families around the turn of the century. With the rise of the automobile, the amusement park began to decline, and in 1929 the Curtiss-Wright Flying Service began carving out facilities there for both land and sea planes.

out, syrettes of morphine. Take the tip off and stick it in. Quarter-grain, it was.

I started on heroin in the late '40s after I got out of the service. That's when I got hooked. The first time I used heroin I was up in Harlem. I was with this broad, she was a junkie. We were in up in her room, and she got off. I said, "What the hell are you doing?" She said, "Oh, shut up," and she took the spike and hit me. This was no mainline she gave me, this was a skin pop. I felt a little funny, but not that much.

The next time I snorted the heroin. I learned to snort up there in Harlem. I could buy it there myself on the street from black dealers. That's when the blacks really got into it. I'd snort it and think nothing of it. I was working, driving a truck. It didn't bother me until, say, around '49. I started to feel that I would want it. I didn't get a real big craving for it, but I was starting to miss it. I'd had a taste of it, and now I was really wanting it. That's when I got the habit, what you'd call hooked. Hooked real good. I started to buy, buy. I didn't give a shit about the job—I quit the job. Then I was just trying to make it one way or the other.

This may sound stupid, but when I noticed I was hooked, it was just like a cloud went over my brain. It's not your body, it's your head, it's your brain that's befogged, you might say. Now [points toward the interviewer], *your* mind is clear, *you* never used anything. Your mind is like it was when you were born. My brain isn't like yours right now, because you have no veil on your mind.

When I first started using heroin regularly, I was driving the truck. When the heroin went away, it was just like snapping your fingers: that's the way my mind cleared. Your eyes got clear; you could look at people when you were talking; you understood. You came back. You came back into the circle again, back into the realization that there was something in your head that counted, that did something to you.

When I really got hooked, I didn't snap out of it like you would after a drunk. There was a permanent change. It was just like somebody taking a bag and putting it over your head. You could see, and talk, and all like that, but . . . it's on your brain, your mind. It does affect your body, your bloodstream and stuff like that, but it's mainly in your head.

SAM

We have mentioned that, during the nineteenth century, many American addicts were victims of chronic disease. They learned, through a physician, pharmacist, or patent medicine vendor, the trick of relieving their ailments with a little opium or morphine. When their symptoms recurred, they took some more, eventually reaching the point of physical dependence. Once they recognized their condition as narcotic addiction, they were ashamed and highly secretive. Association with other users was the last thing they wanted.

Sam is a throwback to this pattern. In fact, the very anachronism of his case makes this interview of great historical interest. Sam's feelings and experiences approximate those of a large "lost" generation of medical addicts who left few written and no oral records. Born in New York City in 1912, Sam was the second son of a prosperous Jewish merchant. By the time Sam was twelve his father was a millionaire. But Sam was unhappy and alienated, bouncing from boarding school to boarding school, eventually dropping out altogether. (However, he continued the habit of reading and acquired, as this narrative makes clear, a formidable self-education.) After a bachelor fling he reluctantly went to work for his father and, with equal reluctance, entered into an arranged marriage in 1933. Then came the migraines.

It's not given to us to remember pain, to relive it. If it were, I don't think there'd be a live person on earth. But I can't emphasize too much the pain of migraine. Women doctors who have experienced both say that migraine is close on the heels of childbirth as the worst natural pain.

My attacks would last, almost by the clock, fifty minutes. I would live from minute to minute. I remember calling my wife up at four o'clock in the morning sometimes and telling her, "I can't make it. I can't get through the next twenty minutes." I remember walking naked through my apartment with my hands to my head, saying softly, "Oh, God. Oh, God. Oh, God." That's all I could say, hoping that I could get through another thirty seconds.

I built a home on Fire Island. The walls, of course, are very thin—all structures on the island are wood. Sometimes when I had a houseful of guests I would have a migraine at three in the morning. The ones you get at night, when you're sleeping, are the worst because you can do nothing to anticipate them.[6] It's the pain that wakes you up; then you're in the middle of an attack. I would go immediately into the bathroom, turn the water on full, put a little chair in front of the basin, and scream into the water so that my guests shouldn't hear what I was going through. I'm very ashamed of these attacks. I'd be screaming into this water, just trying to count the seconds—that was the ferocity of these attacks. They terrify me to this day.

Beyond all question migraine is a psychosomatic disease, much the same as asthma or hay fever or allergy. It is an emotionally induced disease with a physical expression. There were three factors in my life that were

6. Classic migraine headaches are preceded by premonitory signs called an "aura." These signs are usually visual, and a sleeping person could easily miss them.

producing migraine—I figured this out after I don't know how many hours of just sitting with my head in my hands, doping it out, thinking, "What is giving me migraine while someone else doesn't get it? Why do I get it?" One factor was a woman with whom I was entangled; another was my unhappiness with my wife; and the third was my hatred of my father, and the loathing of the work I was engaged in. I hated our family business: it no more represented me or what I am capable of than if I were a farrier. Suppressed rage—that's as good an explanation for my migraine as any.

I had these headaches in the late thirties, but they weren't diagnosed as migraine until about 1945 or '46. Little was known about migraine then. I was tossed around from doctor to doctor—I must have seen between thirty and forty, not only here in New York but all over the world. The diagnosis ranged from "headache" to "Horton's headache" and "histaminic cephalgia" and other names with which I'm no longer familiar. The medicines prescribed were everything from aspirin up to and including cocaine block. They would take a Q-tip about six inches long with the cotton end soaked in medicinal cocaine, as a local anesthetic, and shove that up through the nose into one of the six or seven entrances to the head. When it reaches your eyes—you think it's the top of your head—you start getting nauseous and you faint. It's the most hideous . . . it's almost medieval. But it did no good. Nothing did any good. And the expenses of this were considerable: there was no Medicare, no hospital payment such as we have today. You had to bear the entire cost.

They did endless x-rays on me—they must have weighed five or six pounds. Impossible angles, under huge machines. Then they wanted to check for an aneurysm, which involves opening the skull and injecting a dye into one of the veins. At that point I said, "Stop. I've gone as far as I want to go, and nobody's going to open my skull"—because it was known then as a calculated risk, much the same as a frontal lobotomy. I wasn't about to enter into that area of medicine.

One diagnosis I began to hear quite a bit was Horton's headache.[7] I asked, "Well, who's Dr. Horton? Can't get any higher than that." So I went to see him at the Mayo Clinic. There was a lot of red tape to go through: it was weeks after I arrived at the clinic before I got to the exalted Dr. Horton. He told me that he could only diagnose me when he saw me in an attack, and wanted to know when I would have an attack. I told him I didn't know: I could have one talking to him or have one in the middle of the night, there was no regularity. I said, "But I can produce an attack,

7. Named for Dr. Bayard T. Horton, this condition is known today as cluster headache. It is marked by severe, throbbing pain on one side of the head, usually around the eye. The attacks come in bunches (hence "cluster") during periods of susceptibility but disappear during periods of remission. Like migraine, cluster headache can sometimes be triggered by drinking alcohol.

providing that you'll guarantee that you'll get me out of it. Just give me
an ounce of whiskey, or any liquor, any alcohol, and twenty minutes later
you've got your attack." Because even a sip of beer would produce—to
this day, it still does—a migraine.

He gave me an ounce and a half of good bourbon, which I drank.
Twenty minutes later by the clock I said, "Start giving it to me, here
it comes." He produced a hypodermic and injected me in the arm, the
shoulder, and the hip. I was getting more and more frantic, but he could
no more reduce the pain of this headache than drinking plain tap water. I
think there was some histaminic preparation in that hypo, which was the
basis of the Horton headache remedy. He wouldn't admit it, but it was
obvious to anybody who had witnessed this little scene that his treatment
was no good. He said, "We'll try something else," or whatever. At that
point I was screaming, I threatened suicide. I told him and the others that,
if they couldn't cure me, I was going to kill myself. I was quite serious. I
could no longer stand this pain.

Then somebody else at Mayo, not Dr. Horton, gave me enormous
injections of vitamins. Later they decided to give me Demerol. If I recall
correctly, they gave me a five-piece glass syringe—that's how old it was
—and taught me how to sterilize it. I would put it together religiously
every time I needed it, and I would take Demerol, vitamins and Demerol.
The instructions were sort of vague: just "when I thought it would help"
or "when I thought I needed it." I didn't think it extraordinary at the
time, although I do now. I can only assume that they were aware it was an
addicting medication, but, as to whether they warned me or not, I simply
cannot remember at this remove.

When I had a migraine and couldn't take it any longer, that's when
I would take the Demerol. It must have helped me. But I did not stay
with Demerol very long: maybe a year or two years. Then, in the course
of yet another visit to yet another doctor—he was French, I remember
I was very fond of him. He took my medical history, and I mentioned
the migraine. He said that, as long as I was injecting myself, he had a
wonderful treatment for pain, and he gave me a prescription for a drug
that is so rare that I doubt even today there are three pharmacies in New
York that have heard of it. The name of the drug was Alvodine.

The effect of Alvodine was far more satisfactory than Demerol's. The
Alvodine gave me relief from my migraine, but it had the added benefit, so
to speak, of euphoria. Not producing nausea was another bonus. Demerol
would produce nausea, which is one reason I used it as rarely as I did.
Having a migraine and vomiting, though they are many times companions,
is something I wouldn't wish on anybody.

It's not so much that I physically needed the Demerol. I wanted it, as
against needing it, and there is a difference. It brought about a feeling, a
lassitude—it satisfied a feeling of being a person again instead of a thing.

It satisfied a certain *peace*, that's the word, a peace of mind. At these times I would like always to be alone, so I could be very thorough with whatever I was occupied with: writing, or straightening my home, or reading, or just being quiet. The Demerol satisfied that desire to get things done in a neat and orderly way. But with Alvodine, the desire was for euphoria. All this in addition to relief from the dreaded migraine pain.

The realization that you're hooked doesn't come as a revelation; it comes as a slow awakening. You begin to analyze: "Why did I take that last injection? Did I take it because I had a migraine? Or did I take it because I *thought* I had a migraine? Or didn't even think I had, but because I wanted the injection, invented the need for it? Or did I really have a migraine and really need the drug?" You don't know which is which. It goes in a circle and you finally don't know and don't give a damn.

I can't tell you when I first experienced withdrawal; that came later on. What I felt was more on the order of a fright. The thought of not having a little supply of drugs for the next day or the next week induced panic more than physical withdrawal. I started having this feeling with the Alvodine, because of its rarity and because it was becoming increasingly difficult to get.

Now, mind you, there's nothing dramatic about this, it's not a curtain suddenly lifting. At first I didn't know I was addicted; then I couldn't believe I was addicted; finally, when the realization sank in and I had to admit it, then the process of lowering self-esteem started. It was a lessening of confidence; a growing awareness that I was becoming, or would soon become, a derelict, that I was sinking into something over which I had no control. But I didn't seek out the company of other addicts. On the contrary, I shunned it. I kept this dark secret to myself. I was ashamed of it.

I regret using these drugs because of the mess I'm in now, because I've got a methadone leash around my neck. But they did help the migraines. They got me over some hills which I doubt now, with hindsight, I could have gotten over without some artificial aid. Here was *something* that produced a positive result, as against the endless number of medicines I had been encouraged to take over the years by this army of doctors to whom I had gone.

I'll tell you about the methadone, but there's a step we have to climb before we get to that. About twenty or twenty-five years ago, sometime in the late fifties, a well-meaning friend introduced me to the joys of Seconal. He called them "saggies," there's a hundred names for these things. We were going into a party—on Fire Island parties were endless, one followed another and it would be a four-day drunk. But I couldn't drink, so I would feel very much out of it. How to get drunk without taking alcohol? How to get into the party? My nature is such that, when I'm high, I enjoy myself more, much as people who have cocktails in them enjoy themselves more at a party. Well, one afternoon my friend gave me a Seconal. I said, "You're giving me a sleeping pill when we're going into a party and this is supposed to make me feel good?" He said, "Take it." I took it, and I felt good. I learned that it was the threshold, the point at which you take the barbiturate, that makes the difference. If you swallow it, take your book, and you're comfortable in bed, you'll doze off. If you take it before going into a noisy party and your intention is to get high, you'll get high. So this is self-induced, although I don't pretend to understand the mechanics.

One Seconal gave place to two, then four. Then I began to experiment, as people will. The Seconal gave way to Tuinal, then Placidyl, and then the whole army of these barbiturates. In my instance the barbiturates never precipitated a migraine, and I covered the field pretty well. I went to Mark Cross and had a little case made for me with twelve vials, six on each side. It was custom-tailored. I called it my "how-do-I-want-to-feel-today kit." I kept it with me always. It was very funny in those days: I'd open it and people would get hysterical, because there was every color in the rainbow in those glass vials. It was a laugh. They'd say, "Wait till you see Sam's how-do-I-want-to-feel-today kit! It's a riot!" And I'd open the damn kit, we'd clean up some of the dust in there, lick our fingers, and grab a handful of this or that. All my friends, then and now, are in show business. They are a far more easy-going clique than the officegoer; they accept these things far more readily. Sharing the pills with them made me more socially acceptable in their group. They'd come to me, knowing always that I had plenty of them.

I entered the methadone treatment about 1967 or 1968. By that time I was capable of consuming, I would say, twenty pills a day, of whatever kind or strength. I would mix up "cocktails" of these damn things: four Placidyls went together with six Seconals and five Tuinals and whatever the hell else was handy in my little case. I didn't need physicians to get these pills: the pharmacies were most helpful. I would pick up the phone and order as many as a thousand pills at a time. I'd order three hundred red, three hundred rainbow, and three hundred Placidyl, and they would be in my hands in seven to ten minutes. In bottles, all mixed together. There was no interaction between the narcotics and the barbiturates that I was aware of, although obviously something was happening to my viscera and my mind.

There were drugs that I was taking that I haven't even mentioned, because I'd forgotten them. I was addicted for a while to a hideous drug called paraldehyde. Once you smell it, you'll never forget it; and once you taste it, you'll live with it for the rest of your life. It's a very old standby, a very old drug. Once you take it, it's days before it gets out of your lungs. You *stink* from paraldehyde. You walk into a room, and in two minutes people empty it.

At that point I was taking a combination of pills, Alvodine, Demerol, paraldehyde, and I probably took another one that I've forgotten. There was a sort of a pride; I could still keep my head up a little bit. I was not yet a "junkie"—the commonly accepted convention of the dope fiend, the man lurking in the street with a dirty hypodermic in his pocket, who shoots up in a doorway. Mine was a private problem. I wasn't a junkie. I was a "narcotic addict," if you please, or some other pretty, polite term. All the while not realizing—or perhaps realizing, and not even admitting —that I was a junkie, as I realize today and admit.

3.

Hop

Although today narcotic addiction and heroin addiction are virtually synony-mous, this was not always the case. The smoking of opium, or "hop,"[1] was an important source of addiction well into the twentieth century. Hop was triply se-ductive: it was pleasurable; it was risqué; and it was high-toned. Hop was to the 1920s what cocaine was to the 1970s: a rich man's drug, a favorite of hustlers and partygoers flush with cash and searching for thrills.

Hop was not originally a society drug. In the mid-nineteenth century it was associated with an unholy mix of Chinese coolies and the dregs of the white underworld. Its reputation was so bad that Bathhouse John Coughlin, a Chicago alderman not known for his aversion to vice, declared himself against it. "I know their methods," he said, "and opium-smoking don't go in the First Ward."[2]

It went elsewhere, though, and remained a popular biracial vice, especially in cities and towns with Chinese communities. Beginning in 1909, however, Con-gress passed a series of laws designed to curtail the importation and manufacture of prepared opium. Hop could still be purchased, but the price was higher and the danger greater. Faced with these problems, the hoi polloi among the regular smokers began switching to heroin and morphine, both of which were cheap and legal prior to March 1915, when the Harrison Act took effect. The two groups that remained loyal to hop were the Chinese and the more successful whites. That was the situation when our interviewees entered the picture.

A sense of disappointment runs through these narratives. It was not so much

---

1. Drug jargon, like language generally, changes with time. For many years "hop" has been used to refer to any narcotic. As early as 1940, in *Farewell, My Lovely*, when Philip Marlowe wakes from a stupor in a locked room and finds needle tracks in his arm, he grits his teeth and says, "Okey, Marlowe, . . . You've been shot full of hop and kept under it until you're as crazy as two waltzing mice." For Marlowe, hop equals dope. But not for our antediluvian interviewees. They always used the term "hop" in the narrower sense of opium prepared for smoking. We follow their usage.

2. Dick Griffin, "Opium Addiction in Chicago: 'The Noblest and the Best Brought Low,'" *Chicago History* 6 (1977), 113.

*that they blamed the pipe for leading them into addiction as they resented the fact
that it became harder and harder to obtain hop during the 1930s and 1940s. This
scarcity was often blamed on the growing influence of a new and predominantly
Italian generation of suppliers then gaining greater control of the narcotic traffic.
These suppliers preferred to import and distribute heroin, which was more potent,
compact, and easier to adulterate than hop. Thus even die-hard smokers, white
as well as Chinese, had to switch to heroin. It was that, or do without.*

LOTTY

I was a coal miner's daughter. I was born February 9, 1910, in Charleston,
West Virginia. There was nothing there but a company store, not even
a roller skating rink. No movies. We had a house that belonged to the
company—we paid so much rent. And they had what they called scrip;
you'd go to the store and you'd draw scrip to buy your groceries, your
food, your furniture.

There were six of us in all, but my oldest sister died very young,
seventeen. She got married and had a child eleven months later. She and
the baby both died, because these coal mining doctors are all drunks and
quacks, you know.

My mother was a Sunday school teacher, and we were Baptists. She
was part Indian and had a very bad temper. I thought at one time that
I hated her, but I can understand now that she had all those little kids
hanging on her coattail.

My father was a foreman in a coal mine. He was a wonderful man,
but he liked to show off. They carried those big guns, and he'd have two
every time he went out of the house. One night he got in a quarrel. They
shot him in the back when he turned around.

That left me the oldest; I was thirteen, so I had to get a job. I got a job
in a grocery store first, and then my cousins taught me the switchboard,
so I got a job as a telephone operator. I was the night operator; I went to
school half days. I had one and a half years of high school—they called it
eighth and ninth down there. I went to Gary High School in Gary, West
Virginia.

I saved up about eighty dollars and, with the clothes I had on my back,
I came to New York. I was fourteen; that was 1924. I just thought maybe
I'd get a break here. There was nothing there, it was all little towns. It's
bigger now—Charleston is about two hundred thousand now.

When I came to New York I didn't even know how to go into a restaurant to eat. I really didn't. I'd always been taught to sit at the big table. I'd
go to these cafeterias and places and I didn't know what to do, how to eat.

I checked into a hotel near the station. It was quite expensive. I looked
up auditions and I went to one. I was very lucky: I met a French girl and

she taught me to dance a few steps. And I got the job, first audition I went to.

I'd always wanted to be in show business. I worked in the Golden Slipper, the Seven-Eleven, the Black Cat. These were nightclubs. I was —what do you call it?—the "pony" in the chorus line. I hadn't stopped growing, and I was only about this big. So I was on the end, and it didn't matter what I did, if I kicked my heels high enough.

Then I met a boy, he was in show business also. He said, "Baby, you'll never be a dancer. Let's take up singing lessons." So I took up singing lessons, and I became a singer. I'd been here about a year or so when I met him. He was very talented. He could do anything: he could draw, he could make his own furniture, paint—he was really marvelous. But this boy went with a show and he was drowned. He was seventeen and I was nineteen at the time of his death.

I never had heard of such a thing as dope, because this girl's mother used to come and pick us up after we were through for the night. She saw that we didn't get into any trouble. Her daughter took me home and, as soon as the mother saw me, she said, "Ah, she's just a little baby"— because I was, you know. She said, "Don't be frightened, I'm not going to put you out." She gave me the other bed in her daughter's room. All during the late twenties I lived with them. Every dime I made, she put in the bank. When I left her she gave me every cent she had taken, every nickel of my money. I was just lucky, one of those lucky people. If it wasn't for them, I don't know what would have happened.

This woman was pretty smart. She was a poet. Her first husband had TB and he died. Then, the doctor she took him to, she married him. She had two children by him. So she became a real lucky gal, because he was from a wealthy Italian family. They had an eight-room apartment and a big grand piano and everything. They were in the textile business.

I was a pretty good singer. At that time they didn't pay much. I made seventy-five dollars a week, and when we sat with someone we got tips. I was making a lot of tips; sometimes I couldn't find them all, they'd be all over, twenties and fifties. I'd promise I'd meet them later—you know how the racket goes. It was during Prohibition; these were speakeasies. You had to open the door, and the guy never knew where he was even. He was too drunk. He even signed blank checks.

I worked in a place called "The Key." They had Hawaiian rooms, the Blue Room, this room, that room. Upstairs the man and his wife lived: it was a big, private home. They just had everything there. If a girl got a little tipsy, they'd take her up in one of the rooms and put her to sleep. In that particular club the liquor was very good because the people were brokers and big shots, really big men.

The cops left them alone—they got paid off. Then we had one cop, he was real nasty. He'd come and he'd break everything in the place: all the glasses, all the liquor, even the piano and the musical instruments. I'll never forget his name: it was Brannigan. He'd say to me, "The reason I'm not taking you, I know you're not booked here. You can't go out with a man." We were booked as entertainers, not to go out with the customers.

I sent my mother money every week and managed to keep the family together. My sister married a hillbilly who was no good. He let the children practically starve. My mother wrote me a letter about what he was doing to her. So I brought them to New York.

I left the woman who was looking after me. Her daughter got married —that's the reason I left. I was too lonesome, because we used to go to fraternity dances and had a lot of fun together. We all wore a size-three shoe: if she bought herself three pairs of shoes, she'd buy me three pairs of shoes. She was real lovely to me. I imagine she's dead now. I haven't seen her in about twenty years, because when I got on drugs I didn't feel like it.

I moved out after the '29 crash. When I went on my own I got a job in another nightclub. I made out pretty good. It was a speakeasy, in a way, but a high-class one. One night they brought in Mervyn LeRoy, and he said, "What a gorgeous girl!" He asked me if I'd ever had a screen test. I said, "No," He said, "Would you like to?" I said, "I don't know how to act." He said, "Well, how about coming out and take a try at it." He had me out to Hollywood twice, probably two weeks each time. But I didn't dance well enough. He came right out and told me I'd never be enough of a dancer.

When I came back I started going to parties. This was probably about two years after the crash. They had a lot of big stars that were on opium. They'd put a mattress on the floor. They wore beautiful silk pajamas and had a big can of opium and a big pipe. They'd roll the pills and everybody would pass it around. They didn't think anything of it. If they got sick they'd take a bottle of medicine and put opium in it; when they'd take a dose they'd put a spoon of water back in. They'd reduce themselves if they had a habit.

The boss of the speakeasy asked me, he said, "Why don't you go out and have some fun one of these nights?" The party was held on Riverside Drive. There were big stars there and gorgeous people. They looked at me and said, "What kind of silk pajamas do you think she should wear?" One said blue and one said green, and another guy said, "Green, a light green." We laid on a big satin mattress in the middle of the floor, and we had dishes of all sorts of fruits and candies—hard candies, in case you got dry from smoking.

The first night I was there, I was jumping around like crazy. I didn't know it would make you sick afterward if you jumped around. But I didn't get sick, and they were amazed that I took to the opium so well. They said, "This girl's going to be a junkie." I said, "What's a junkie?" They said, "That's when you get on the white stuff." They thought that was terrible, you know.

I loved it. I'd jump around and get the grapes and the candy. I don't know, it was a wonderful feeling—you'd feel like you were walking on eggs. It was really marvelous. But I had no idea I was going to that kind of a party when the boss asked me. I never knew what I was getting myself in for.

FRIEDA

At eighty-one, Frieda was one of the oldest methadone patients we interviewed. Something of a medical miracle, she was still in good health, despite chain-smoking cigarettes and nearly sixty years of narcotic addiction. She remained in her Bronx apartment, even though most of her white neighbors had long since fled to the suburbs.

I was born in 1899 in New York City, on the Lower East Side. We were a poor family, just getting along. My parents were born on the other side, in Russia. My parents were Jewish, but they were not religious people. My father was a cigar maker, my mother was a housewife. There were six children; I was the youngest of the six. We had four brothers, and two girls. The last four children were born here: two in Europe and four here.

I went to public school and I went to high school. I didn't graduate from high school; I went there about two years. I was just tired of school, that's all.

I went to work as a cashier in a restaurant. I worked at that a couple of years. I was married in about 1920. I had one son. I was with him about two years, then I divorced him. He was tight, a very stingy man. I couldn't stand it. I had the baby, and he'd go into a restaurant; he'd eat, and I'd stand by the window and look in and watch him eat. That's the truth, God's honest truth. Two years I was with him and that was it.

I first started using drugs after I was divorced. I was smoking opium, that's how I started. It seems that we all went to a party—they called it "a party." We all went there and we laid around. We smoked. We had fruit, candy, and everything. These were boys and girls, just friends. I knew there was going to be opium at the party. I just wanted to see what it was. I felt good. I felt nice. I was calm. Some get sick, some don't. I didn't. All I felt was a good feeling. I kept on going, every night. I didn't think of the danger; I didn't think of nothing. I just smoked every night until I got hooked.

It was easy to come by, two dollars a little toy. Three for five dollars. People on the street were selling it, and at night we went and we smoked. I smoked with people like myself, all white people—I never smoked with any Chinese. These were men and women, about half and half. Some were working, some weren't. I never asked them their business.

It's true that they weren't like the junkies in the street. It was much nicer to smoke opium than to use H. Nicer people used to smoke opium. There was a man, he was a clothing manufacturer. He just wanted to smoke once a week. Every Saturday night he would call me up, and he'd have two chorus girls, and we'd check into the hotel, and we'd lay down and smoke. I was a chef: I used to know how to make the pills. I'd get twenty-five dollars every time I cheffed for him. But that's not how I paid for my own opium. He treated us; he bought us candy and perfume and other things. And when I got through I went home; he stayed there with the two girls.

It just happened that I knew how to chef. I tried—I started playing with it, and played and played until I got to know. Did you ever see an opium pipe? It's a bowl and a stick, and then you had a little lamp and a *yen-hok*. The *yen-hok* makes the pill, it's like a knitting needle. You'd pick up a little hop from the tin, and you'd put it over the lamp and roll it and roll it. Then it gets bigger and bigger, and you stick it right into the pipe. And then you puff on it. [Takes two imaginary draws.] But not everybody could do that.

Lots of times I bought my own opium. Everybody did. We all chipped in: I'd buy it one night, then somebody else would buy it the next night —we always had it. I always smoked in a group: we had about six, seven people. Why? Because it was nice. It gave you a nice lift, you felt good. It was just one of those things. I enjoyed doing it with friends.

I always smoked with the same group of people. Every night at twelve o'clock we'd congregate, and we'd go up to somebody's hotel, or up in a rooming house where somebody lived, and we smoked. Sometimes you put towels with water on the door so the fumes wouldn't go out.

Then I couldn't get opium no more. That was years ago, God knows when—about 1930, 1935, somewhere in there. I just couldn't buy it no more. When I couldn't get opium, I took heroin. I was skin popping. It's true that opium was bulky and that heroin was easier to smuggle in. At that time heroin was cheap: it was twelve dollars an ounce. In fact I used to give this one a little bit, that one a little bit—you know, those that didn't have nothing.

When I was smoking opium I didn't look down on people who used the needle; I never bothered with them. When I started using heroin it was all right, it wasn't bad—but I liked opium better.

I was married a second time, in 1940. This lasted eight years. I was using heroin at the time—my husband knew. He helped supply me with money—he was a very nice man. He worked for his brother. They had an egg business down in the egg market. But he committed suicide. For no reason at all. Had money, had everything. He was just melancholy. One

Sunday morning I got up and I found him on the kitchen floor. Sleeping pills, he took a whole bottle of sleeping pills. I found them in the kitchen. After that I went to work for a telephone answering service. I worked seventeen years, and nobody knew that I was using stuff.

We were living in the Bronx when he killed himself. We moved there in 1940. That's when I started to use Dilaudid. I lost my heroin connection on the Lower East Side. I got the Dilaudid from doctors. I got my needles from a druggist in the Bronx. He knew me for years. He must have known I was addicted. I never said nothing, but I used to cash my Dilaudid prescriptions in there, so he knew.

I entered the methadone program because I couldn't get Dilaudid. The doctor got a call from an agent who told him not to give it to me anymore. So he stopped. That was in 1976. I heard people talking about the methadone program, so I figured I'd better go and check in. I want to stay on methadone. At my age, if I got off I'd die, I'd never make it.

I'm happy. As long as I've got money and can play numbers, I'm happy. The whole day is spent playing numbers. I play numbers every day. There are three or four places right in the neighborhood. I don't play for much, two dollars a number. So, if I hit, I make eighteen dollars. But I still play. If I make a few dollars, I play again, and I wind up losing, I wind up with nothing. Every day, I'm losing, losing, losing. I play a four, a five comes in; I play a five, a four comes in. But it keeps me going, you know —something to do.

LAO PAI-HSING

Lao Pai-hsing, also eighty-one years old, was born in Hong Kong at the turn of the century. The son of a tobacco merchant, he received some education before going to sea aboard a Standard Oil tanker around 1920. This is a translation of portions of an interview conducted in both Pidgin English and Cantonese.

I was a fireman on the ship. I sailed to England, then to America; I first saw New York City in August 1921. I wanted to stay, but I couldn't because of the immigration laws. But I came back about 1924 and worked in different restaurants, first as a dishwasher, then as a cook. I made sixty dollars a month, but I spent the money on smoking opium.

I started smoking opium on the ship. The crew was Chinese. The opium made me high. I also found out that it helped me work, it gave me energy. Without the opium I'd get sleepy, low. I couldn't work as usual. I developed into a two-time-a-day smoker. I smoked before I went to work and after. If I didn't smoke, I'd sure be sick.

I was an addict, a steady smoker, when I settled in New York City. I'd smoke, go to work, come home, smoke again. I went to four or five different smoke houses; one smoke house was in Newark. They were for Chinese people only: we didn't trust white people. I smoked a toy a day, same as on the ship. You could buy a small toy for two dollars.

Sometimes you couldn't get opium, maybe no ship had come in. So I changed to the white stuff—heroin. This was when I was about thirty-five years old. I bought it all over the place—uptown, downtown, Chinatown. Later, I even went to Harlem to buy it.

At first I put some in my nose—I sniffed it. But putting it in the nose used too much. The price got too high, so I started to skin pop. Yes, I was afraid of the needle. When I was smoking opium—oh!—I'd see someone using the needle, I got scared myself. But I learned from other people how to prepare it, to put a little stuff in a spoon, and take it out with a dropper, and to put the needle down here in my arm. It was better than opium; it kept you longer.

I got my needle in a drugstore. I was sure to keep it to myself. If you use somebody else's needle, they may be no good, they may be sick. I also kept my needle in alcohol.

Then why is there a scar on my arm? I had an operation for an infection. But it wasn't from another person's needle. Sometimes my connection wouldn't come, and I had to buy bad dope, dirty heroin. That's what caused my arm to swell all the way up to the elbow.

MEL

Addicts who started with the pipe generally ended up on heroin. Almost uniquely, Mel reversed the pattern—at least for a while. Mel was born in 1915, the only child of poor black parents. When he was about six years old his natural father died; shortly after that, his mother remarried.

I grew up in the South Side of Chicago—they called that the Black Belt. I went to school there, as far as the eighth grade. I didn't do too well. I was very poor in math and history and things of that sort. Very poor in them subjects.

I left there in 1930: January 15, 1930. I was about fourteen. I left because of family discrepancies; my home life wasn't too good. I had a stepfather, you know, and we just couldn't make it. I had a fight with him. Then there were certain things I wanted, and it seems that I was never able to get them. And I felt as though I was somewhat a burden. So I just made up my mind to get away. I felt as though I could probably go out and try to take care of myself—I thought I could.

I left there and I hitchhiked here to New York City. I'd heard so much talk about it from elder associates. It sounded like it was a good place to make a start; great opportunities here for a person. So I said, "I'll try it."

The first night in New York I just walked around. I met a couple of other fellows; they were in the same circumstances I was. They were probably a little older than me, so naturally I put my age up, I upped my age to eighteen. At that time I looked older than I actually was.

They introduced me to Father Divine. I guess you've heard of him; he was a great clergyman here at the time.[3] He was very helpful to all the blacks, whites, and whatnot. He had these establishments, and he would hardly turn anybody away. If it was in his power to help, he would. His food was fifteen cents, and I mean you got a full meal: chicken, potato salad, greens, and biscuit. I stayed there and got my lodging and food; I worked around the premises, helping here and helping there, for my keep. I stayed there about two or three months. After that I started drifting here, drifting there—you know how it was.

I never was a drinker. I saw too much of that in my family life. But I had been smoking marijuana, even in Chicago. I was about eleven, twelve, something like that. You could buy it from the Mexicans and the Philippine kids. I continued to smoke reefer in New York. It was cheap. You could get it for a nickel. They had a guy here, he had what was supposed to have been the best. I've never had anything like it since. He's dead now; his name was Mezzrow. He used to sell it three for fifty cents. He's the only one I know that maintained that price from the time I got acquainted with him in 1931 until he died: three for a half. I'd been smoking other types of marijuana, what they called "panatellas." But this here to me was the best I had *ever* had.

I figure I smoked about an ounce or a half-ounce a day. About a half. The majority of time I'd have company, but then I enjoyed smoking it alone. These were mostly theatrical people and people in other walks of life in general. This guy might be a working guy, this guy might be a thief, this guy might be a . . . it was a mix of characters.

I didn't start messing with stuff until I was about sixteen. I mean hard stuff. I found out about it through the type of people I was hanging out with, the same people that smoked pot. A lot of them I knew in Chicago— I was surprised to find them here. They had their connections and people they knew, so they would introduce me to this and to that, and that was it. So, after I got around to where I knew how to get me a halfway decent dollar, I wanted to do like everybody else and be right on in the crowd.

3. Born George Baker, Father Divine was a charismatic black preacher who gathered his impoverished disciples into communal "heavens," where they were able to obtain cheap food and shelter. "The trademark of the movement was the banquet. Devotees would sit down to the table at his most important 'heaven,' located at 152 West 126th Street, and feast on twenty kinds of meat, five salads, eleven relishes, fifteen kinds of bread, six desserts, six different beverages, and cheeses and cakes 'as big as automobile tires.' For all this each disciple paid only fifteen cents" (Edward Robb Ellis, *The Epic of New York City* [New York: Coward-McCann, 1966], 535).

I wasn't working; I was just hustling around. I was able to get, as I got older, fifty or sixty dollars a day. At that time that was good money. I was running a crap game and other little things. After that I got a connection and I started selling a little marijuana myself.

The very first time I sniffed heroin I was nervous. Nervous and anxious. I had, oh, a sense of curiosity—I'd heard so much about it. I wanted to be like the big guys, like my buddy. He seemed to be doing so well. It didn't bother him apparently. He showed me it wouldn't hurt me. I didn't know how destructive it was. They never tell you the bad side of nothing.

So I didn't have no fears, no real extreme fears about it. In 1932, I think it was, the stuff was extremely good. It wasn't like it is now—trash, nothing. I think I snorted about as much as the crushed butt in that ashtray there, just about five grains. The next thing you know I started feeling itchy, kind of groovy like, and then I went into a stupor. After that, being a tender, I started throwing up. I hadn't done it before, my stomach and whatnot wasn't used to it. I started perspiring, and the fellows they thought something was going to happen to me, like an O.D. I was going into this deep stupor, and I felt like I was helpless. But, anyway, I came around. And it wasn't as bad as I thought it would be. I got high all right. But it gives you that sluggishness, it puts you into that lackadaisical thing. You just don't have no push for nothing; you just want to sit down and think or whatever.

I sniffed heroin for a while; then I got introduced to the needle. They told me that's much quicker. I started off skinning it. I didn't know nothing about no tying up, doing it myself. I'd seen others doing it, but I didn't do it. Some of them thought I couldn't do it, and, the first time I did, this guy he shot it for me. He tied me up and hit me. That was in the middle of '32. I started sniffing in '31; by '32 I was on the spike. Then, after that, in 1933—shit, I was smoking then.

With opium, it's something like marijuana: you don't get that quick rush like you do with heroin. See, when you're smoking, it's a soothing thing. Like you sit down and smoke a cigar, right? You take your cigar and you inhale it and you enjoy it. You let your smoke out gradually.

The smokers were the better class of the hustling type. I met these people through parties and things. They were neatly dressed, oh yes. That's what makes opium so great: it sort of stimulates your dignity, your pride. You never seen a greasy hop smoker. He's very neat, immaculate: he wants everything just here, just there.

There were some smokers affiliated with show business. They had various occupations: this guy was a drummer, this one a singer—you understand what I mean. And the better class of hustler, in order for him to associate with them, he would have to make a certain standard of living himself, dollar-wise.

I never went back to heroin during the period when I was smoking

Interesting point.

opium. It was sort of like a classified [*sic*] thing. Say I'm an opium smoker, you're a heroin user: I felt a little more superior to you. I'd be disgusted with you because, when you're using that needle, you're looking at all that blood and everything. It seems filthy. But the opium user is a lot different. Why, he's got a man—a chef—he comes and cooks for you, cleans up, everything is done. There's none of that dirt around you.

When I started smoking, it was like I'd moved into a fancy suburb. I'd come up from the slums into a mansion domain. I got to the place where I could stick my chest out and say, "I'm one of you, now." It was a status symbol for a hustler, like a big car or a diamond pinkie ring.

Smoking is not an everyday thing. You make arrangements. Like, I'd say, "I'm going to go lay down for two days, Tuesday till Thursday." Then I'd cancel all my business appointments—bam. So those two days I'm going to smoke. I may not go smoke no more for the next two, three weeks. When I wasn't smoking, I kept some *yen-poks* around the house. You get up, you take your coffee, throw your *yen-pok* in there. You drink it, you do it that way. Some eat it. Sure, I ate *yen-shee*. I knew some kids that had *yen-shee* habits.

That's what made opium so beautiful: there's so many ways you can use it, without anybody knowing. You don't need a lot of apparatus. It's not a dirty thing. The only thing dirty about it is when you're cooking raw opium: you have to lock up everything because the scent is so strong. You got to keep everything in close because it stinks. Stinks terrible.

I learned how to chef for myself. I learned how to cook, to use the *yen-hok*. The *yen-hok* is a needle about nine, ten inches long. If you can't afford one, or maybe you've broken your pipe, you had to learn how to make one, what you call a homemade joint. Then you'd take a small milk bottle or a vaseline jar and hook it onto a board, put your oil in there, and put the flame to it. That was your lamp. Now you've got your pipe and bowl; you take your *yen-hok* and dip down into the mud. You run it over the fire and you turn it, turn it until it gets good and hot. Then you take it from there and put it on the bowl of the pipe and roll it into a pill. You stick it down into the hole, stick the needle through, pull the needle out, and turn the pipe over the flame. That's what they call "laying on your ear." Or "taking it on the hip"—same thing.

The Chinese and the whites didn't usually smoke together. But I smoked with Chinamen; I had some very good Chinamen friends. I went twice to a den with nothing but Chinese; that was in 1933. When I did time I got acquainted with one of them in the penitentiary. I was what you called "captain of the house": I was the head man to see that the dormitory was kept clean. Chinamen are very clannish. Over in this part of the dormitory would be all the Chinamen; over in this part of the dormitory would be the whites; over in this part the blacks. Not that you were compelled to be discriminated; they did it because that's the way they wanted it themselves. We all mingled together, played cards together, had dinner together, and whatnot. But, as I say, the Chinese were very clannish: they don't associate or get acquainted too quickly. But they couldn't avoid me, because I'd have to see that their quarters were clean. So I had a chance to really know them and, knowing some of them, learning their ways, their likes and dislikes. A couple of them were opium smokers and, when we got out, we passed along addresses.

We smoked together in a room in Chinatown. The couple of times I smoked with them, all of the Chinese smokers were men. I was never messing with their women. On a couple of occasions, when I smoked with a mixed group of whites and blacks, a woman would be there. Not often; it was mainly men. I'd say my consistent association was mainly black. This was up in Harlem.

I started dealing in 1934. I was selling heroin, coke, morphine. I had a bankroll. I found a guy that handled it by quantity, so I just went and bought some. I bought me an ounce or two. I'd make three, four hundred dollars a week. That's one way I'd support my opium habit.

I was selling from Thirtieth Street to Thirty-fifth Street, about five blocks on the West Side. I sold from my apartment—you know, telephones and things like that. Somebody would call me, and I'd send somebody over there and find out what it's all about—bam, bingo, and that's it. But I wasn't selling on the street, no. People would come to my apartment and make an arrangement.

When I first started dealing I had Chinese and Jewish connections; later I had Italian connections. It was a beautiful thing when the Chinese and the Jews had it. But when the Italians had it—bah!—they messed it all up. They started thinking people were just a bunch of animals—just give them anything. They took out the true substance of the drug. They started diluting it to a weaker state. I mean it was nothing but pure trash —you had more chemical in there and less narcotic. They took all the purity out and the price went up. They're still getting away with it. What they call "pure," they'll give it to you and you're still getting scrambled eggs. We know there ain't no such thing as pure, hundred percent heroin; they might get 85 percent, tops. You don't get no pure *nothing*.

The last time I smoked was in 1935, just before I went to the penitentiary. I got busted for sale and possession. This was during the time of the Harrison Act. The feds and the state busted me. I sold to a stool pigeon; then he handed it over to the agent. They gave me a proposition: do I want the government to handle it or the state to handle it? Being my first experience, I feared the government, so I accepted the state. If I hadn't, I could have gone to Lexington for eighteen months. But, to duck the eighteen months and to keep from having a federal record, I chose the state record. I had a three-to-five-year sentence. I got out in June 1939. June 19th. I got back on heroin—I didn't have sufficient contacts for opium, and financially I wasn't able to take care of it at that particular time.

Then they had a panic during the war; from there we went to morphine, whatever you could put your hands on. I used Dilaudid and Pantopon, boiled down P.G., ate *yen-shee*, if it could be found. The morphine and other drugs were mostly stolen—that's when a lot of drugstore and hospital burglaries started coming into play. I made croakers, too. I even stole a few scrips, stole a pad and then forged them. Once you get the formula it isn't hard to do. And at that time a lot of the doctors were even doing under-the-table business. They'd rather do it that way than have their place broken into or torn up. That was their idea of cooperating.

AL AND EMILY

Al and Emily were the only married couple we interviewed. We set out to tape them separately but, as things developed, they began to interrupt, correct, and elaborate one another's stories. Since the sessions evolved into a joint interview, they are presented as a joint narrative.

Emily was dying of throat cancer. Game to the end, she kept answering questions until pain overwhelmed her and she could speak no more.

Al: I've been mostly on my own ever since I was a kid. I must have been two or three years old when my parents died—I don't even remember, to be frank with you. My grandmother was the one that raised me. She told me that my father was a tailor, and that was about all I ever knew. My parents were born here, but their people came from the old country —I'm the third generation. The old country was like Russia, Poland; my father's, my mother's parents came from Poland. They settled in San Francisco; I was born there in 1904. Then they died and I came back East to be with my grandmother. She lived in New York, in Eldridge Street, on the Lower East Side. I was an only child—I was the only one of my relatives living in her house. But I had aunts and uncles close by, they used to come and visit quite often. I haven't seen them since I was a kid, so I can't even remember them too well.

It was a religious household. I used to go to synagogue on Fridays —she made me go. There was the old Rumanian synagogue there, on Rivington Street, Rivington and the corner of Eldridge. As a matter of fact, when I was thirteen, I was bar mitzvahed there—"confirmation," I guess they call that among Gentiles.

She made me go to a rabbi for about three years, a private rabbi, a tutor. I went to two public schools on the Lower East Side, but I didn't even go to school that much. I graduated, I think it was, in the third or fourth grade; I didn't go no further. I was all by myself. I ran my own life, nobody to take care of me. Just my grandmother—to her I was everything, do you understand? And that was the whole thing.

When I was about ten years old I used to go around with some fellows who were pickpockets. I knew them from the neighborhood—it was a little rough in them days; it was a tough neighborhood. It was a little mixed around there, Italian and Jewish kids. We used to work the subways, Fourteenth Street and up. Whenever they used to get the wallets, or whatever they got, they'd give it to me, because I was a little kid, and I was very fast on the run. We had a special meet on the Lower East Side in a restaurant on Delancey Street. I would meet them two or three hours later and, whatever I had, I would give them, and they'd give me two, three dollars for myself.

One day, I had about three or four wallets. I went home first, and I opened up the wallets. That was the first time I did that—I was afraid, to be truthful with you. But I opened them up and I saw there was a lot of money there, like three, four hundred dollars in one wallet, five hundred in the other. So I took more than half for myself. When I met them, I gave it to them. One said, "Is that all?" He must have had an idea; he must have looked. So they never took me with them no more. But it was all right; I had a little experience, so I went with another crew. They gave me 10 percent, 5 percent, every day. Then I went with another crew; I got 20 percent; I let myself in.

Then I became a thief. I was a pretty good thief in them days. I was twelve years old, but I was a big kid, a pretty smart kid. I was very bright. Even then, I always looked ahead. Education to me didn't mean anything —I got it all on the street.

I worked with other people. There used to be a section on the Lower East Side with lots of cloth, silks, and woolens. We used to go around there at night with a horse and wagon. We would break in and take the stuff—they had a place to get rid of everything. I used to make myself a hundred dollars, two hundred dollars every time we went out, which was sometimes once a week, twice a week, sometimes once a month—it all depended. That's how I raised myself up.

I gave my grandmother a few dollars from this money, but one time I gave her a little too much. She wanted to know where I got it from. I told her I was working. So I made a mistake there. I only gave her like a dollar a time from then on.

I was ten years old, less than ten years, when I started to smoke opium. As I said, I was around all them guys that stole. Everybody that used to steal in them days used to smoke opium. They were the wise guys. Prohibition and all that stuff was around, and this was around and that, so they all went to opium. So I became what you'd call a wise guy—I became an opium smoker. Then I became smarter, and I used to go to Chinatown to buy it. I got a connection with a chink down there, and I used to buy a half a litchi nut full of opium for a half dollar, and sell it for a dollar. That's how I made my little income, see.

We'd smoke in people's houses on the East Side, anybody's house. I knew friends; we used to go over to their house and stay there two days, three nights, three days, whatever you wanted. Somebody in the crowd knew how to chef—they would chef for us. We would smoke for a while, then go out and steal for a while, then come back and smoke some more. It was an everyday routine, mostly everyday, unless I had a little money. I wouldn't do nothing for two, three months sometimes, if I had enough money to keep me.

I didn't become addicted right away. As a matter of fact, to become addicted with opium, you've got to smoke for a long, long time—continuously, day and night. You can stay in the house for a week and continue to smoke. You smoke, get up and eat something, lay down and sleep, get up, smoke again. I smoked on and off for years, a couple of years continuously before I became hooked.

I got arrested one time. They took me to the flats in the old Tombs. I met some friends of mine there. In the back they had all these people that were breaking habits, opium habits. I never knew nothing about junk —well, I knew a little, but I never knew any junkies then. I used to see them chinks on the ground breaking habits. They used to sit bent over for days and days. Then I got very sick, and I knew. I must have been about fifteen, sixteen years old, and I knew I was in trouble. I was hooked.

Emily: I was born in New York City on Suffolk Street in 1912. My mother had eight children; I was number three. I had two brothers. All the rest were sisters.

Life was all shooting and tough guys. They'd break into my mother's house and put the lights out and steal the bulbs, and I had to fight with them. I took care of my brothers and sisters—I was the tough one in the house. My mother was a super; I had to help her out. My father worked as a presser. He made maybe nine dollars a week. So I had to get up in the morning and help them put out the barrels and clean the toilets. If the landlord was coming I had to wash the whole building, and the floor. It was a four-story tenement. All the toilets were in the hall, and we had to clean them if the people didn't. I wouldn't let my mother and father do it—I did it. I put on the rubber gloves and I cleaned them.

I went to P.S. 140 on Norfolk Street. I got as far as 8A, 8B in P.S. 91—that was on Forsythe Street. I left school at the eighth grade, then I went to continuation school. I studied cooking [laughs], how to be a good mother. And I'm a very good cook; I cook, I bake.

After that I became a sales girl on Clinton Street. I was selling dresses. That lasted about two years. At sixteen I became a checkroom girl. I worked in the Havana Madrid, my first job as a checkroom girl. I first made the union and became a tough broad with Lepke's sister-in-law. You've heard of Lepke?[4] I knew them very well. When I got married I lived at 72 Suffolk Street, right where they hung out, and they used to come up to my house for coffee, or sit down and talk, you know.

I was first married when I was about sixteen, seventeen years old. His name was Seth. I divorced him because he had a habit to hit. It was nothing to punch me, or I would punch him—you know, we were like childhood friends . . . It's too intimate.

Seth was, let me see, older than me two years—he was about eighteen when I married him. He worked as a moving van driver. We had a son, Manny, born in 1931. He was a year and a half old when I divorced his father—my mother-in-law was my witness. I was married to Seth altogether about two years. I had an abortion, the first baby. I worked during the marriage.

I became involved with drugs after I got rid of Seth. A friend of mine introduced me. She said to me, "Look, Emily, you got trouble. I see the way you walk. I see when you come home in the morning"—I used to play blackjack, my out was to gamble. So I used to lose all my money. So she'd say, "Come on, we'll lay down and smoke opium." Well, I'd heard of opium, but I'd never smoked it. So I went down to the hotel on Fourth Street and Second Avenue. I laid down there and, the first pill, I got very sick. Then every Saturday night—I was off Sunday—I smoked.

In the thirties it was all rich people, all wise guys, who smoked. I knew so-and-so was a big shot, so-and-so came up to smoke on Broadway—he had his own apartment, lived in a penthouse. We used to go there every Saturday before I moved to Coney Island. One of them owned a trucking company. In the union he was a very big shot, in the garments union and the truckmen's union. Lepke I don't know as a smoker, but Gurrah I knew was a smoker. And then there was some guy that worked for Lepke-Gurrah—Dinny. He had his own place on Broadway and Eightieth Street. Eightieth Street, Seventy-Ninth Street, where all the rich

Gambling as an outlet.

---

4. Louis "Lepke" Buchalter was a shrewd and ruthless gangster whose interests ranged from labor racketeering to narcotics to the infamous Murder, Inc. Although his build was slight and his manner retiring, he quietly ordered the executions of dozens of rivals and loose talkers. (It was Buchalter who coined the word "hit" as a euphemism for contract murder.) Eventually, however, several of his henchmen broke under questioning, providing prosecutors with enough evidence for a murder conviction. Although he managed no fewer than six times to avoid execution through stays and legal maneuvers, he finally went to the electric chair on March 4, 1944.

Lepke's chief ally was Jacob "Gurrah" Shapiro, a squat, two-hundred-pound enforcer who specialized in beating rebellious union members and intimidating their bosses. Demoralized by Lepke's execution, and suffering from diabetes and heart disease, he died in prison on June 9, 1947. The New York Times, in reviewing Shapiro's career, described him as "loud-mouthed, hoarsely guttural, thick-lipped, given to exaggerated gesticulation. He people then lived . . . [free associating] Park Avenue . . . Mazie, a showgirl . . . what's-his-name, Pretty Amberg—his brother got killed in New York, from the jail. And then his brother, Pretty.[5] I was very friendly with Pretty. I knew the day he was going to get killed because I heard it from the guy that I was with in the room. I wanted to tell him, "Gee, Pretty, don't be in this-and-this today," but I figured they'd know it came from me, because I was the only girl there where we were smoking. They trusted me with everything.

I smoked once a week until I was about twenty-one years, until I met Al. I went with him for about four years, five years, before I got married. I didn't want to get married until everybody said, "He's so handsome, he wouldn't marry you in a million years." I said, "I could marry him in two minutes." Which I did. I got married in Maryland——

Al: Hey, what's going on here?

Emily: He was a pushover.

Al: [Laughs.]

Emily: To me, anyway. [As if in confidence.] He went out with a school-teacher for six years.

Al: [Teasing.] Hey, we're going to get thirty dollars for this.

Emily: Big deal! I'll buy you you-know-what.

Al: [Laughs.]

Emily: So we got married in . . . 1939.

Al: No, before that, Emily.

---

was the Donald Duck of the New York underworld, constantly out of temper" (June 10, 1947, 56).

5. There were four Amberg brothers, three of whom died spectacular, violent deaths. On November 3, 1926, Hyman "Hymie the Rat" Amberg, a robber and murderer, tried to shoot his way out of the Tombs with the help of two accomplices. When the attempt failed and the men were trapped in the prison yard, they turned their smuggled pistols on themselves and blew their brains out. Nine years later, on November 20, 1935, Joseph "Joey" Amberg, extortionist, loan shark, and narcotics dealer, was lined up in a Brooklyn garage with his driver, Morris Kessler, and executed St.-Valentine's-Day-Massacre-style. Then, on October 23, 1935, Louis "Pretty" Amberg's hacked remains were found in the back seat of a burned-out automobile. His claim to underworld fame was the invention of the sack murder, in which the victim was pinioned in a heavy bag with his arms and legs tied in such a way that his movements would progressively tighten a wire noose around

Emily: 1938. In '38 we got married in Maryland. I told you I went five years without getting married—I didn't want to get married.

I smoked every week with him, and then came twice a week. We used to smoke on Broome Street. We used to lay down there and give the woman ten dollars—she used to chef for us. I said, "Why should I give her ten dollars?" Then we moved out to Coney Island and got our own room. I said to him one day, "Look, Lena knows I smoke"—Lena was the landlady—"I'm going to learn to chef if I drop dead. I ain't going to give nobody ten dollars to chef." And I learned to chef [claps hands] the first night I laid down.

I bought mainly whatever I needed. I didn't have a pipe—the woman, she wouldn't allow this, because the cops on Coney Island were knocking on the doors. So I got a bottle and made a pipe. I went to the drugstore and got a tube. A straw wouldn't let the heat go through; it would bust. I had to get glass. I got a glass tube and a baby nipple and a little bottle, a number six Pyrex bottle. I put it on and made like a pipe.

Al: I explained to them about that in [another part of] my interview.

Emily: But you had to have a certain needle to make the hole, because it wouldn't go through—the Pyrex bottle is very strong. Finally I made the bottle. I went into Woolworth's and bought a size fourteen needle—like a crochet needle. Very thin. And I made like a *yen-hok* to chef. I cheffed myself, and every night we smoked.

Al: Through her cheffing, I learned how to chef. When our kids were small, I used to smoke opium in the house. We had this colored girl with us—she knew what it was all about. As a matter of fact, she came from the South. Her husband went to the chair in Harlem, and I happened to be in a certain place at the time in Harlem, and she came up there crying. She never knew her way around. My wife was with me; my wife felt sorry for her and we took her home with us. She remained with us ever since —for twenty years she worked with us. Her husband was electrocuted for murder, but she never knew nothing. She was a legitimate girl, lived and raised her kids in the South. It was the first time she was in New York, when I saw her.

---

his throat. (Pretty's charred hands were bound with wire and there was a sack over his head—perhaps an ironic gesture.) Several gangsters were mentioned in connection with the Amberg murders, including Al Stern, Arthur "Dutch Schultz" Flegenheimer (who himself died a short time later), Benjamin "Bugsy" Siegel, Louis Capone, Martin "Bugsy" Goldstein, and the hulking Harry "PittsburghPhil" Strauss. The last four named were linked to Lepke through Murder, Inc. There was also speculation that the killings were part of the growing rivalry between Italian and Jewish gangs.

She was a smart girl, because she would say to our children, "You can't go in your father's bedroom because he's taking his asthma medicine." I had asthma, and that was my out for asthma. But I thought I was kidding them kids; later on they told *me* what I was doing. I didn't ask them at what age they knew, but they must have known at an early age, because they were too smart. I thought I was kidding them, telling them I was taking my asthma. Every time I was in there it was, "Hey, Pop! You taking your asthma?" I said, "Yeah." [Laughs.] It was very funny.

You'd be surprised: wealthy people smoked opium, millionaires, rich people. Down in the garment center years ago, there were clothing suit manufacturers—they all came from the East Side originally—they knew what it was. Union leaders used to smoke. I don't know if they were hooked. They used to come down, like, once a week to smoke. They had what they called a once-a-week habit. There was a guy out in Jersey—my wife might be able to remember his name—he had a big factory out in Jersey. He had a liquor store years ago in the East Side; he sold that and went into the manufacturing of clothing suits with a nephew of his. He used to smoke continuous, then he became what you call a twice-a-week smoker: Wednesday and Saturday. He went to Florida later on and died down there. I never see anybody that I knew years ago; they're all gone. They died or went to junk.

It wasn't all rich people who smoked. It was a mixture. Mostly thieves and knock-around guys, we called them: they're the ones that smoked opium. And there were people who knew what it was all about, who came from a neighborhood where they had smoked years ago. Then they made money, they went into business, they happened to make it good, and they kept on smoking—once a week, twice a week, whatever they wanted. But the criminals who smoked were neat. You couldn't tell, I mean, you always kept yourself just right.

Women smokers were rare. I can't give you a ballpark figure—it's impossible to figure that out. But they were a very small minority. Billie Holiday used to smoke before she used junk. She used to come to my house when we lived on the East Side and sing to my kids. That was back in the thirties—'38, '39. She really went down the hill with heroin, but when she was smoking opium she kept herself very good: made all kinds of money, she was never late for an appointment, she always took care of business, singing in clubs and everything. She was a great singer; she used to sing Jewish songs to my kids. My son, she used to sing to him all the time—she loved him.

I saw her when she was in real bad shape. She asked me once to do her a favor, which I did. At that time it was a big favor to get her junk. I got her a connection; I got her someone that I knew well. I didn't make no money in it. I gave her to the party that was doing business at the time. And I never knew that she was using junk. She confessed to me, she told

me the truth. She couldn't get nothing, and I was still smoking at the time
—as a matter of fact, I offered to take her to smoke with me. She said,
"Ah, it wouldn't help me." I said, "Why not?" She told me she was using
junk—once you use junk, it doesn't help. I gave her an introduction to
this guy that I knew well, and I don't know what happened to her. I never
saw her again. This was just before the war, I imagine—'39, '40, maybe
it was.

I smoked in Chinatown many a time. I think in the thirties I used to
smoke there. I went down there a few times; I saw some Chinese that I
knew and they offered for me to come in and smoke, and I went along
with them. They used to show movies in them days. They had what they
called "dens." I used to go to these guys' homes—it looked like their
home. Like, you had to walk a half of a mile in the back of a restaurant,
in and out, anyway, until you got there. It was a nice furnished house—
apartment, rather. You'd go up there, lay down on the floor, and there'd
be six, seven chinks and myself, and I had a friend with me most of the
time.

The Chinese and the white smokers didn't usually smoke together.
They never mixed together. Somehow or other there was always friction
between them. You see, years ago—I'm going back sixty years ago—the
chinks used to have braids behind their hair. Most of them worked in
laundries. The tough guys in the neighborhood, mostly Italian kids, they
were very nasty, a lot of them. A lot of Jewish kids the same way. Irish kids
too. They used to cut their tail off behind them and hold it for ransom;
they were looking to buy it back. See, a lot of people don't know that—
they've never seen this in a movie. But that's what they used to do: cut
their hair off, hold it, and they used to buy it back. Twenty dollars, fifty
dollars, whatever they could afford. That's why they always hated them
kids, for doing that to them. Maybe that was the reason.[6]

But there were quite a few chinks who, once you got to know them,
were nice people to deal with. It was a special privilege for me to smoke,
sure. Nobody could have gone there—very, very few people. But I knew
them since I was a kid: that's how I got very friendly with them.

I've never been to, I never saw, a *den*—I mean, I've never seen what

6. The *queue*, or plait of hair dangling from the back of the head, was introduced in
China by the Manchus after A.D. 1644. At first it was worn as a sign of submission to
the Manchu rulers, but gradually it became the national hairstyle and a matter of great
pride. After the Revolution of 1911, however, the queue was condemned by progressives as
decadent and un-Chinese, and once again became a political symbol. While the progressives
reached for the razor, the more conservative Chinese tucked their queues into their hats
and cast anxious glances over their shoulders: queue-cutting episodes were common in
China, as elsewhere. The difference was that, in America, queue-cutting was generally an
act of extortion or harassment, rather than an anti-imperialist statement.

they used to show in the pictures as dens. We used to go into a neighborhood where the guy had an apartment and we used to smoke. That was our den. But a lot of people, some rich people, thought, "I'm going to a den," and they'd go to Chinatown. They'd lay down in a Chinese den, they called it, with beds one on top of another. They'd lay there and smoke or something. I've seen, years ago, these women who used to come down to Chinatown for some kind of thrill. I never bothered with them, but they looked to be very well-spoken women, and they looked to be very wealthy women. They had chauffeurs, most of them, waiting for them in the car.

One danger of opium is that it gives off a distinct odor. To avoid that danger you take a wet towel—say, you go to a strange hotel to smoke, you've never been there before. You take a room for the night: five, six, seven of us would come in there. We'd take towels, wet towels, and put them over the openings around the door. That would eliminate the smell from going out.

The outfit was bulky. You had to have the pipe—the stick—the opium, the gee rag, and the top part of the bowl, and the things to clean it after you were through smoking. The *yen-hok* is the thing you used to clean the bowl. You'd take the bowl off the stick, then you'd clean it out, and use the powder again, resmoke it.[7] Or you can cook it again: if you can get enough stuff together you recook it, and it comes back to opium. That's one thing about it: there's always something to do with it.

Once I was caught in the act, years ago, on Second Avenue. There were ten of us in the house. The cops came in, but they didn't know what it was. It was a nuisance charge. There used to be a court on Second Avenue and Second Street, I think; we went there and paid a two-dollar fine. We gave phony names and that was that—I was gone.

When I first started smoking opium it was a half a dollar for a little litchi nut. Then they had toys, it used to be two dollars a toy—a little ointment jar full of opium. They used to sell that for two dollars, or three for five. I used to buy that off guys in the street, three toys for five. Then, later on, Second World War, right after that, it became five dollars for one toy, then ten, then fifteen, then twenty. See, years ago, the Jews had power, so it was very cheap. In '37, '38, I bought, for a friend of mine whose brother was a junkie, an ounce of morphine, pure. Twelve dollars I paid for it, wholesale. An ounce, a pure ounce, of morphine. It just shows you—what would that cost today?

When the Italians took over, when they became the real bosses of the

7. Although Al may have made do with the *yen-hok*, most smokers scraped the bowl with a separate instrument called the *yen-she gow*. *Yen-shee* is the residue of the smoked opium.

junk business, they started raising the prices up. After World War II I saw
more of the heroin, and the opium decreased. They gave the excuse that
a pound of opium would bring them more money in the market if they
extracted the morphine out of it. They could realize more money that way.
That's why they never bothered to bring the opium—it was bulky. About
like that of morphine or heroin [indicates small amount with fingers] was
equivalent to the same amount of money; why should they bother with
the bulk of opium?

The Italians stepped on the H much more than the Jews, and they
charged more money. It happened before the war, but you weren't about
to see it—just a few people saw it. Like I saw it, and maybe a few more
people like me—like, if this guy was a dealer, he saw it in them days.
But the average man in the street didn't know what was happening. He
didn't know until after World War II, when they branched out good and
they took everything over. As a matter of fact, the old timers that used
junk—nothing else, they used to steal and use junk—would pass the
remark many a time, "Jesus, it's too bad the Jews ain't around to handle
it again." Because they were lenient with the price, they never charged
those fabulous prices they charge today. The Jews were much easier on
everybody. I never dealt in drugs, but I imagine if a guy was dealing in
drugs and he was buying from them steady, if he was short, they'd go
along with him. Not like these people who'll kill you right away.

In the thirties—toward the end, nearer to the forties—the Jews started
fighting amongst themselves. And the Italians were getting more powerful
there, see. They came out with this "donski" business. "Donski" is an
expression they used; it's a don. It's their way of talking family. Every
neighborhood had a guy who was the boss. It could be a kid sixteen years
old, just because his father was Don so-and-so from the old country, a
Sicilian or whatever it is. And, so, if a guy in the neighborhood was doing
something, if he was a bookmaker, he had to kick in a percentage of his
business to this kid from the neighborhood. He thought, "Who's this guy
that's sixteen years old? I've been around for forty years, been doing this
all my life. Who is he that I should give something to?" Well, you had a lot
of trouble in them days. A lot of guys got killed that nobody knew about.
These kids were brazen, they'd stick their chest out just because their
father had made them donskis.

Also, I think in the early forties, they were selling them donskis. These
big wops, the bosses, were selling, like, lieutenantships. It was like degrees
they were selling. This guy wants to be a donski? . . . He gave out maybe
five thousand dollars . . . he had a whole neighborhood to himself. *This*
guy wanted to be a donski? . . . They gave him a badge, or whatever they
called it—he paid maybe seven thousand. *This* guy, he knew him better—
he paid three thousand. That was happening.

When I was around smoking opium with these guys, they weren't donskis, they were just lieutenants for the bosses. They became junkies themselves because they were kids and they wanted to see what it tasted like. So all these wopskis that became junkies were from the families who sold junk years ago.

A couple of guys I know, Jewish guys, used to be junk dealers. They never bothered nobody in the neighborhood, we never knew what it was. They never created no scenes in the street. When people did their business, that was that. Then something happened to the children of some families. They believed . . . in the Jewish religion, like it's a curse on them, because they were selling narcotics to people, the sin fell upon their children. So they stopped right there and then. I know a couple of cases where that happened—they never sold any drugs any more. So, amongst the Jewish people, it got lower and lower. That's when the wops came in power. They became so strong that they became real bosses, you see. Now, they can make a phone call to any part of the country. They can call from New York, say, to Miami and have something done in a minute. That's how powerful they are, one to another. It's all one clannish gang, like. All one.

Jews stopped selling [handwritten margin note]

The Italians still controlled the traffic in '58, when we started shooting up. They were as big as ever—they were getting bigger and bigger. The wops from Italy had all the connections; the port of Marseilles in them days was a depot for junk.

Emily: Lucky Luciano was the biggest.

Al: I remember Lucky when he used to sell decks in the street. Lucky Luciano used to sell decks for five dollars.

Emily: He killed a couple and became a big shot.

Al: I remember him well. Dewey was the one that sent him to prison——

Emily: He was *makkes*![8] He worked for Gurrah and Lepke, until he killed a couple of——

8. *Makkes* means "nothing" in Yiddish. Charles "Lucky" Luciano, christened in his native Sicily as Salvatore Lucania, began his criminal career as a thief and small-time narcotic dealer. But, after he arranged the 1931 murders of Joseph "Joe the Boss" Masseria and Salvatore "Boss of Bosses" Maranzano, he emerged as one of New York's most powerful gangsters. He and Lepke had a large interest in the narcotic traffic during the early 1930s. In 1936 District Attorney Thomas E. Dewey managed to convict Luciano on sixty-one counts of compulsory prostitution, and he was sent to Clinton Prison at Dannemora for thirty to fifty years. However, because he cooperated with the Office of Naval Intelligence in arranging security for New York's docks during World War II, he was paroled and then

Al: Emily, excuse me. You talked about Lucky going away—Dewey sent him away. I did a bit of shylocking, too, in them days. Dewey sent me away for shylocking, sent me away before Lucky.

Emily: Well, Dewey sent away Lepke, who got the chair. That was the biggest. And Gurrah died in the crazy house. These were the biggest Jews.

Al: He wanted to be the big boss, that Lucky. He was the whole drug connection. And he was nothing, he used to be in the streets—like today, they sell junk in the streets. He had a place in front of Reynolds and Delancey Street. That was his spot there.

Emily: Lucky used to sell to the hoosiers.

Al: They'd come by there and he'd sell them decks, the size of a cigarette box, for five dollars. Then he became one of the big bosses. Amongst the wops I don't know how they do it, but they get higher and higher. Yeah, they've got everything today. The whole thing.

I was smoking opium during World War II. To me, it wasn't harder to get, because I had them connections—I told you I knew solid people, people in business that I could depend on. The element I was in, I was always able to get it up to the last minute. I got opium when the *chinks* couldn't get opium.

Later on, after World War II, it was very hard to come by. But I had some very good friends of mine—in fact, with one very good friend, I don't think I paid for my opium nine times out of ten. The guy wouldn't let me pay for it. He was in the trucking business in the garment center —I was on the payroll there for quite some time. He'd say, "Go ahead, Al, it's all right." Yeah, I knew a lot of people around there who smoked for years and nobody knew about it. Even their wives didn't know, a lot of them; they ran away from their wives. But with me, it was different. Whatever I did, my wife did. We did everything together. We stayed away from street addicts pretty much. Only towards the end, when we had to score junk, we started to mix in the street. We lived in the South Bronx in them days, around '68 or '70, I guess.

I don't remember when I started skin popping—around '55, towards

deported to Italy in 1946. He maintained his ties to narcotic dealers and financiers in the United States, and allegedly became a key connection for overseas heroin, most of which was processed in and distributed from Marseilles. Details of Luciano's parole and deportation are in Rodney Campbell, *The Luciano Project: The Secret Wartime Collaboration of the Mafia and the U.S. Navy* (New York: Macmillan, 1977).

the end, '56, somewhere in there. Most of my friends went over to junk well before '55, '56. I first went to the doctors. I got Dilaudids. It's junk, but it's drugstore junk. It's very good.

I never took a mainline in my life. I just took a skin pop. I think the fact that I never mainlined helped me stay alive. A mainline is disgusting; I've seen the way they used to play with the blood and all that. They used to go into a nod—I'm afraid of it, I just dread it. When I'd see how they looked I used to run away. I'd just be glad to get my little skin pop, feel all right, not sick, and then I was satisfied.

We used the Dilaudid whenever we were able to get it, whenever we were able to make the doctors. Sometimes we were disappointed: the doctor we had an appointment with, he'd be afraid to give us any. We found the doctors through friends of ours, one would tell another. They were all in New York City—one or two in the Bronx, in the beginning. Then they somehow quit, the ones in the Bronx. I just had one doctor left, this woman doctor who was a drug addict herself.

This went on maybe four, five years continuous with the Dilaudids. Running around to doctors knocked hell out of me. After all, I was getting older, and it was tough making money, tough getting around to make money to score.

When the Dilaudids ran out I went to heroin. I used the heroin maybe three, four years. I was shooting it, skin popping. I don't think I ever shot junk with anybody. I'd take it home. I'd buy the needles in the street too, but I'd come home and sterilize them and then use them. I'd never use them in the cold, like.

I was looking to break; I didn't know where to go. Previous to that I was trying to get on this methadone program, but people that were on the program told me, "It's a long wait, two to three, four years' wait." It made me feel pretty bad. So, finally there was a guy and his girl on the program; he spoke to this woman doctor, Joyce Lowinson. She was very interested in us, she was interested in helping those who were looking to break. About two or three weeks later, this guy came with a letter and said, "Go ahead, Al, you and the wife go down." We had an appointment in the hospital; we went into the methadone program within a couple of days. It's been a life saver, absolutely a life saver. Without it, I don't know where I'd be today, believe me.

Emily: When I became a junkie, I lost my life. There's nothing like a pipie. They kept themselves immaculate—dresses, furs. I had a diamond, black mink coat. I had a mink stole, a Persian stole—whatever fur was, I had it, because you wanted to look good. Nobody even knew I was a pipie. When people found out I was a pipie, they couldn't believe it. Instead of a pipie, they said I was a junkie already—which I never was, then. There was a million times difference between heroin and opium users, a million times.

I like to be neat. Al too. God, there's nobody cleaner than him! He's crazy clean. That's the truth. The hankie's got to be just so. I mean, you wouldn't find junkies like that—not because it's me or him. Thank God I've kept my cleanliness until now.

4.

The Needle

Heroin users may have been a caste apart from the hop smokers, but they were not an undifferentiated group. An important distinction had to do with the way in which they used the drug, whether by sniffing, subcutaneous or intramuscular injection ("skin popping"), or intravenous injection ("mainlining"). The mainliners were those who had reached the most advanced and deadly stage of heroin addiction; the sniffers were generally neophytes or dabblers, and the skin poppers were somewhere in between.

Since about 1910, when heroin surfaced as a recreational drug in American cities, sniffing has been the preferred method of new users. Like most Americans, they initially feared the hypodermic, which they associated with painful "shots" —vaccinations, novocaine injections, and the like. Sniffing appealed to them because it avoided the needle altogether. It also bypassed the digestive tract, which was a slow and sometimes unsettling way of getting opiates into the system.

Sniffing had its drawbacks, however. Like cocaine, heroin would ultimately destroy the septum, or partition, between the nasal passages; it would literally put a third hole inside a user's nose. Sniffing was also a relatively inefficient way of administering the drug. Injection produced a stronger feeling of relief and euphoria, and produced it more quickly. Mainlining produced the strongest feeling of all.

Users often picked up the trick of mainlining from veteran addicts, but sometimes the discovery was accidental. Buck, a Harlem junkman and mugger, was a cocaine and heroin sniffer who graduated to the needle after he became addicted. "I went to the needle because I just couldn't stand sniffing up my nose no more, and I wasn't getting the kick out of it I was supposed to get out of it," he explained. One day he "discovered mainlining accidentally. I was skin popping and I didn't know I'd hit a vein in my forearm. I got a rush. I felt good behind it, and scared too because I hadn't had that kind of feeling when I was snorting. Then I just kept on shooting." Pleasure mingled with surprise or fear was a fairly common reaction to the first mainline shot. "Boy, that gave me a rush to my head," recalled another addict, "I was going crazy back and forth in the room." Remarks like this are conspicuously absent from accounts of medical addiction in the nineteenth century. When addicts could purchase uncut drugs they had no need of intravenous injection. If they had injected pure morphine into their veins, it might well have killed them.

Heroin mainliners were also in jeopardy. An unusually strong bag could trigger a fatal overdose. This was a constant risk, since the addict usually had no idea of the purity of the drug he was sending directly into bloodstream and brain. The survivors we interviewed were wary of this danger, and tried to minimize it by regularizing their intake, being careful about their suppliers, or by procuring medical narcotics of known strength. They also managed to escape most of the serious needle-related infections that ended the careers of so many of their peers: hepatitis, endocarditis, syphilis, and tetanus. But, despite their precautions, they could not avoid the almost inevitable problems of long-term intravenous injection: abscesses, scarred and swollen arms, and collapsed veins. Sometimes these problems became so serious that they were forced to seek out treatment. Buck, for example, eventually entered a methadone program because "I couldn't find no vein. I got tired of sticking and getting nowhere. You can't find no vein in my forearm—you can't even see it. Nothing. Or in my back. I can't find nothing. And I'm not going under my arm, or in my neck—I'd rather quit entirely."

Mainlining was an indirect consequence of the police approach to narcotic addiction. Outlawing heroin and restricting access to other narcotics created a black market; like all such markets, it operated without external quality controls. Ruthless criminals took advantage of the situation and, just like the bootleggers who watered their hooch or poisoned it with methanol, they adulterated the heroin or mixed it with dangerous stimulants like strychnine. (This is more than just an analogy; most of the big-name narcotic traffickers of the 1930s, 1940s, and 1950s were experienced bootleggers from the Prohibition era. Tampering with the merchandise was nothing new to them. It also helped that their big market was among addicts, who would settle for practically anything.) The worse the heroin, the greater the temptation to mainline; the more widespread the mainlining, the greater the chance of medical disaster. This was the rule during the classic era, and it is still the case today.

The law aggravated the health risks of addiction in another way. Many places, including New York, had laws against the possession of hypodermic paraphernalia without a prescription. The medicine-dropper-and-needle "works" addicts used to inject themselves were hence illegal, and this created a dilemma. To keep one's own works was to increase the likelihood of arrest and successful prosecution; but to share a set with a group of users was to increase the likelihood of infection. It is our strong impression, confirmed by the interviewees' comments, that the surviving addicts resolved the dilemma in favor of medical safety. It was the junkies who chose to play bacteriological roulette in the shooting galleries. This was not an invariable pattern, however, nor is it easy to quantify. The addicts themselves admitted that there were times when circumstances forced them to share their works with others.

Finally, the relationship between punitive laws and needle use was circular.

The thought of injecting drugs disgusted the public; it made addicts seem even more perverse and demented, more like the fanged creatures editorial cartoonists drew and labeled "the dope evil." By underscoring the deviancy, even the subhumanity, of addicts, needle use reinforced the antinarcotic consensus.

ARTHUR

Arthur was born in Harlem in 1914. His mother was from Puerto Rico, his father from the Virgin Islands. "We weren't rich and we weren't poor. My father always worked; we always had our Easter suit; we always had a big tree for Christmas and a lot of Christmas toys. We were a close, happy family." After graduating from high school, Arthur started to work in a grocery store, ultimately rising to a managerial position. But he also began leading a double life, experimenting with the drugs that were becoming increasingly common on the streets of Depression Harlem. He drank bootleg liquor, smoked marijuana, and then discovered heroin in 1935.

I was old enough to know better: I was age twenty-one when I first started to use heroin. At first I snorted it, because I was deathly afraid of a needle. You couldn't come near me with a needle. I could snort, and snort, and snort, though. The guys said, "You're going to eat out the lining of your nose, you're going to get adenoids," and all that. But I wouldn't ever stick a needle in me.

Every day I had to go to the bank at one o'clock to make the deposit from the store where I worked as a clerk. I'd go and make the deposit, then I'd go up to this place and buy a deck for fifty cents. It was at 131st Street and Seventh Avenue. I'd buy a fifty-cent deck, snort up my deck, and go back to work. A deck would last two days, that's how strong the stuff was at that time, in the thirties. You could take half of it, and two guys would get high off it, and then save up the rest. You wouldn't want no more until tomorrow. If drugs come back like that, I don't know what'll become of these methadone programs.

There were a half a dozen people on the street selling it. They were elderly black men, in their forties or fifties. They would be in a poolroom, on a street corner, in a doorway, mostly in the street. I imagine they got their drugs the same place I got it later, when I advanced. Instead of buying decks, I started buying half-ounces, then I started buying ounces over on the east side of Harlem.

You didn't see no kids selling or using drugs. If a kid came around, fifteen or sixteen years old, they'd chase them. They'd say, "What do you want? Get out of here! You want a lollipop or something?" The kids were definitely not involved in the thirties or forties. They would chase them away, see.

Different scene.

I snorted for about two years. Everybody else in my clique—about ten, twelve people—was shooting except me. One year I said, "Let's have a Thanksgiving party. I work in a grocery store. I'll bring all the food if somebody will cook it." That's just what I did. I got everything wholesale, or below sale. So I came with a big box of food and somebody—"Fats" was his name—fixed a big Thanksgiving dinner, and everybody sat there, and we ate. At the end of dinner, somebody said, "Let's do something for Arthur now." "Do what?" They said, "Let's give him a little pop"— that's a shot, a skin pop. I said, "No, no, I don't want nobody sticking a needle in me!" They said, "You won't feel a thing." I said, "No, I'll keep snorting my number." Then I said, "All right, just one time." So I took off my jacket and I put my head down so I wouldn't see the needle. I said, "Go ahead, go ahead," and I felt somebody fooling around with my shoulder a little. I'm still hollering, "Go ahead, go ahead," and then everybody started laughing. I said, "What the hell are you laughing at? Go ahead." He said, "Man, I stuck you five minutes ago." I said, "You stuck a needle in my arm and I didn't feel nothing?" He said, "I certainly did." Well, needless to say, since then I kept shooting too, because that's better.

I took some time before I began to mainline. But I did, and now I don't have a hitable vein in my body. That's what kept me out of the armed forces in World War II. I received several cards asking me to come down to a pre-induction exam. When I finally went, there were about five or six attempts to get blood out of me. But at that time my arms were swollen, my veins were collapsed; they couldn't get blood out of me anyplace. My missus, who died in '45, she was standing there with my clothes in her hand. It was ten o'clock at night, and we had been there since the afternoon, and everybody had stuck, stuck, stuck. They kept saying, "Dr. Payne will get him." So they called Dr. Payne. When Dr. Payne came down, he turned out to be a big, black dude, like Joe Louis, with a bald head. He stripped my clothes away. He said, "Sit on one of them operating tables." He got those focus lights, and put two focus lights on me. All the nurses and the attendants were gathered around. He said, "Get me a small needle. A small needle, a hypodermic, and a syringe." He began going over minutely my arms, my legs, my back. I could see beads of perspiration breaking out on his head. He didn't stick me once. He might have realized I was an addict, but he didn't mention it.

I got my works in a drugstore. I had help from my dearly beloved mother, who was a legitimate diabetic. I used to go to the store with my mother's diabetic card and buy insulin, which she didn't need. I'd say, "A bottle of insulin and two half-inch, twenty-six gauge hypodermics." It was a game I played with the druggist. He'd say, "Why don't you take a dozen? The cost's cheaper." I'd say, "A dozen? How much does a dozen cost? All right, give me a dozen." My mother already had all that she needed, so I'd take my dozen. I'd give them to my friends or I'd sell them. It didn't cost nothing. They used to cost thirty-five cents on the street. Now I understand they cost a dollar and a half.

I very seldom sterilized the needle. We'd just use it until it got dull and then we'd throw it away. Once in awhile I'd put it in the pot and throw water in and let it boil for a couple of minutes, but this is something that's not even worth mentioning. I usually tried to keep my own set of works apart, but if somebody came in and they didn't have any, I'd let them use it. If I had just gotten off, I let them use it. If we came in together, well, naturally, it's my works, I'm going to get off first.

I never got hepatitis or tetanus. But I have numerous scars covering three-quarters of my body, all except my arms and above my neck. From my neck down to my knees is generously covered with ulcer scars. I shot in my arms, but at a minimum. It was because of my work in the stores, so people wouldn't know.

Nobody knew. I never looked like an addict. I never hung out with addicts; I never associated with them. It's just to take care of business, you know, quick, here's the stuff, give me the money and—bang!—gone. You'd never see me on the corner, you'd never see me in the poolroom, you'd never see me in the bar. It's strictly business with me.

Out of every ten of the friends I started to shoot up with in Harlem, nine of them are in the cemetery. Why did I survive and my friends die? Because I've always considered myself an addict, and not a dope fiend. The big difference to me is that a dope fiend, if he has a barrel of stuff, he's going to sit right here and shoot and shoot and shoot and shoot. But I got off four times a day: seven o'clock in the morning, one o'clock in the afternoon, seven o'clock at night, and before I went to sleep. And I always had a shoe box practically full of stuff—I could use all I wanted. But why should I? I couldn't, because I was conducting business for these people. I had money to count. I had deposits to make. I had to order all the merchandise. I've always been deeply involved in business.

On Saturdays and Sundays, that's when I would get tore up in the house. I'd get a little coke with the girl that I'm with, and we'd have a lot of fun. About six, seven o'clock Sunday night we'd stop, because you had to be straight for Monday morning.

I did have trouble getting stuff to shoot during the war, though. There were no drugs in New York during World War II, no drugs in Philadelphia, no drugs in Chicago—there were no drugs on the East Coast. *No drugs.* We traveled around in "wolf packs." Somebody would come and say, "There's some drugs on Forty-second Street!" We'd yell, "Taxi! Taxi! Taxi!" Everybody would run down there; as soon as you'd get there, it was out. Then another group would come and say, "There's some drugs up on 131st Street and Madison Avenue. Somebody's got something that came through." Everybody'd jump in cabs and run up there. . . .

We boiled down paregoric, used pills. We used to take Nembutals, mix it up, and shoot it. That would knock you out. I used to take three; my old lady would take five, and she would fall out. I'd just lay her back and then, when we'd come to, we'd do it all over again. [Laughs.] They were very cheap, twenty for a dollar.

The quality of heroin was much worse after World War II than it was prior to World War II. There were spots, you know—some shipment would come through, the word would get around. During the late forties I was able to get a little bit of heroin, but the quality was so weak I had to augment with other things. I used Dilaudid during this period; I used anything I could get to maintain, to function normally every day.

I got the Dilaudid by making doctors. Old doctors, located in Manhattan and the Bronx. They'd write a scrip out for you; most of them knew what was happening. I had one particular doctor who I used to make, not for Dilaudid, but for barbiturates. You could only go once a month. I had a book, and I would list five names in it, one for each day of the week. I would go and put this book in front of him and he would write a prescription: "Mary Jones, thirty Tuinals, take one a night at bedtime; John Brown, thirty. . . ." He'd give me five different prescriptions, see. And I'd give him twenty-five dollars. That's what he used to charge.

I used to get Dolophines from doctors, too. Same thing: at that time it was five dollars a prescription. Some of them would write, some of them would throw you out of the room. They'd yell, "Get out! Get out! Get out! I don't want blah, blah, blah." It's hell trying to make doctors. You go to about ten, and you're lucky to get two that will write.

JACK

Jack was born in Jersey City in 1909. His mother was a German immigrant; his father was second-generation Irish. Jack was an only child. Due to his father's drinking, his parents separated when he was three years old. His mother was later remarried to a German national living in the United States.

My mother and my stepfather opened a restaurant in Jersey. They were building a hanger for the *Graf Zeppelin* then, I think that was 1920 or '21.[1] They sold the business and they went to Germany. I went too. My stepfather made a lot of money, but he went broke through the inflation over there. It was nothing like this inflation today; it was unbelievable. What they were doing was taking a fifty-thousand-mark bill and just

1. The hangar, which was then the world's largest building, was actually erected in 1919–20 and housed the airships *Shenandoah* and *Los Angeles*. The *Graf Zeppelin* was not launched until 1928.

stamping over it "five million marks." That's how fast the inflation was. And he traded most of his money in for ninety-eight marks to the dollar, which was like giving it away. What kept our heads above water, more or less, was that my mother held back some money. When we'd go to the store, they knew we had dollar bills, American money. [Laughs.] They would rather have a dollar bill than their own money, because it just kept getting worth less and less all the time.

I didn't continue my education in Germany. I went to school a few times, but the language barrier was too much, because my parents spoke English at home. I learned German eventually—you know, a kid will learn anything—but by the time I did learn it, I never went back to school, which I left when I was ten years old.

I started using heroin in Hamburg around 1925. I heard about it by hanging out with fellows my own age down on the waterfront. I didn't even know what it was at first. We used to get a little package—we used to chip in. It came to about a quarter apiece for the four of us. We used to sniff and throw the rest away, instead of getting caught with it. It didn't cost anything.

Everybody got sick the first time. It's a nausea, but it's a pleasant nausea. I don't know how to explain it. You get slightly nauseous in your stomach and, for some reason or another, it just comes up. As soon as you vomit, then you feel real good. You see somebody vomit, then they have a big smile on their face. It looks ridiculous, it really does.

I came back to this country in October 1926. I couldn't get along with my stepfather, no way. When I was seventeen I went to the American consul, told him I wanted to come back. He got me a spot on a ship where I had to work—the *Westphalia*, that was the name of the ship. I had some stuff with me to take care of my habit, enough for thirteen days. Somehow or other I got into contact with my father, my real father. He met me at the pier. He didn't recognize me, but I recognized him. He died the following year. He was drinking heavy, went out in the rain, got soaking wet, and got walking pneumonia. Forty-two years old. One thing about him though: he was not the type of alcoholic who was down-and-out or dirty; he was no wino. He was very neat. In fact, he tended bar. The only way that you could tell he had drinks in him was that he [*sotto voce*] spoke very low, just like a whisper. [Laughs.] I never saw him stagger. If he didn't talk, I would've never know that he'd been drinking. I didn't drink myself. Whiskey and heroin, they don't mix.

I lived with my grandparents in Hoboken. My father lived there too, on and off, until he died. I went to work for the Commercial Cable Company. I was still using heroin, but the job wasn't enough to support my habit. As the price went up, I didn't have the time to go to work. So I quit the job and started dealing, around '32 or '33. Somebody, a Jewish fellow, gave me a proposition to deal for him. When I started I was paying thirty-five or forty dollars an ounce—cut—and making sixty-five one-dollar packages out of it. So I was doubling my money. I was a street dealer, more or less, but I'd try to get it in bulk so I wouldn't have to handle it that many times. In 1933, when I got arrested by the federals, I had a hundred ounces of stuff in the YMHA on Ninety-second Street and Lexington. I did fourteen months in Leavenworth for that.

I didn't use the needle in Germany. I started using it in this country, when the Italians got the stuff and they started to cut it. That was in 1929, when Arnold Rothstein got killed in the *Times* Building, in a card game. He was shot by an Irish guy by the name of Willie McCabe. From then on, that's when the Italians infiltrated. Because Rothstein really had them bulldozed—listen, them Jews were tough bastards, believe me, I'm telling you, they were. And them Italians, they stayed in their place as long as he ruled the roost, as long as he was there they didn't butt in. But, once he was gone, that's when they started to infiltrate. But it wasn't overnight, you know; they didn't give that up overnight. There was a lot of money involved in that. So, probably, infiltration was gradual.[2] And when they got it and they started to cut it—not too bad at first, it was still 40 percent. But gradually it got weaker, and weaker, and weaker. After the war, that's when it really started to go down fast.

In the thirties I was skin popping. I didn't start mainlining until the stuff got real bad, during the war. Previous to that, you didn't have to. I started shooting with a group of friends, but I'd also shoot by myself —it didn't make any difference. But, later on, when the narcotic squads started to come into effect, and things got a little tighter, people became more isolated. Like, everybody didn't trust one another.

I learned to use the needle from watching other people. We didn't use a syringe. We used a medicine dropper with a bulb on the end. Or you could take a nipple from a baby's bottle, or from a pacifier. Pacifiers were the best. See, the advantage that you had with a pacifier, especially if you shot intravenously, was this: you'd take your needle and leave an air

2. Arnold Rothstein, gambler and narcotics financier, was shot in the Park Central Hotel on November 4, 1928, and died, without naming his killer, two days later. Although there was much speculation, no one was ever convicted of the crime. William "Tough Willie" McCabe was Rothstein's bodyguard.

Jack's story is corroborated by the 1964 Senate testimony of federal narcotic supervisor Charles G. Ward: "The bulk of the narcotic traffic in New York is controlled by the five major families of the Mafia. . . . Many years ago, going back into the 1920's, it was a different picture. The Jewish racketeers of New York almost exclusively controlled narcotics, but back in the 1920's, the leader at that time was Arnold Rothstein. He was murdered and the advent of the Italian racketeers taking over began. As time went on, they became more entrenched. . . . They outmaneuvered [the Jewish mobs] with muscle. They killed quite a few of them, and forced them to do their bidding" (U.S. Senate, *Organized Crime and Illicit Traffic in Narcotics: Hearings before the Permanent Subcommittee on Investigations of the Committee*

bubble in the bottom; the minute you hit the vein, the air bubble would bounce up, and you knew you had it. Whereas, with the syringe, you have to draw it up to see if you've got it. I remember one time a doctor broke his last needle, and he didn't know what to do with this guy who was having a heart attack. So I told him, "Well, give me the point. Just stick it in and put a dropper over it. And it will go in that way."

You know, drug addicts were once a lot more sanitary than they are today. I used to throw the needle in alcohol. I didn't share the needle with other people, not unless it was a girl I was living with, maybe. I'd share with her, but I would sterilize between the shots. I always lived with a woman, but I was never married. Personally, I never had any trouble having sex. I had a seven-year run—and I'm not bragging—where I had sex once a night. This woman, who was also an addict, would not let me go to sleep. I could do this because I was cautious with heroin; I used it to stay at a level. If somebody gets too much heroin, it's just like somebody getting too drunk. Using and abusing, there is a difference.

They'd have pieces in the paper, "SICK ADDICT BURGLARIZES ROOM, RAPES WOMAN." That's ridiculous. A man who's sick is not going to have any sex. If you don't have the heroin in you, all your nerves are on edge. In fact, you have multiple wet dreams. Sometimes you'll just turn over, your penis will hit the mattress and—boom! No thrill to it: it just runs out. If you approached a woman when you were sick—boom!—it would be over with before you even entered her. You couldn't do it; it's impossible to do anything when you're real sick. And when you're high, you wouldn't go to the trouble, because your sex drive's not that urgent—unless you're sleeping in a bed with a woman, and you're up against her, or something like that.

At first, during the late twenties, it wasn't hard to keep up my habit. I was buying an ounce for fourteen dollars. But then there was a panic that started after this country got into the war, in 1941. Security tightened up with the ships coming in. It just kept getting worse and worse and worse. I couldn't deal during the war. I lost my connections. Everybody did, more or less. The only ones that were dealing then were the people who really had it, and they would put the price up to where they wanted it.

You supported yourself anyway you could during the war: stealing, whatever. Anybody that's been a drug addict has done some kind of stealing, I don't care who they are. Sometimes I'd find some work, but when I was unemployed I'd end up shoplifting—department stores mostly.

We made doctors for Dilaudid, morphine. It was a constant hassle. One time I went to a doctor—I had been to thirty doctors that morning.

on Government Operations, Part 4 [Washington, D.C.: G.P.O., 1964], 912–13). But for a different version of these events, see the interview with Ralph Salerno in ch. 8.

It was very hot, and there were about twenty people sitting in his waiting room. I wasn't even going to bother, with that many people; I just sat down to rest. I was exhausted. Then he came out, looked around, and said, "You, come here." I went into his office. He said, "What's your trouble?" I said, "My trouble is this: I'm addicted, and I'm sick. I've got no drugs and no way of getting them." He said, "What do you use? . . . Here." He wrote me out a prescription, five grains of morphine. And he says, "That will be three dollars. Come back next week."

Now this man was very good: he done it to help me. I went to him for about six or seven weeks. One night, at one o'clock in the morning, I got a phone call from him. He said, "Listen, I've been called up to go in the service. Come over now, if you can." So I went over—I didn't ask any questions. He had twenty-six weeks' prescriptions written out. He said, "I'm not going to give you these; I'm going to put them in a drugstore and tell them to give them to you as the dates fall." [Laughs.] I don't think that doctor was out for money. But after that six months was up, I went to other doctors. It was a constant hassle.

Most doctors willing to write script were greedy. There were a few like this doctor I described. Usually the ones that did it out of compassion were older. I can understand why. Say a doctor was fifty-five or sixty years old; he had his money made, if he was going to make it. He wasn't at the beginning of his career. And they did it because they felt sorry. I've seen them turn people down and call them back and say, "Here," and not take no money.

Whether or not these doctors were addicted is hard to say. But you could tell, the minute that you went in, whether the doctor wrote or not. If the doctor didn't write he'd say, "You're wasting your time with me." If they would write, they would sit down and talk, hem and haw. There were more doctors who would write outside of New York, especially down through the South and in country areas. When things were tough at the beginning of the war, we used to go to upstate New York, right along the Canadian border, from one town to another. The majority of those doctors would write for you, especially if you used the excuse: "Well, I'm on my way to Kentucky. I ran out of medication and it's too far to go. I'll be sick on the way." He'd say, "Well, how long are you going to stay?" "As soon as I get any medicine, as soon as I get straight, I'm leaving." They'd write just to get you out of town. It seems like the police departments went along with that. They'd say, "Yeah, give him a prescription. Let him cash it and go. Get rid of him."

In Jersey and Connecticut you could get paregoric and needles without a prescription. It was an all-day thing, to go over there and get paregoric. You'd take the paregoric and dump the bottle in a flat pan, put it on a gas stove, turn the gas up, and put a match to the top. The further you boiled it down, the better off you were. Most people put it in the

Frigidaire. When it cooled off, the paraffin came to the top. The opium—supposedly all opium—went to the bottom. What they'd do is make a hole in the paraffin, stick the dropper through there, draw it up, and shoot it intravenously. The reason for shooting it intravenously was that, if that stuff got in your skin, it would burn it like somebody stuck a hot poker in your flesh. It was very painful.

It really became hard to keep up a habit after the war, because that's when habits started to cost you thirty, forty, fifty dollars a day. A lot of people who couldn't support their habit would lend out their works for a few drops to get high, or let someone use their room. They would have a set of works up there. Unless the owner cleaned them out, some guy might be in a hurry, he'd say, "that's all right," and—shish!—inject himself. That's how they get the infections.

I'm very conservative when it comes to narcotics, because it is a poison. Maybe that's the reason I'm alive yet, because I was very, very careful about never taking too much—you can always take more, but you can't take it out. I would only shoot up twice a day in the thirties. That's all. Listen, some people—we called it a needle habit—used to go to the cooker every two hours, and take a very little bit at a time. Whether they done this purposely or not, I don't know. They had a fixation with the needle.

You probably get different stories from different people, and they're probably telling the truth. Everybody is different. Would you believe I knew this person that had a habit with the needle and was needle-shy? She had a habit on the needle, and I used to have to grab her and hold her in the corner and fix her. She couldn't put a needle in herself.

DUSTY

Dusty, a light-skinned mulatto, was born in a Philadelphia suburb in 1918. He went as far as the eighth grade but then left school and got in trouble with the law for stealing and till-tapping. While working as a bartender, he made contact with two black middlemen, who persuaded him to start selling decks of heroin. His first experience with heroin, in 1939, was a bad one: a jealous rival deliberately gave him an overdose. "I was so sick I throwed up in technicolor; I felt like nails was coming out of my throat. I was blind for three days." So he went to some friends he could trust.

Drug addicts in Philly at that time were very rare, and you never knew they were drug addicts. You didn't see nobody sittin' and noddin'. They'd get their dope, go home, and get off. They'd sit and nod for a few minutes, then they'd drink a cold drink or something, and then get up and go out and hustle. Men were programmed this way; they weren't like this new group of drug addicts today that'll take a brick and throw it through your car window because they saw a leather coat in there. These men were professionals at what they were doing. If you were going to try to be something, you would try to be like one of them. You would sit and talk to them about it: "Listen, I want to play this shot. How do I do it?" Pickpockets, five or six of them, would show you. And they would let you practice on them. These were the type of men who told me I'd been given an overdose. So I started using with them.

I had Patsy and Jimmy show me how to do it. I said, "I'll never let nobody else stick a needle in my arm as long as I live. It's like giving somebody a pistol to shoot you with." So I talked to them, and they let me tie up and get off in front of them. I used just a little, small amount, but I felt it.

After that I shot up by myself. I learned everything I could learn about it before I did it again. I got my own private needle. When I would sit down to get off, I had a bottle of alcohol, and water as hot as I could stand it in a metal container, and then I had a glass of plain faucet water. Before I stuck the needle in my arm, I would dip the needle in the alcohol, then the water; then I'd use my handkerchief or something to wipe it with alcohol. I shot in this one vein from here to here [points to arm] for twenty years; that's what you call "the pit." On white people the vein turns blue; on black people it looks like a scab running up and down the arm. This was the only place I shot for twenty years. I was very careful. I didn't let anyone else use my works. My *wife* didn't use my works. Back in them days, everybody had to have their own. If you asked a person to use their works, they got offended. Everybody carried their works on them, until the head of the narcotics squad in Philadelphia finally got what he wanted, and they could lock you up for a mark. See, you could have a pin mark from where you stuck yourself from fixin' a button on your shirt, and, if they took you down and the doctor said that was a needle mark, you were a positive drug addict and you got time in Philadelphia. And don't get caught with no paraphernalia on you, or you're going to jail anyhow, whether you have a mark or not. All of this happened in the early forties. That's when addicts started leaving their works, or hiding their works somewhere.

It took me about three weeks to get hooked. People asked me, "How long you been getting off?" So I said, "Every morning when I get up, I get off." They said, "Don't you get off before you go to bed?" I said, "What am I going to shoot dope for and go to sleep? I don't need nothing to make me sleep." That was my habit until I got greedy, over here in New York. I'd get up in the morning and take a shot; I'd be so busy buying and selling that I didn't have time to be sitting down and getting off every half hour. Then the quality of the dope was such that you didn't have to get high every five minutes. Today people shoot five, six, seven, eight quarters of dope a day. Back then, nobody could shoot no quarter of dope, because it was *dope*. Listen, I don't know what this stuff is out here now.

They told me, "If you shoot dope three days in a row, you got a habit." The people I was closely associated with told me that. But I always thought they were trying to set me up, so I wouldn't get high and then I'd give them some. So I went to talk to my friends Jimmy and Patsy. I said, "How do you know when you're hooked?" Patsy says, "Dusty, just wait and sleep past your get-up time one morning. Then you'll find out if you've got a Jones or not." I said, "What do you mean, 'I'm going to find out?'" Jimmy went to tell me something, but Patsy shook his head. I said, "Wait a minute, man, let him finish. What are you trying to prove?" Patsy said, "I'm just telling you, if you want to know, get up at twelve or one, instead of your normal time of eight o'clock." Hustlers in them days got up like working people.

One morning I did sleep in; my mother and a friend of hers had gone out shopping. It was no big thing really, but I got the idea what it would be like. The phone rang, and I had to go from upstairs downstairs to the phone. When I jumped out of the bed, I started feeling like, "What's wrong? Why can't I run?" When I got downstairs and started talking on the phone, I kept finding myself moving into something, and the person I was talking to said, "What's the matter?" I said, "Just a minute." When I came back, he said, "What's the matter?" I said, "I had to go to the bathroom. Man, what a smell!" He said, "You did your thing yet?" I said no. "What time do you generally do it?" I said, "Between seven-thirty and eight." He said, "It's almost two o'clock, man. You better do your thing if you don't want to throw up." I said, "Oh, you people make something out of it that it ain't."

I went to the kitchen and started frying me some eggs. I puked all over the place. I don't know if it was the smell of the grease or what. I began to feel nauseous and blah, so to speak. I just didn't want to do nothing. You feel sluggish, and when you lay down, the more you sleep, the sicker you get. So I got up and took a fix. It was like a cure-all, and then I knew.

I lived next door to a doctor. I could get any medical book I wanted. I would talk to him, say, "Let me read this." He asked why. I wouldn't lie— I told him the truth. I said, "I'm messing around, and I want to know this, that, and the other." I read up on addiction once I realized I was hooked.

I wasn't a greedy drug addict. I was a skeptical drug addict, but not a greedy one. A greedy drug addict is a person who will never refuse drugs. If they've just finished taking off, and they're sitting there with their head between their legs, and somebody comes in to get off and says, "You sick? You need something?" the greedy drug addict will say, "Yeah, man." But for fifteen years all I ever shot was one deck of dope a day.

I see kids out there today whose arms make them look like they've been shooting dope since they were infants. I used to just ball my fist up, squeeze my arm like that, and hit. You see, I never sat and shot dope just to see the blood go up and down. Once the dope got in me, I took the needle out, cleaned it up, and got away.

But when I started shooting speedballs, that caused a problem. I had to go in different places, because coke collapses your veins. You can hit one vein, and ten minutes later go back and you can't get a hit in it. When I started shooting speedballs I began getting very noticeable tracks. But that didn't stop me, because it's the only way I got the sensation that was vaguely similar to the one I got when I first started shooting heroin.

When I first started shooting heroin they were cutting it with bonita, and coke with epsom salts. Then somewhere between . . . [pauses] 1948 and 1960 it took a nosedive in quality and in the chemicals that they cut it with. This guy Florida Jack was the first man who sold dope with quinine in it.[3] People began to get that rush from the quinine, and if they didn't get that rush from the quinine the dope wasn't no good. They got so that they would get down, get off, get the rush, and ten minutes later they were sick.

3. According to Dr. Milton Helpern, former Chief Medical Examiner for New York City, quinine was introduced as an adulterant sometime in the early 1930s, following a malaria pandemic among addicts sharing contaminated needles ("Epidemic of Fatal Estivo-Autumnal Malaria . . . ," *American Journal of Surgery* 26 [1934], 111–23, 142; "Causes of Death from Drugs of Dependence," in C.W.M. Wilson, ed., *The Pharmacological and Epidemiological Aspects of Adolescent Drug Dependence* [Oxford: Pergamon, 1968], 222). Some have suggested that quinine was implicated in the sudden, gruesome heroin "overdose" deaths that were noticed around 1943, and which accelerated during the 1950s and 1960s (Edward M. Brecher et al., *Licit and Illicit Drugs* [Boston: Little, Brown, 1972], 110, 114).

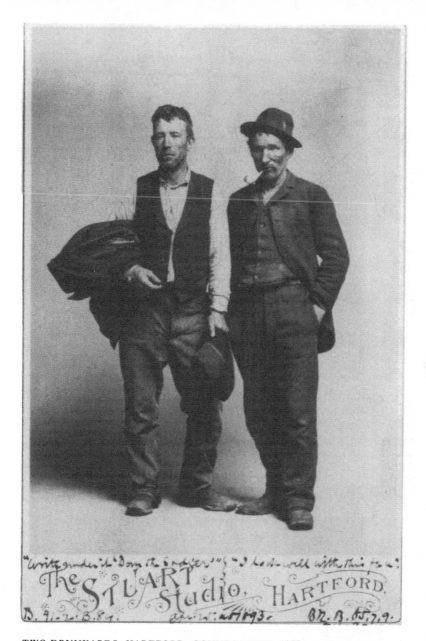

TWO DRUNKARDS, HARTFORD, CONNECTICUT, 1893
These men were paid a quarter apiece to be photographed; their benefactor was John James McCook, a reformer who was convinced that drink was the major source of the "tramp problem" and other social ills. McCook and his contemporaries did not generally think of narcotic users in these terms. By World War I, however, addicts had come increasingly to resemble the alcoholic stereotype—male, rootless, disheveled, dangerous. *The Social Reform Papers of John James McCook.* Courtesy *Antiquarian and Landmarks Society, Inc., Hartford, Connecticut*

118

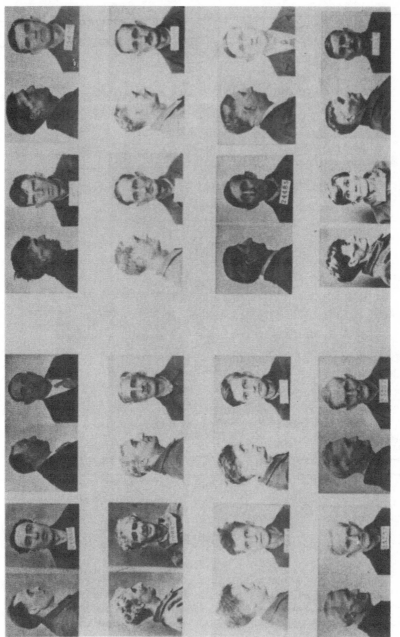

ADDICTS BEFORE AND AFTER IMPRISONMENT, ABOUT 1927

These photographs were probably intended as an exhibit for the 1928 congressional hearings on the establishment of federal narcotic farms, the point being that addicts' health and appearance improved after a period of enforced abstinence. *Drug Enforcement Administration (hereafter cited as DEA)*

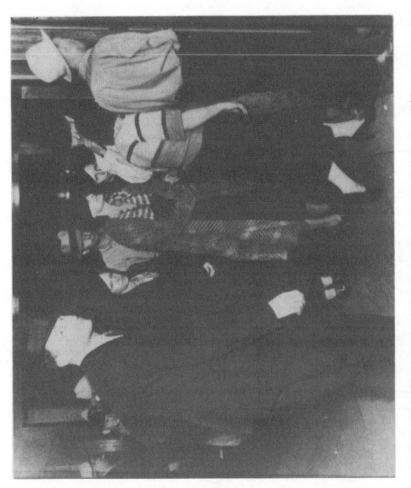

ROUNDUP OF SUSPECTED NARCOTIC-LAW VIOLATORS, FT. WORTH, 1936
Narcotic agents and local police lead arrestees into the Federal Building for questioning. Note the absence of black suspects: narcotic addiction in the mid-1930s was still predominantly a white phenomenon, especially in the South. *DEA*

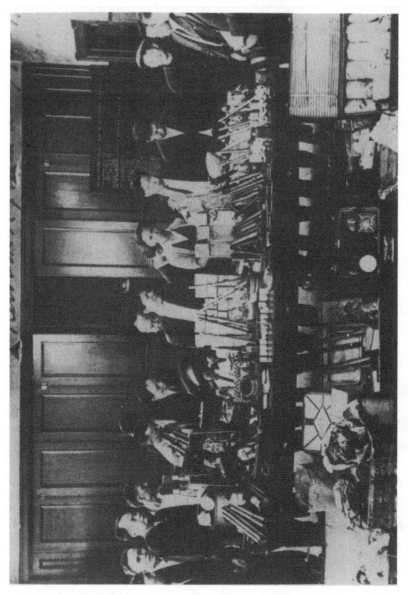

OPIUM SEIZURE AND DEFENDANTS, NEWARK, 1927

Indicted proprietors of opium dens stand behind seized smoking paraphernalia and large packages of opium. Opium smoking, which was identified with Chinese immigrants, fallen women, and the white underworld, was the target of local, state, and, in 1909, federal legislation. *DEA*

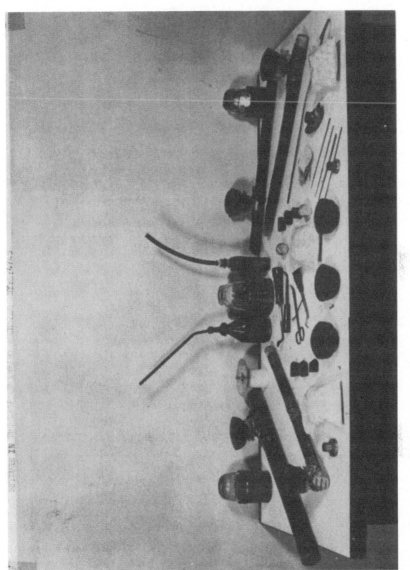

OPIUM PIPES AND PARAPHERNALIA

Opium pipes could be elaborate works of art, or homemade contraptions of bottles and tubing. Shown are various implements for manipulating opium pills, scraping *yen-shee* from bowls, and trimming the wicks of lamps; small tins containing hop; and white cubes of what appears to have been morphine sulfate. *DEA*

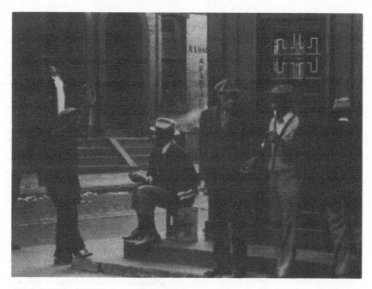

GHETTO HEROIN TRANSACTION

Heroin use among urban blacks increased steadily during the 1920s and 1930s, and then very rapidly after World War II. This surveillance photograph was probably taken in Philadelphia; no date is given. *DEA*

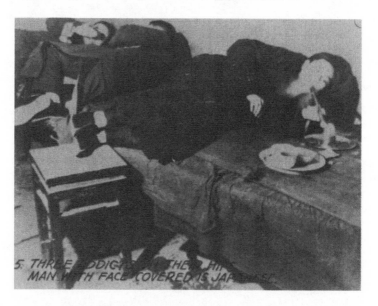

OPIUM SMOKER TAKING A DRAW

The heat from the lamp ignites the pellet of opium in his tilted pipe. Although this photograph is undated, the handwritten caption accompanying it suggests the late 1930s or early 1940s, the period during which Anslinger repeatedly accused the Japanese of fostering narcotic addiction to further their imperial ambitions. *DEA*

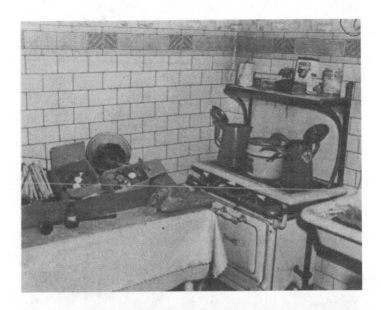

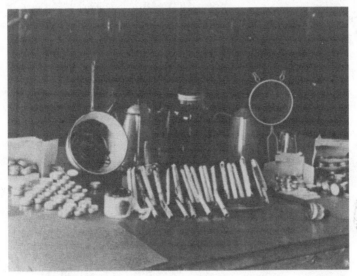

"COOKING" CRUDE OPIUM

"I would boil it down until it looked like a black sauce," recalled Jerry. *Above:* the operation *in situ. Below:* everything neatly sorted out. The purpose was to take crude Persian opium, in the white sticks, and refine it until it was suitable for smoking in a pipe. *DEA*

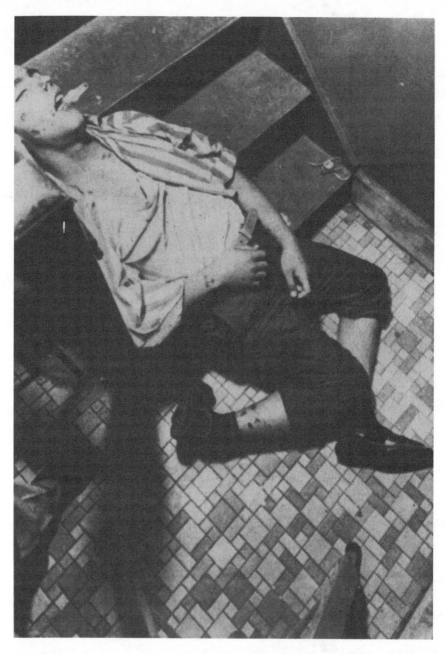

OVERDOSE VICTIM
A fate our interviewees managed to avoid. This addict's companions made a crude attempt to revive him after he collapsed, but then abandoned him in a tenement house stairway. His "works" are on the bottom step. *C.W.M. Wilson, ed.*, The Pharmacological and Epidemiological Aspects of Adolescent Drug Dependence (*Oxford: Pergamon Press, 1968*).

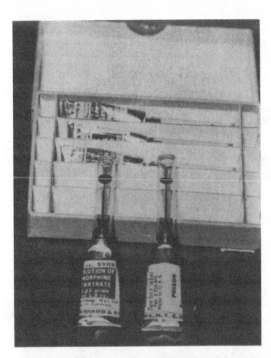

SYRETTES OF MORPHINE TARTRATE
Intended for use in battlefield or emergency conditions, addicts sometimes stole these from medical kits or purchased them from those who had. *DEA*

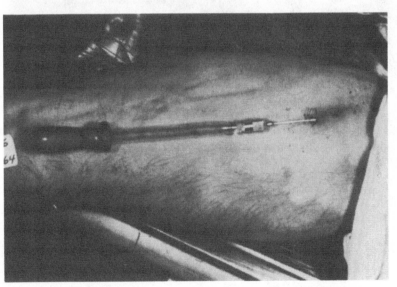

DEAD MAINLINER'S ARM
The reason hop smokers dreaded becoming junkies. Intravenous injection was both dangerous and revulsive, and served to reinforce the dope fiend image. Even William S. Burroughs conceded, in *Naked Lunch*, that "it's a wildly unpretty spectacle." *C.W.M. Wilson, ed.,* The Pharmacological and Epidemiological Aspects of Adolescent Drug Dependence (*Oxford: Pergamon Press, 1968*).

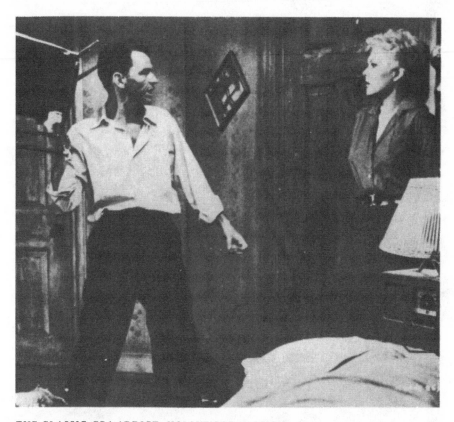

THE CLASSIC-ERA ADDICT: HOLLYWOOD VERSION
Frank Sinatra played Frankie Majcinek, a.k.a. Frankie Machine, in Otto Preminger's *The Man With the Golden Arm* (1955). Nelson Algren's 1949 novel of the same title ends with Frankie hanging himself in a Chicago flophouse; in the movie he kicks cold turkey, is rid of his neurotic wife, and walks away with the B-girl, Molly, played by Kim Novak. *Courtesy, Otto Preminger Films, Ltd.*

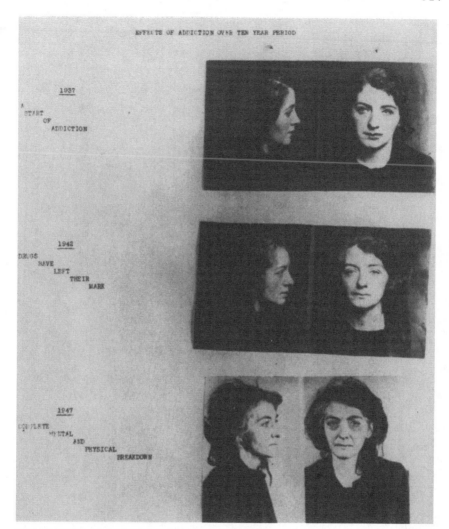

THE CLASSIC-ERA ADDICT: OFFICIAL VERSION
Whether dealing with statistics or photographs, federal officials sometimes lent reality a helping hand. These pictures were retouched to exaggerate the effect of ten years' narcotic use (1937–47), most notably by adding bags beneath the woman's eyes in the lower right-hand photograph. There is no doubt, however, that most addicts' lives were stressful and unhealthful. *DEA*

PART TWO:
IN THE LIFE

5.

Scoring

Once addicted, classic-era users had to obtain narcotics on a regular basis or endure the pains of withdrawal. There were no ambulatory detoxification facilities and no maintenance clinics; they either scored or they became ill. This duality was the dominant fact of their lives and shaped every aspect of their behavior.

There were two principal sources of narcotics: doctors, who could sometimes be persuaded to write prescriptions for a fee, and street dealers, who were the retailers for the illicit market. Morphine and synthetic opiates could be obtained through the former, adulterated heroin from the latter. One interesting point that surfaced in the interviews was that the addicts tended to specialize. Some confined themselves to making doctors, others to purchasing heroin from dealers. Once they had the knack and the connections for scoring from one source or the other, they stuck with it, at least until an unforeseen event disrupted their routine.

One such event was the shortage occasioned by World War II. As Arthur and Jack mentioned in the previous chapter, and as John describes in this chapter, illicit narcotics became increasingly scarce and expensive during the early 1940s. Axis occupations in Europe and Asia eliminated several traditional sources of heroin and opium, while submarines and strict wartime customs inspections made smuggling difficult. Anslinger had also been busy buying up most of the Near Eastern opium crop, both to insure a military stockpile for the Allies and to keep such invaluable medication out of enemy hands (whereupon German researchers developed methadone, the synthetic opiate that would boomerang on the Bureau of Narcotics twenty years later).

The combination of disrupted smuggling and preemptive purchases created a massive "panic" among addicts; by 1942 street heroin was about 2 percent pure, if it could be found at all. We spoke to a few people, like Teddy, who said that they were able to purchase heroin regularly during the war, but this was exceptional. Most addicts accustomed to black market heroin had to switch to other drugs or quit altogether. Those who lacked the skill or patience to make doctors often resorted to robbery and burglary—"everybody with a white coat, everybody even remotely associated with medicine" was liable to be held up during a panic.[1] *Another expedient was to boil down and inject paregoric, the camphorated tincture of opium still widely available without a prescription in the early 1940s. Once druggists caught on, they began profiteering. One midwestern pharmacist upped the price of a gallon of paregoric to $165, or about thirty-three times the wholesale cost.*[2] *He did not want for customers.*

JOHN

John was born into a black family in Norfolk, Virginia, in 1915. His parents moved to Baltimore briefly, then to New York City in 1926.

I started using drugs in the thirties. This was more or less an experimental thing. I had been smoking marijuana when I was a youngster, seventeen, eighteen, nineteen. In Harlem you can buy anything—you just have to know where to buy it. When I was a kid, we used to go to a reefer pad and buy it and smoke in the pad. We'd sit there listening to a jukebox or a phonograph. We'd listen all day. We'd spend maybe six, seven hours in there smoking. This was, I suppose you'd say, being "cool" or "cooling it." Most of the people that were considered to be in the life smoked marijuana—the night people, people that were considered "down," such as gamblers, numbers people, prostitutes.

At that particular time marijuana was the only drug you found in the reefer pads. There was a separation between marijuana and the heroin. The coke was separate too. You'd go to another place, and you'd sit down, and coke would be put on a plate. Coke, and whiskey. This was a different type thing. I went to these pads, but not too often though. There were mostly pimps and prostitutes there, and gamblers.

I was about twenty-three when I first used heroin. In the block I came out of, 143rd Street, there was a group of older fellows, and most of them, I suppose, had habits. We used to wonder about them, why they were so much higher than we were. We were smoking the best reefer around, because we were smoking meserole, and during that time, anybody that

1. Claude Brown, *Manchild in the Promised Land* (New York: Macmillan, 1965), 353.

2. "What's Cooking?" *Newsweek* 25 (April 9, 1945), 99–100. See also Gerard Piel, "Narcotics: War Has Brought Illicit Traffic to All-time Low but U.S. Treasury Fears Rising Postwar Addiction," *Life* 15 (July 19, 1943), 82–94, and Douglas Clark Kinder and William O. Walker, "Stable Force in a Storm: Harry J. Anslinger and United States Narcotic Foreign Policy, 1930–1962, " *Journal of American History* 72 (1986), 919–21.

smoked meserole, they smoked the best reefer in New York. Mezzrow was a man's name, and the reefer took his name. He was a musician.[3] Like I said, this reefer was so good that it was assumed to be habit-forming, that you had to have a stick when you got up in the morning. So we'd wonder why these other guys, these older guys, were so much higher than we—they'd be sleeping and nodding. After probing, and talking to them, and asking them, they finally took us to one of the pads one night where we could buy some horse. We went to the pad, and the guy gave me my first shot. In the hip—I never snorted.

This heroin pad was in a hotel room—I suppose you could say it was an apartment, because this guy lived there. He sold dope for a living. You'd go up there, he had the works there, and you'd get off. He had about eight or ten sets of works on the table. It was more or less like a shooting gallery of today, where you'd go in and there'd be maybe six or eight, ten people there. He'd clean the works as you finished with them. He'd clean with water, hot water. He always had several glasses with water in them. He'd start off with one glass and go down the line and shake it out—which I don't suppose was very clean, considering. But that's the way it was done.

The guy that brought us there, he would hit me and my friend, and we'd leave. I got one shot a day, damn near every day. A shot was fifty cents. Even though I was a pretty good hustler, it wasn't cheap. In the thirties, when things were bad, fifty cents was a lot of money. Girls on the street were selling their bodies for fifty cents.

After about eight months I stopped going to these places where you could get a shot in a pad. I started going downtown, down around San Juan Hill, and buying my own stuff, taking it to my house, and using it myself. I had started experimenting with vein shots. I bought my needles from people on the street. I'd cop down at San Juan Hill because I could buy a half-ounce of heroin for seven dollars. I'd get more for seven dollars than I'd get spending fifty cents a pop. If I'd buy seven or eight dollars worth of stuff here, in Harlem, for fifty cents each, I wouldn't get half as much as I'd get from the seven-dollar half-ounce.

I don't know whether anybody would be able to understand it, but it seems that one addict would recognize another. If I would come in the

3. Milton "Mezz" Mezzrow was a white, Chicago-born jazz clarinetist heavily influenced by the New Orleans style. He was also well known as a dealer in Harlem, and was imprisoned in 1940–42 for selling marijuana. Mezzrow's motto: "Light up and be somebody." In his autobiography, he explained that *mezzroll* described "the kind of fat, well-packed and clean cigarette I used to roll (this word later got corrupted to *meserole* and it's still used to mean a certain size and shape of reefer, which is different from the so-called panatella)." See Milton Mezzrow and Bernard Wolfe, *Really the Blues* (New York: Random House, 1946), 212, 215.

block down there, if I'd go to Sixty-second Street, we'll say, and stand on the corner a little while, somebody would walk up to me and ask if I would like to score. That's how I was able to make a connection.

At that time I'd say the dope was running about 64 percent, 67 percent pure. There wasn't too much chemical in the dope; it was more dope than chemical. But that half-ounce wouldn't last too long, because I always had a lot of hanger-on-ers, people that I'd take care of. Say five of us could sit up all night and, if we had the stamina, we could shoot up all night on that one half-ounce. And I'd have some for when I woke up in the morning.

The price of heroin went up during the early forties though. I told you that, prior to the war, I used to pay seven dollars for a half-ounce, which made it fourteen dollars an ounce. Then a fellow here in Harlem started selling quarters—he broke an ounce into quarters, and he would sell it for five dollars a quarter, which made it go up to twenty dollars an ounce. For a while there wasn't any heroin around; all the dope was taken up for the soldiers. When it came back the price had soared: I used to pay twenty dollars an eighth for it, after things let up a little bit. Now, this was a big jump, from seven dollars a half-ounce to twenty dollars an eighth. But, if you're an addict, you're going to buy.

Big jump in $ but industry demand.

When there was no heroin available, I used prescription drugs, like everybody else. You must remember that, during this time, you were grabbing at straws. You'd be burned quite often. So I started using Dilaudid and Pantopon. I got them from scrip cashers, people who make a hustle of cashing doctors' scrips. I'd buy the pills I needed from them. About '40, '41 I also started using morphine sulfate—no, not morphine sulfate —morphine-atropine. The morphine sulfate didn't give me the boot I wanted, so I had to break an atropine tablet too. Sometimes I'd speedball, using coke and morphine together. The morphine came in vials. They would sell on the street for twenty dollars. If I went up to a guy who had three vials, or five vials, I'd give him a certain price—maybe he'd knock two dollars off each vial, or something like that. I really couldn't say whether the prescription-drug habit was more expensive than the heroin habit. I bought more than the average person that was around me, and I spent just as much on one as on the other.

The scrip cashers I bought from were black, but I know that whites had croakers that they used to go to—a "croaker" is a doctor. They would go to him and get whatever they wanted, or whatever they used, and sell it on the street. I knew a fellow who was a veteran of World War I. I used to buy morphine from him. He had some particular type of ailment that allowed him to have access to all the morphine that he could use. He told me that one of the people that used to write for him was the Commissioner of Health of Connecticut.

In 1942 I went into the army, even though I was addicted. I had started mainlining in the late thirties, and I had the normal marks of the average addict. When I took the physical, twenty-eight doctors suggested that I be rejected. But there was a captain who decided whether to accept you or reject you, and I had had an argument with him when I first came in. He didn't like my tone, and I didn't like his tone. I must have said something like, "Listen, you don't have to talk to me like that; I'm not in the army— yet." He said, "Oh, I don't? You'll be in the army when you come out." So I went along the line of physicals. All the doctors that examined me recognized the fact that I was an addict. They suggested that I be rejected from the army. But this captain had a hard-on for me. He accepted me into the army over the objections of all these doctors. I even went back to the doctor in charge after this guy accepted me, and explained it to him. He got the other doctors, and they had a conference, and they all agreed that I shouldn't be accepted into the army. But I was anyway. I got my order to report to the induction center in June 1942.

I spent most of my three years in the army in and around New York. I didn't maintain my habit as such, but whenever I came out on pass I'd buy me some drugs. I had some money from gambling, and whatnot. I'd take the drugs back to camp and make them last for two or three days. I also used tartrates, which they had in medical kits. If you got a wound on the field, they'd shoot you up with this. If you weren't an addict, I guess it was ample. With me it was nothing—I could shoot two or three of them. I had my own works in the army. I slept in a room with another guy; when he was out I'd close the door and use the room to inject myself with drugs.

When I came out of the army in '45 I was still buying prescription drugs on the streets. The heroin came back, I guess, about '46 or '47. It was more expensive, and it was a lower grade. It was about 50 percent more expensive than before World War II. A quarter was about fifty, sixty dollars. But I preferred the heroin to the prescription drugs. If I was a rich man, I'd use heroin until I died.

MIKE

Mike was born in 1906 into a "very religious" middle-class white family. He spent his early years in a Boston suburb, then moved to New York City when he was about eight years old. An excellent student, he received top marks in his class and won a scholarship to a Catholic military school.

They gave me a job as custodian of the gun room. Everybody did some little thing, especially the scholarship students. But in the middle of the room they had three pool tables, and I was forever playing pool, pool, pool, every day. I became so good at it that I became a professional pool player. Being young like that, I thought it was a good thing. I dropped out of school in the fourth year. About six months after I quit school I left New York. I became a pool hustler. This was about 1923—I was seventeen when I left home.

When you're a pool hustler, you're actually a student of human nature. You have to say the right thing at the right time. A dummy can't do this; you have to have certain brains to do this, or experience. As I went from town to town—and I've been in every town in the United States over twenty-five thousand—I developed a technique of talking to different types of people. The honest man—you can't win any money from an honest man. You find a few up in Maine, New Hampshire, Vermont. Then there are people who are greedy and have larceny in them. They're the kind I'd win most of the money from, because they're trying to beat *me*. I'd tell them that I didn't play as good as I really did, make conversation, and this and that. But you win the bigger money when they send for the town champion, or the county champion, or the best player in that vicinity. Now they think for sure he's going to beat me, and they all bet on him, and I win. After I win, then it's the next town.

You don't win a lot of money on the road. Some years you'll make good money, other years very little. I averaged about ten thousand a year—that was in hard times. Ten thousand was like thirty thousand today. In Texas I once won twelve thousand in one day, and in Norfolk, Virginia, I won eight thousand in one day. But that was very unusual.

I started using drugs after I got in an automobile accident in Miami, Florida, when I was about twenty-five years old. Miami was sort of my headquarters. The accident wasn't too bad, but I had pains in the back. The spine was bumped up a little. So I went to a doctor. He gave me medicine for the pain. I'm not sure whether it was Darvon, but it didn't seem to help. I couldn't sleep. I was getting terrific pains in the back. This is no lie—this is the truth. Finally I got so bad that he gave me a little morphine, small amounts, to stop the pain. Course he meant right —he stopped the pain right away. This was only for about two weeks, so I could sleep.

About a month later I still wasn't well yet, but I was all right, I didn't need anything. I met this girl and, to make a long story short, I started living with her. She had been a nurse. I didn't know it, but she was also a morphine addict. When I met her, I wasn't using. I had been, but at that particular time I decided to quit. But, when I lived with her, I went back on it again. I wasn't in pain at that time; the back had healed up.

To make money playing pool I had to go on the road and keep traveling from town to town. When I traveled, I'd have to go to a doctor in the town. These were mostly smaller towns, not big cities. Sometimes he would write a prescription for morphine, sometimes not. If not, I went to drugstores, and I got three or four bottles of paregoric, which at that time you could buy without any prescription. I found out how to get all the alcohol and camphor out of the paregoric. I'd cook it down and get everything but the narcotic out of it. You have to inject it into a vein, you can't "skin it," as they say. It ruins your veins: the camphor in there burns them up somehow. Within five years you have very few veins left if you take it every day.

Drug addicts know how to lie good. I would tell a doctor I had trigeminal neuralgia of the face. Of course it wasn't the truth; I was lying. But the doctor would write a prescription for morphine. I told him I had taken morphine for that, and it was about the only thing that stopped the pain. It is very, very bad pain, you know. So some doctors feel sorry for you, and they write it. Others won't. They tell you, "I'm sorry, I can't write for any drugs." If they didn't, as I said before, I'd go to a drugstore and get some paregoric.

Doctors in the southern states would prescribe much quicker than doctors in the northern states, for some reason. I don't know exactly why; I never did find out. Also, an old doctor would be more likely to give you morphine—by far. I'd say nine out of ten old doctors. They seemed to understand the problem more. I don't know if the doctors I saw were themselves addicts. But I do know this: everytime I went to Lexington there were always three or four southern doctors there as drug addicts, for a cure. I never saw a northern doctor there. 'Course Lexington's in the South, in Kentucky.

They gouged me: they charged me more than ordinary for a prescription. Sure. Some of them charged twenty dollars—at that time it was only three dollars for a prescription. That was for sixty half-grain morphine tablets, or quarter-grain at times. They were greedy, and they thought that there was no risk attached to it, that my story was probably true. You know, in small towns a lot of doctors don't make too much money. They would know that I wasn't from the town, nobody would find out in the town—only the pharmacist—and that I'd be leaving there in a week or so. They were protected more or less, they thought. That's what *I* thought. But it was no sweat for me, because I was making a good income.

Some doctors would give it to you out of compassion, at cost. Not too many, but some. Some of the old timers, I think, really cared more about doing what they believed in. They knew they were right—they *thought* they were right, I don't say they *knew* they were right. I needed it. I would be sick without it. It was medicine—and they wrote.

When I was in New York City in the 1930s, you could buy heroin from pushers, which I didn't want. I was always afraid of heroin. It was too powerful for me, maybe, or I was afraid they didn't know how to cut it right and they might put something in there that would hurt you. I had a friend of mine die from it—not from an O.D., but from the way the heroin was cut. But there were occasionally morphine sellers. They got it from a legitimate source somehow. I think they got it from doctors that were addicts themselves—I'm not positive. But I never stayed in New York too long anyway. I couldn't make money in New York. I was pretty well known as a top player, and once you're well known, you can't make much money unless you're on the road.

My contention is—and the doctors in Lexington told me this is the truth—that if you use morphine moderately it does not hurt your body in any way. It helps your body, because you're calm all the time, your nerves are settled. If anything, morphine made me play better. Although I can't say positively, because I played so good anyway. It steadied your nerves. I was calm. No matter how large the crowd, or how much I was betting, I never got nervous. But I attributed that to my experience, because this happened so many times I was beyond the stage of being nervous. I knew exactly what to say, what to do. I knew I couldn't lose. These town champions had no chance with me.

BRENDA

Brenda married her second husband, a con man and morphine addict, in Chicago in 1951. They began traveling with a carnival, earning good money by operating several concessions. Like Mike, they specialized in making doctors in the various towns they passed through and for years remained aloof from the street dealers and their customers.

I met my husband at the club the first time, but I really got to know him when I met him a second time at this doctor's office. We were both there late at night, nine-thirty. There were fourteen other patients in the hallway waiting for him to show up. He was late. He never arrived until eleven o'clock that night.

This doctor was a writer. He was a Greek; he spoke such bad English that I took it for granted that he hadn't been here too long. His office was in a very poor, a very tore-up neighborhood. It was considered the skid row of Chicago.

Everyone in that hallway was waiting for a narcotic prescription. These were all white people. There were older women, women in their fifties, like I am today. This is what amazed me. The men were the same: late forties. These were very home-like, very family-type people, not loud or boisterous. They were quiet, clean, neat. Today people say, "that person's a drug addict" by appearance, or people will see a group and say, "they're all junkies." It wasn't anything like that. These were just people to see a doctor, and you woke up to the fact that you were all there for the same thing.

After we all got together and talked, the pharmacy downstairs would get a call to stay open until all the patients were seen, which was sometimes one-thirty in the morning. You could look across the street and the doctor would be in his car necking with some young girl, while all the people were up in the hallway waiting, half of them sick. You could see they were withdrawing.

The doctor's charges were really excessive—this is what the conversation was all about. He would charge different people different amounts. He introduced me to Dolophine, what we call methadone today. It was 1949. He told me, "You won't have to take morphine. There's a new drug, it's a synthetic from Germany," and went on to explain the Dolophine. He would give me a prescription for a 20cc bottle of liquid Dolophine. Eventually, my future husband and I were getting prescriptions from him every day. I would get a bottle and he would get a bottle. We injected it. It was a 20cc bottle, 10 milligrams to a cc. It was an enormous amount of Dolophine but, like everything else, I didn't know it, and my husband didn't know it, so we ended up taking a whole bottle every day. By the end of six months we had quite a habit.

It was thirty-five dollars for two bottles. Don't get me wrong now, I'm saying thirty-five dollars for the prescription. But there were other ways, financially, that you got to this person. There were other gifts of money given to him. He let it be known what he wanted. Once he got to know you, he laid his cards on the table: that he wasn't there for no doctoring, that he was there to write prescriptions, but he was going to be paid, and paid well. And a hundred-dollar bill would go into an envelope and be given to him. Quite often.

Why did we continue with this doctor? Well, once 1950 hit, things with doctors started to become a little difficult. They weren't as open. You couldn't find that many. It was easy up to that point; after that doctors who would write became scarce. It seemed that there were more addicts coming from nowhere, just popping up. Heroin addicts. Doctors that would give you prescriptions before would start saying, "No, no, I'm getting afraid. Too many people are coming for prescriptions." You see, when heroin became very heavy, and people became addicted to heroin and then couldn't get it, they would go to a doctor. When the doctor's office became overcrowded with people looking for narcotics, along with his patients, it became very fearful to him.

Once we began to travel with the carnival we were in every different state, so we would have to find a doctor, maybe two doctors, in the area for ten days. We would both find doctors, but the approach was different. I still felt that it was ridiculous to go to a doctor and tell him a story that wasn't so. I thought you were not only making a fool out of the doctor, you were making a fool out of yourself. Now my husband was quite a con man. He would go to a doctor and tell him he had an ailment and that it was necessary that he have Dilaudid. The doctor would give it to him or not, according to how hard he pressured. I, on the other hand, would tell the doctor that I would go to that I was an addict. It was up to him. If he didn't want to give me the prescription, he didn't give it to me. But I was amazed to find that quite a few did give it to me. Some doctors would say, positively not, and stay with that. Other doctors would ask, "How long will you be in town?" I'd tell them ten days. "I will give you the prescription providing you never come back again," and I would maybe get fifty or a hundred one-sixteenth grain tablets of Dilaudid.

We would find the doctors by just looking in the phone book. It seemed to be the smaller the town, the better the chance of getting a doctor to write you a prescription. This was because of the poverty in some of these small areas of Tennessee, Kentucky, Alabama, Georgia. Doctors were older, needing money. Money played a part, a big part. If the doctor would just write you that one prescription and tell you never to come back, he would charge you maybe three dollars. But if you found a doctor that would write and not say anything or question anything, you would go back in two or three days and see if he would give you another prescription. If he did, you knew that this was a doctor that would make any prescription for any amount, providing you offered enough money—fifty dollars, a hundred dollars, depending on the doctor. You had to know people; it took me a long time to see this.

We were in Canada in '52, just right across from Detroit, in Windsor. The doctors seemed to look upon narcotic addiction in a different way. My husband went on to Quebec. I didn't. According to him it was much easier to not have to go into any long, drawn-out illness. When he would go in to talk about his "sickness" the doctor would tell him, "You don't have to go through all this. What are you looking for?" and cut him off immediately. Evidently there was a much more liberal attitude in Canada.

We had an apartment in Chicago. Most of our winters were spent there. Fall, spring, and summer we were on the road. Winter wasn't no vacation: we would come back to Chicago, and he'd either be working at night in the club, or I would be down there. He ran a gambling game in the back.

The Greek doctor wasn't the only doctor I had in Chicago. I had three, four, five around the city and in the suburbs. There was one doctor in the suburbs that was known as a writer. Just about everyone that used narcotics knew him. When I first went to his office for a prescription, I couldn't believe it. I introduced myself and I told him what I was there for. He asked me, "How many do you want? You know it's going to cost you two dollars a pill." I said, "Do you mean you're going to give me the pills here in the office and not a prescription?" He said, "No. How many pills do you want me to write for. It's two dollars a pill." Then I realized here was a doctor you could obtain any amount from. All you had to do was have the two dollars for each pill and he would write a hundred, two hundred, whatever you needed.

I returned to this doctor two years later in a very bad financial situation. I was going back out of town, needed two hundred pills, and had enough money for a hundred. I had given him a lot of business and thought surely he would give me the prescription when I came back into Chicago. But he said, "Well, you have a ring on your finger. Just leave the ring." This was hard for me to take, because I didn't want to part with that ring. But I did.

He was a man in his seventies. The narcotic people had been in on him and told him they had seen some of his prescriptions in a few drugstores, and that he was overwriting and he would have to stop. But he completely ignored this and continued on. It went on for about three years. He was never arrested until finally, about 1955, they took his narcotic license away from him.

When I go back in life there were a lot of people, and a lot of doctors, that were wonderful to me. By the same token, I met some horrors. Once I was arrested in a raid on a doctor's office. This was in the West Side of Chicago in 1955, 1956, around in there. This doctor, to me, was the most wonderful man I had ever met. He was a wonderful man, that's all I can say. I was kept in jail for three days and tormented, really tormented. They came to me with hypodermic needles with water in them and the police would tell me, "If you will tell us how much this doctor gave you on prescription and how many prescriptions he wrote for you, we'll give you a shot." In other words, they waited for all the withdrawal to get me at the worst possible stage.

I think this was a crossroads in my life. I told myself over and over again, this man was so wonderful to me that there'd be no way I would . . . I would rather have died than say anything against him. All I could say was, "He didn't write a prescription for me. He never gave me anything." I stayed with that, and they put me through a living hell.

The reason I think I had to stand up so much for this doctor was that, at first, he didn't want to write for me. I was sick, and I really broke him down, broke him down in such a way that his attitude was, "There, but for the grace of God, goes my own daughter." He had a daughter about my own age. No way could I ever hurt him.

The doctor had a good reputation, and this was all harassment more than anything else. It ended up in 1960. This doctor killed himself, but he had a brain tumor. He was in Florida with his wife. He committed suicide. And killed her too.

EDDIE

Eddie was born in New York City in 1911 and grew up in the Bronx. His father was an Italian fruit and vegetable dealer, his mother a housewife. He went

through the eighth grade of school, then left to help his father sell produce—and
score drugs.

My father was a drug addict. He was addicted before I was born. He was
born in Italy and came to this country when he was a little boy, maybe nine
years old. That was around the turn of the century. He was sixteen or
seventeen when he got addicted. He had a headache one day—so he tells
me—and he took a snort of heroin. And on and on, and he got addicted.

My mother was never addicted. Never. My father wasn't addicted at
the time he married my mother—it was after. His addiction bothered her
for a while, but she got used to it. He didn't try to hide his habit from the
family, not as we got older. In fact, I used to go and get it for him.

I started to cop for my father in the 1930s. I copped for him mostly in
Harlem though; the Bronx was never noted for a drug place. Harlem was
the main place. I'd buy from guys in the street. They were Italian, all Italian—the ones I knew anyhow. These were just knock-around guys, you
know, guys that didn't want to work and figured that they'd get into it and
make money like that. They were selling to colored guys and everybody
else. I'd usually go to a couple of people that I knew very well. If I didn't
see them, I'd go to someone else—but everyone I went to, I knew.

The price of heroin in the thirties? I used to get a half-ounce—I
wouldn't say it was pure, but practically pure—for maybe fifteen dollars,
eighteen dollars. My father had another guy working for him who was
also an addict; they used to use it together. It would last the two of them
maybe a week and a half, a week. So it cost my father about nine dollars
a week. He was able to hold on to his job—he was noted as the best
wholesale grape dealer in the business. They all used to say, "Jesus, for a
junkie, your father's a hell of a man. He works, he's brought up a family."
We always had a car and stuff like that.

My father knew that I was taking a chance going to Harlem and buying
drugs. He didn't want me to do it, but I'd do it because I figured he'd get
arrested because he'd look like a junkie or something, while I wouldn't.
People would let me in their house where they wouldn't let him in. They
would trust me more than they would trust him because I wasn't addicted,
and they knew I was a nice fellow, and if anything happened I wouldn't
say anything. If they sold to my father, and the cops nabbed him, they
were afraid he would squeal: the cops would put him in the corner for an
hour and he'd probably tell them everything they wanted to know. But if
they were dealing with me, they knew there was no chance: I wasn't going
to be kicking cold turkey in prison somewhere and spilling my guts.

But I was never arrested. It was strictly a business deal. I'd give the
money to them and forget about it. That's all. I was never tempted to try
his heroin. I never even thought about it. I became involved with drugs
later, in 1955. I'll tell you the truth: I was working for some people, mixing

kilos. The people who got me involved were Mafia guys—I hung out with
a lot of people that knocked around and stuff like that. They knew about
my father's habit. They were telling me how much money you could make
—just cut it, get so much a week, and this and that—I figured it was easy.
So I done it. But I mixed without a mask on, which was very stupid. And
the fumes actually got into my system. It's easier to get addicted that way
than any way else.

The first time I knew I was addicted to it was when I was in Florida.
I got down to Florida with this friend of mine, and we got the chills, and
our bones hurt, so we went to see somebody. A doctor, a masseur didn't
do us no good. We met a friend of ours in the junk business. We told him,
"Gee, we've come from New York, and we feel this way and that." He
says, "Come with me." He went to the drawer and took out a package of
white stuff. We snorted it then and we felt fine. Then we knew we were
addicted.

My father was still alive at the time. Just before he died in 1960, he
knew that I was shooting up. But no, we never shot up together. Never.

6.

Hustling

The addicts' need to score constantly, whether from medical or street sources, translated into a constant need for cash. To get that cash, they had to hustle, usually by committing crimes like shoplifting or burglary. Sensational headlines to the contrary, few addicts were involved in major heists, since that sort of crime required time for planning, and time was a luxury they did not have. Addicts preferred hustles that were less lucrative but more dependable, and that could be practiced on a daily basis.

The relation between addiction and hustling was at the heart of the critique of the antimaintenance regime. For liberal rationalists, indifferent or hostile toward the symbolic functions of narcotic laws, addicts were essentially victims. They were victims in a double sense: not only did their social circumstances (e.g., being born into a broken family in the ghetto) predispose them to addiction, but, once addicted, they were forced to commit all manner of crimes because the government had shortsightedly denied them access to cheap narcotics. The laws were unjust and counterproductive and should therefore be changed.

The conservative rejoinder to this argument was that addicts were criminals anyway, that they had repeatedly broken the law before becoming addicted, and that the real source of mischief lay in some combination of their moral, psychological, and class characteristics (i.e., bad, abnormal, and lower). Moreover high prices, while they might aggravate addicts' behavior, nevertheless served to keep narcotics out of the hands of ordinary citizens. Rather than regarding expensive, adulterated heroin as a liability, the Bureau of Narcotics routinely cited statistics of high price and adulteration to show that its enforcement efforts were working.[1]

In one sense, the narratives in this and the following two chapters prove the liberal critics' point. There can be no question that the sheer volume of crime reported by our subjects was related to their daily need for narcotics, even though narrators like Al or John freely admitted that they were hustlers before they

---

1. For example, the remarks by Bureau spokesman Malachi Harney in *Comments on Narcotic Drugs* (Washington, D.C.: Bureau of Narcotics, 1958), 56.

*became involved with drugs. This is not to say, however, that strict narcotic
laws were necessarily counterproductive in some ultimate, utilitarian accounting.
The unambiguous message they broadcast—narcotics are bad for you—doubtless
deterred many people from using them.[2] But no one knew how many had been
so deterred, or how to compare the social savings they represented with the more
tangible social costs of addicts' crime. This, in retrospect, was one of Anslinger's
principal problems: he was dealing in prevention, which is always abstract. His
opponents were dealing in unpleasant urban realities—stolen purses and rifled
mailboxes—which they could plausibly link to the policy of narcotic prohibition.*

AL AND EMILY

Al: I never did any work. I stole all the time. Between '20 and '30 I was
in a higher bracket—I was a safe-cracker. Today they have electronic
systems—too much for my brain. I have no education. I didn't crack safes
in homes, though. Funny thing about homes: I have a tendency toward
the family. I never wanted to hit them places. I never stole in a house in
my life. I stole in lofts where they manufactured jewelry. Rhinestones—
right after World War II, rhinestones were at a premium. They came from
Czechoslovakia.

In the twenties I was stealing with other fellows. In the thirties it was
the same way, but I went into a higher bracket: I went for different kinds
of jewelry, gold, silver. In lofts, all lofts. Neckties we stole. There used
to be a firm called Sulka Neckties, they used to sell for ten dollars a
necktie during the Depression days. We didn't have a hard time during
the Depression; we always had a little.

I was doing the same thing during the forties, stealing all the time. In
the fifties I was down in the garment center; I had a poolroom and I was
booking down there. I was doing very good booking—booking numbers
for myself. You run into an element of people—do you know what I
mean?—you know one another. I used to go to the Garden. We went to
college basketball games three times a week. We used to go to the fights
every Friday night. Now, you meet all different kinds of people there, you

2. Although, paradoxically, it attracted others. "I know from my own experience that
when I was at West Point," recalled Ulysses Grant, "the fact that tobacco, in every form,
was prohibited, and the mere possession of the weed severely punished, made the majority
of the cadets, myself included, try to acquire the habit of using it" (*Personal Memoirs*, 1
[New York: Charles L. Webster, 1885], 65). Several commentators have made the same
point about narcotics, that illegality has added to their mystique. The difficulty, which still
plagues prevention efforts, is in computing what might be described as "net deterrence": the
number of persons repulsed by punitive laws and negative propaganda minus the number
whose curiosity is thus aroused.

get to know people, and you make customers out of them. They bet you on whatever you're doing—baseball, sports, horses, anything.

In the sixties I was still booking, and we had dress shops. We had three at one time, two on Southern Boulevard and one on 149th Street. We went into the business because my friends around the garment center knew everybody there. There was a guy who was the president of the Cutwork Association. They deliver dresses from one house to another place where they sew them and then bring them back—they call that "cutwork." We were talking, so this guy says, "Why don't you open up a couple of dress shops? Open one dress shop there, and I'll give your wife places to go to pick up wholesale, less than wholesale." So he took my wife to all these manufacturers down in the garment center, and my wife used to buy the dresses from all the wholesale houses. They would send the packages of dresses to a friend of mine's place, and I would pick them up for the store. But we gave that up when we were spending more money on junk than we were taking in.

Oh, yeah, I ran card games too. I guess I forgot to tell you, that was my main source of income. I ran card games for over twenty years in the Bronx, since the war till about '68, '69, when I stopped. My income— I'm ashamed to tell what I made a week from these card games. I used to make two, three thousand a week for small card games: seventy-five cents, a dollar and a half. We had games going day and night—we had a game going for a year without a stop.

Emily always loved to gamble, even to this very day. She used to take care of my card games for me. Many a time she'd give a woman or a man there—it was a mixed game, men and women we had—she'd give them twenty dollars for a seat. There was no seat in the house, maybe we had two tables going. It was five-card poker in them days, see, and you got seven players. She'd give twenty dollars so they could go home, and she'd take the seat to play.

I gambled because I had to sometimes. If the game got short, I'd sit down and hold the game, keep playing until a few more hands came in. The game would get stronger and I'd go away. I'd prefer to be the house; I'd rather not gamble. I didn't like to gamble, but sometimes you can't help yourself. Although with her, it was different: she loved to play cards.

When she lost money it didn't mean anything to me. Even in the beginning, when I first met her, I was a dealer on the Lower East Side. The little while I worked as a dealer, during the thirties and the early forties, I used to earn, say, for one night's work, fifty, sixty dollars. You know, that was good money in them days. I was able to support my habit and my wife's habit, but up till then the only habit we had was the opium habit. It wasn't too bad. But later on, when we had a heroin habit, I couldn't take care of my business. Because, somehow or other, I was always looking for stuff—stuff was always hard to get, and there were some people I wouldn't buy it from. There was stuff to get, and the prices kept going up high, and there were always panics, and, whatever money I had, I couldn't keep up with it. We lost our businesses, and I lost the card games—not that I lost it, I just couldn't take care of it, do you know what I mean? The dress shops we blew, we lost that, we couldn't take care of that because of the heroin. And it wasn't much of a habit; we were very conservative, because we skin popped. We weren't the type that was very hungry. We'd take stuff just to feel all right, yeah, to feel normal. We'd use between us maybe forty, fifty dollars a day, tops. I hear stories of people using eighty, a hundred, two hundred dollars—I don't know how. I can't understand it.

Emily: Never in my life was I arrested. Never in my life was I in jail, outside of visiting him. He was arrested for booking; Dewey sent him away. He was arrested about five, six times. The first sentence was from seven and a half to fifteen; he did exactly four years in Sing Sing. That was in the thirties. When he was in Sing Sing, I worked as a checkroom girl. I could have gotten into any place, because I formed the union, I organized the Village. The first thing was all the tough guys owned these nightclubs. The Nineteenth Hole, I organized. Then Ernie's, I organized. Then the Village Inn, I organized. I used to be an organizer with Lepke's sister-in-law. She was a tall Irish woman. Through people like Lepke and Gurrah I got jobs as a hat checker, and then I organized the union. I used to be in the union, until I got jobs myself. When the union was formed I got myself a job in the Village Inn, uptown, it was on Fifty-some-odd street. Then I went downtown, because there were more people that I knew who went there to nightclubs. I followed my people wherever they went. I mean, people that I knew I could get fifty dollars from in the checkroom when Al was away. See, Al was very much liked by them. So they used to say to me, "Where you working, Emily?" I'd say, "I'm working at . . ." They'd say, "Oh, come on down, I'll be at this-and-this on that day and I'll get you to Tony Bender and Tony Bender will get you into the Nineteenth Hole." Tony had the first place in the Village. He was married to a Jewish woman. And then Johnny Roberts was partners with Tony Bender; he had the Village Inn. I got in there.[3]

3. Joseph Valachi on Johnny Roberts: "He was partners with Tony Bender in different clubs, Hollywood Restaurant, the Village Inn. Whatever Johnny used to do—Tony was partners with him." Later Roberts (born Robilotto) shifted his allegiance to Albert Anastasia and became a high-ranking member of the Carlo Gambino family. Following Anastasia's murder in 1957, Roberts agreed to make a comeback (revenge killing) against those responsible for Anastasia's death, but then backed out of the deal. This was not appreciated. Robert's body was found in Brooklyn, September 7, 1958, "the cause of death being multiple gunshot wounds of the head and face" (U.S. Senate, *Organized Crime and Illicit Traffic*

When Al got out of jail and started running games, I stopped working. I started running games on the phone. They used to call at all hours. We'd be sleeping and they'd call—who needs money, who can get money, you know. Al was put away by one judge. We came in front of him about a million times; he *had* to send him away. He got nine months, nine months concurrently in Riker's Island, the toughest place he did a bit.

Al: I was very sick when I was arrested, but I was lucky: each time the wife got me out on bail. I was able to cure myself, to get off the habit. I didn't have to kick cold turkey in jail. I kicked it in the street. I went to doctors —Dr. Grossman, I went to a number of times. He would get me off the stuff. He had his own way of prescribing some kind of medication. He'd give you pills every day. You had to go every day to his office. No, these weren't dollies. Funny thing about dollies though: I think I was one of the first guys to get Dolophine. I had a cousin who was a medic in Germany. He gave me a handful of dollies when he came back, right after the war, '45. I never knew what they were. He said, "Here, Al, take 'em. See what they are." I had them in my house for about a year. I don't know what happened to them. I know I didn't take them. I must have thrown them away.

We've been in the methadone program about eight, ten years. Before I entered the program I had to go back to stealing. To make ends meet I had to do something, though I hated to, because my kids were big, and we were away from the kids, we just drifted away. It got so bad for me— I'd never done this in my life—I used to go to these stores to steal meat. We'd steal meat, me and the wife, and sell it so we could buy junk. That's how bad I was toward the end. It's got to get you that way—I mean, you can't make enough money. If you had a million dollars you'd go through it. All the money in the world can't keep you in junk.

Once I got into the methadone program, I stopped everything. I was living again; I got back to my old self. My family, my children were different. My daughter got us an apartment in a lovely neighborhood. My son acted different. Everybody was different. Methadone saved the whole situation.

J O H N

I was arrested for stealing during my last year in high school. I was about eighteen or nineteen, maybe twenty. I started off stealing generally in Harlem, stealing from delivery trucks, delivery men, stealing various

in Narcotics: Hearings before the Permanent Subcommittee on Investigations of the Committee on Government Operations, Part 1 [Washington, D.C.: G.P.O., 1963], 348–50, 361).

things that came into the area, and selling to the people in the area. I went away for about a year to New York City Reformatory. That's in Goshen, New York.

I finished high school in the reformatory, and I got the idea to go to college when I came out. I went to school in West Virginia, an all-black institute. I went at the insistence of my mother. She wanted me to have a better education, better things, a better life than she had. She figured schooling was a way to get it. But I didn't graduate. I just went a year and a half. I suppose I had too much money; I had no interest in college. Too much money, too many girls. I was rather spoiled. My people worked very hard to give me certain things, and I think they gave me a little too much.

After I dropped out of school I didn't do anything. I came back to New York. I stayed with my mother. I had a friend, and every day he used to come around and whistle under my window—every morning we got together and went stealing like a person would go to work. I tried to work a little while; I gave it a try anyway. But I'd had too much money from the stealing.

I've always considered myself to be a pretty good hustler. By a "hustler" I mean being able to get a hold of money without working for it. Counting the times I didn't go to jail, I was a pretty good thief. I stole quite a bit of money during my time, and I've had occasion to be liked by different women, and they gave me a few dollars here and there.

I wasn't a mugger or a stick-up man: I'd steal out of railroad terminals, or from the American Railway Express, things like that. It has been figured that, over a period of years, I stole approximately—this is an estimate—seven million dollars. This was figured out by one of the psychologists in Lexington, Kentucky. From the period I started stealing until we talked, she figured I stole about seven million dollars worth of merchandise and money.

I wouldn't steal from stores per se; I'd steal from the warehouses, the railheads. I'd sell it to a fence. I'd get somebody near downtown, in the Thirties or Forties, to buy the entire lot of whatever I had. I'd get somebody either black or white. It didn't make any difference to me: their money was the same color. These were merchants, or people that were like me. He's a thief, but he doesn't go out to steal: he buys from me and sells it at a profit. I let him make a profit off whatever I steal. I was like a wholesaler in business. I think that I provided somewhat of a service to people, in that the stuff that I stole I sold much cheaper than they could get it in the stores.

I was known to quite a number of people. They'd buy whatever I had to sell because I usually would have something nice that they could see and make a profit: clothing, furs, whiskey, cigarettes, anything. I'd steal it today and sell it today. Put it on a truck and sell it—I had my own truck. The warehouses were aware I was doing this, but the point is catching you. And I got caught often enough. I can't even begin to count the number of times I've been arrested. Certainly over ten—about thirty. I didn't realize it at the time, but I think it probably saved my life, being arrested. Because all of the people I knew during that time, the guys that I came along with, most of them are dead.

Mostly I would steal during a period of lull, like when the sun is sinking and there's a change in crew: the day crew is going home and the night crew is coming on. I could walk on any property and they'd accept me as one of the people that worked there. And if I'm moving some merchandise, they would think that I'm working late. On my truck was usually painted some fictitious transport company's name.

I was able to get a legitimate job when I came out of Lexington, and I suppose I got what I was qualified for: I worked in the garment center as a clothing cutter for a while. Financially, I thought it was beneath me. My pay was menial, ninety-some dollars a week. I was able to make much more than that on my street hustle—very much more. I could make, say, two thousand dollars a week, within that range.

There was no price on my habit. All of the money went for that, all except for the essentials of living and keeping my appearance up. I had a car. I was a sharp dresser. The addicts of yesteryear, they had more class. They were more caring. I was an addict, but I wore a suit and a tie every day. I wouldn't come out of the house without a suit and a tie and my shoes shined. I knew some really dirty addicts, but I didn't associate with them. The people I knew, they . . . like I met Billie Holiday. I met her uptown, in an uptown house. I didn't shoot up with her. I've smoked reefers with her, though. During this period that I'm talking about she was younger and then, after she came out of jail, I met her again, when she was on her way down. That's a waste.

I had quite a bit of money, but thieves don't save anything. I've had quite a bit of money go through my hands, and I've never saved a dime in my life. When I was in Kentucky, and the psychologist figured that I'd stolen seven million dollars, I didn't have a quarter to my name.

I'm in a methadone program now, and I have a job. They don't know that I'm on methadone at work. Personally, I can't say that I feel any discrimination because I'm a methadone patient. But I don't tell anybody, [laughs] and I certainly don't put any signs on my back saying, "I am a methadone patient."

I'll tell you something else. There's an entirely new type of person on the methadone program today; as people they're just not my cup of tea. I can very well understand the squares saying that they don't want methadone in their communities. A certain portion of these people will always hang out by wherever the methadone program is. The things they do are disgusting—to *me*—and *I'm* an addict, or a former addict, or a methadone patient, or whatever.

In the beginning there was definitely a different class of patients taken in. Before, people were more mature. Now you have more kids. You have a younger group and they seem to think it's some sort of badge of honor to be on the methadone. A number of them have never used drugs: they became hooked using methadone on the street, where they had to buy it. Eventually they were hooked, they needed the methadone, and they just couldn't get the ten or fifteen bucks needed to sustain their habit, so they joined the methadone program.

M E L

Mel was in prison for most of the years between 1942 and 1969, when he finally entered a methadone program. "You commit the crime, you do the time," he said philosophically. But before serving a long series of sentences, he prospered briefly as an itinerant hustler during the early 1940s.

We traveled outside of New York City during the panic. In a lot of parts of the country they never had a flow of addicts, so they would just imagine that you were a sick person and deal with you in such a manner. A lot of doctors were ignorant really. We used to play small towns, and they would just practically give it to you because they'd think they were helping you.

Most of the time we stayed on the road, traveling from town to town along the East Coast, all up into Erie, Pennsylvania—Coatesville, Pottstown, Chester, mostly places like that, up in the coal mining area. At that time we had girls, and we would take them to these towns, and they would do a little hustling and different things, especially around the mining areas. I didn't call myself a pimp, no. But it's all right to use the phrase.

I wasn't dealing during this time—just hustling ordinarily. Playing little con games, short changing, and whatnot. For instance, I'd take a ten-dollar bill and run it up to maybe twenty dollars. Like I'll go into a store, and I'll take and order an item, and I'll hand him my ten-dollar bill. And, maybe before he gets ready to make the change, I'll hold it and I'll order something else. It's a game of confusion. Then, in the countdown, I'll take and hide my ten and give him a fast count. He'll give me twenty for the ten he done gave me, see. During the confusion he'll forget about the ten he already gave me. I'll take his ten, you understand, and count it —boom!—take the rest of the change—boom!—count it back and make him give me my twenty out of the cash register—I see that he's got twenty there.[4]

---

4. If this sounds confusing, it is meant to be. Confusion is what the con man depends on in this situation. The key is getting (or taking) a ten-dollar bill from the cashier and

I dealt a little three-card monte too. That, and we played hicks—instead of using cards, we used shells. It's all done practically the same way, in a sense.

I was traveling with a regular group of people. We had what we called "the mob." Maybe I'd meet you in this town. Maybe I'd switch up. Maybe you'd played Virginia already, right? So I'll tell you about Philadelphia. So you'll take my team and go to Philly, and I'll take part of your team and go to Virginia. These people were all addicts.

It was a well-paying outfit. Barnum said, "There's one born every day." I made thirty-five to fifty grand a year, I wouldn't be afraid to say. Tax free. How much went to pay for the morphine and other drugs? Who knows. You don't count it, you know. I had a lot left over after paying for drugs, but you're doing other things: you're going to nightclubs, your clothes, your automobile, and whatnot. Yeah, I was living pretty high.

The thing that we appreciated was that we weren't hurting nobody physically. If we didn't get in with our brains, we didn't want it. We used our wits. We didn't believe in mugging or none of that.

Being a con man was a better hustle than being a dealer. You were more respected, even by the police. More so than a dealer because, under them circumstances, you had to become a very mean guy to say no to a person who's ill. It's a pretty hard thing to know a person's sick and then you turn your back on him because you need the money. If he don't have the money, it's no tickee, no laundry. Con men hurt people too, because maybe you're taking someone's life savings. He might not be able to recuperate no more in life. But, as a rule, they generally don't take it all.

Most con men were not drug users. Some few did, but those were the exceptions to the rule. The majority of them were very heavy gamblers. That, and sex. They had the psychological feeling that they were superior to the average hustler. They had a grand attachment to themselves, a vainness. They'd glory in getting together and talking, how they fooled this one and how they fooled that one. They'd talk about the different little tricks that they had to use in order to make the victim lose the money, about how hard it was, and how they had to mellow him down.

Maybe you know this, but con men made more money annually than bank robbers, stick-up men, and burglars. The money's so consistent, see. His money comes every day, where a bank robber, he might have one score this year and no more until next year. But I might take a grand here today, and tomorrow get up and take five thousand. There are more suckers than there are banks.

---

then counting it back to him with some other bills to get a twenty. For a more detailed description of how this hustle, called "the hype" or "laying the note," works, see David W. Maurer, *The American Confidence Man* (Springfield, Ill.: Charles C. Thomas, 1974), 240–41.

ARTHUR

Sometimes the line between a legitimate job and a hustle is very thin. Arthur managed, with the connivance of his employers, to integrate the two so closely as to make them indistinguishable. He became, in effect, a fast-change artist for the A&P.

During the thirties, before the panic, I guess I spent about fifteen, twenty dollars a week on heroin. I was earning twelve to fifteen—the highest I ever earned before I went to the chains was twenty-five dollars. No, my entire salary didn't go on drugs: I had to pay rent too. Where did I get the extra money? I'd steal it from the customers in the grocery store.

I am basically an honest guy, see. I've handled money for corporations all over, even today. I steal from the customers; I never steal from my employers. I'll steal from the customer in a minute—in fact, in some cases with the cooperation of my boss. When I was working on the East Side, my boss would say, "Arthur, you take care of checking. They watch me too much." And the customer would say, "I don't want that Jew to wait on me—he's going to steal my money. You're just like me. You won't steal my money." She'd be better off if he waited on her, because I'm going to screw her out of three or four dollars. I'm pretty good on figures—there were no calculators in those days, there were no adding machines. She would be illiterate: she'd sign the check with a cross. I'd take a big bag, and I would give the kids a nickel box of animal crackers, and I'd take a can of peaches off the shelf, which cost twenty-nine cents at the time, and say, "Here, take this—the boss isn't looking." I'd run it up. I'd write big. I'd make about three columns of figures. I'd make a fifty-cent mistake here, another fifty-cent mistake here, a dollar mistake here. Then I'd take the three totals and make a dollar-, dollar-and-a-half mistake on that. She thought she was getting a little extra, but meanwhile I'm screwing her. Now this money I'd split down with the boss—I couldn't make it without his merchandise.

These were poor people, but they never went hungry. I wouldn't screw them out so they'd go hungry. And they were getting at that time food vouchers. I don't know if you remember that—you had to write on the back everything that they bought.

I never stole from my employer. Without my employer I wouldn't have a job. I had to make sure he makes money so I'd have my job. The same thing with the A&P. If you don't make the money at the A&P, they move you, they move the managers out in a minute. I was selected to be put in stores that were losing money. You see, every five weeks a car would pull up and three guys would jump out. One of them would go right to the register and the other would walk down the aisle, calling out, "Fifteen boxes of corn flakes, twelve boxes of . . ."—they'd take inventory. You don't know when they're coming. If you come out understocked twice in a row, you get a big letter, you have to go to the office which was 149th Street in the Bronx someplace—I've never been there, because I was never understocked. And they ask you, "Why are you understocked?" Then they'd call me and say, "Arthur, I have store No. 204 or No. 207, they're three thousand dollars under. How long will it take you to pull it out for us?" Now, he knows I have to steal to put the store back on the street again. But I've done that for many stores for the A&P. I'd say first, "Where is the store located?" so I'd know what kind of people I'd have to deal with. Whether they're intelligent people, whether they're middle-class people. And, on the basis of that, I'd tell him one period or two periods—a period was five weeks.

So I was able to cut corners to make more money, to pay my rent and everything else. I also used to give my main clerk five dollars extra a week. I'd put down his salary and I'd say, "Here's a little extra." I used to give a little extra, three dollars, to the part-timer. And to the kids who used to come in on Saturday to deliver an order, I used to give all the cakes that was left, and the pies—I'd say, "Whatever you want." I did all right for the A&P. I knew how to run the store to make it look good for the company. You have to make money for the company. If you don't make money for the company, they don't want you. Listen, everybody's in the business to make a buck, right?

Now this wasn't my only hustle. I also sold drugs. When I started, in the late forties, I dealt solely with people in the entertainment field: musicians primarily, singers, dancers. I hurried up and dropped it like a hot potato when a very close friend of mine, Billie Holiday, told me that the FBI had come to her, and to other performers, and told them that they knew of their drug affiliations, and that they were going to ruin her career, and bust the people that were supplying them, and this and that. The prime interest of the people in the entertainment field was their career; they didn't want to mess up their career, see. And this lady was kind enough to come and tell me this,[5] and that caused me to cut loose from my visits backstage to supply musicians, dancers.

I knew Billie when she started out singing in the Hot-Cha Club, 134th Street on Seventh Avenue. That was back in the thirties. She wasn't even using stuff then either. We was all smoking pot. We used to smoke, then

5. Billie Holiday was arrested on a narcotics charge in Philadelphia on May 16, 1947, and tried on May 27, 1947. She received a sentence of one year and one day, of which she actually served nine and one-half months. It is not clear whether she warned Arthur before her arrest, or while she was awaiting trial and singing at Club 18 in New York City (John Chilton, *Billie's Blues: Billie Holiday's Story, 1933–1959* [Briarcliff Manor, N.Y.: Stein and Day, 1975], 112–18).

put the pot behind the sun visor in the car, and sit. The car didn't even have a radio in it. She had a little Victrola and she used to play records in the car. We used to go down to the Village. We used to go way upstate to the White Castle. Not the White Castle hamburger stand; there was a nightclub way up in Westchester County we used to call the White Castle. We used to go up there practically every Sunday morning for breakfast when she finished work at four o'clock in the morning. Her, and another girl by the name of Audrey Thompson who used to work at the Silver Dollar, another nightclub, 146th Street on St. Nicholas Avenue, and my friends Scotty and Freddy. Billie and her mother used to live at 127th Street between Fifth and Lenox Avenues, in a private house, one of those brownstone houses. We used to come home Sunday morning, about seven, eight o'clock. She used to take off her shoes and walk out of the car bare-footed. We used to . . . ah, I think of things I used to do, boy, when I was young and I look at myself and I can't see myself doing those things. When I was younger, you know, then it just was a natural thing to do.

Like I said, she was the cause of me starting to do business with professionals, with entertainers. I sold to Gene Krupa and to this singer . . . I would rather not mention these people's names. They're still around, still making a living. A lot of them were very prominent. I would say this, though, off of the top of my head: 70 percent of people in the entertainment field are involved in drugs. I would say 90 percent of the recording industry is involved in drugs. I would say that 90 percent of the people in the recording business, they pay the artists, the singers, with drugs and money. This I know for a fact because I have been to recording places and saw drugs and money being passed to associates of mine.

When I cut out dealing with entertainers altogether, I started doing business with streetwalkers, prostitutes. I very seldom did business with men. Always with broads. And they're all prostitutes, because the kind of money to keep a habit you can't get a job and earn.

I had eight girls who I used to supply. They were primarily black. There was a white—Mary, she was white. I would say fifty-fifty Puerto Ricans and blacks and a couple of white girls. I was very, very, very particular about whom I sold drugs to. I picked these eight girls because they were the ones I knew who could make that kind of money. I used to sell ten- and twenty-dollar bags only. You had to buy at least fifty dollars worth of drugs; otherwise I didn't want to talk to you. I made enemies of girls who'd want to buy five- or ten-dollar bags—I don't want to do no business with them. But if you bought drugs Monday, Tuesday, Wednesday, Thursday, Friday, and Saturday, I'd give you Sunday free. I don't work Sunday, see.

I bought my drugs from a lot of guys. In Harlem I bought only from

Interesting

black guys or black women. But after 1950 I switched over to the Italians in East Harlem because I got better quality stuff, and the prices were better.

In the forties an ounce would cost a hundred and thirty dollars. In the fifties the same ounce would cost you five hundred dollars: the price quadrupled. An ounce, that's sixteen spoons. Scale weight, you get twenty-one spoons. That's the difference, see. If you buy it from the niggers uptown, they're going to give you sixteen level spoons. But if you go over to the guineas on First Avenue, you get twenty-one level spoons an ounce.

The Italians actually said to me, "Do you want it pure? Do you want one cut or do you want two cuts?" Whatever you wanted. If you wanted pure, it cost you a certain amount. If you wanted one cut on it, it cost you another. Two cuts, three, whatever. And they wouldn't screw you around. They would give you legit what you wanted. If you wanted three cuts, that's what you got. If you wanted pure, that's what you got. I used to get one cut and then take it home and cut it right down the middle, make it two. So every time I bought an ounce I had two ounces. That made me have the best stuff on the street.

And it cost me. The New York Police Department charged me two thousand dollars a month in order to operate between 110th Street and 125th Street, from Fifth Avenue to Manhattan Avenue. That was my territory. I couldn't get busted in there.

NYPD was in

I was on the pad. At that time there was such a thing in existence, they called it "on the pad." Two thousand dollars a month. How do you do it? You could do it. You go outside and you pick a uniformed police officer and say, "I want to see the captain. I want to talk to the captain." That's all. The captain comes to you, in my particular case, I told him, "Captain, I have a few girls who are prostitutes. They all use drugs. I wouldn't want to see them get busted. They stay here with me." When I told him what I wanted to do . . . there was a cafeteria on 116th Street, Solar Cafeteria. The first Sunday in every month, I had to go in that cafeteria. I'd go in and have breakfast, see. At one o'clock on the button the prowl car would pull up. He would go to the counter, get a cup of coffee, and come and sit at my table—I would pick an isolated table. I had my two thousand dollars in my lap and I'm reading the paper. He's sitting there with his cup of coffee opposite me, and I just slipped it under the table, put it on his lap. He never looked at me. He finished his cup of coffee and walked out. There was never no conversation between us.

Then they started shaking me down, even though I'm paying two thousand dollars a month. Once a week, or once every other week, a couple of cops would come and knock on the door. "Who is it?" I'd say. They would mention my name, "Arthur." I'd say to the girls, "Ah, shit, don't worry, everything's all right." So they come in: "Well, Arthur, how you doing? How's everything? Everything's all right?" "Yes," I say, "everything." But

I know what that means. Then I have to reach in my pocket and take fifty, seventy-five dollars and plunk it down. You never hand them nothing, see. You never hand a policeman nothing. You put it down. I said, "OK, girls, let's go next door." I walk out in the hallway and do something, and I come back and there's two officers and, naturally, the money's gone. I can't say nobody took it. I didn't see nobody take it, even though I put it there.

But they started doing that too often. I guess another guy would tell his friend, and he would come up and say, "Hey, Arthur, how you doing? How's things?" These were white cops. There was never a black cop involved in this particular operation.

I actually had two apartments on West 116th Street: one apartment where the girls stayed, and one apartment where I lived across the hall. They didn't work out of their apartment; they just came there to sleep. Every night at eleven o'clock I waked them up. They got their own johns. They were on their own; I had nothing to do with that. I was never a pimp. I hate the word "pimp." I'm a businessman. They buy drugs—I supply the drugs. I supply their clothes—they couldn't buy a pair of drawers. I buy them. I don't go in the store. I tell boosters, "I need some size-four shoes, and need some size-six . . ."—all I want to know is whatever size they wear. And the boosters come in, they bring me clothes—I had more clothes in the closet than you could shake a stick at. You never take nothing to the cleaners. When they wear it once or twice, you throw it out and get some more. The boosters, they bring it in. I give them a quarter-ounce of dope. That's all. To me, it costs nothing, the quarter-ounce. If it was more, I'd give them a half-ounce.

I'd supply their clothes. I'd give them one meal a day. When they'd come in in the morning they'd have breakfast. I *guaranteed* they never went to jail. I *guaranteed* they'd never get any venereal disease. I didn't charge them too much: a minimum of one hundred dollars a night, for the protection and the dope. Sometimes I got two hundred or I got three hundred. I had so much money one time I went to the Chemical Bank right here at 110th Street and I rented a safety deposit box. I used to keep it in there. All this time I continued to work in the store. I was working days and nights. I was Doctor Jekyll and Mr. Hyde. Days in the supermarket and nights on the street.

I did this for two or three years, until the police department told me to stop. One Thursday night a policeman came up to me. Not a captain, not a lieutenant, a policeman. "Look, Arthur," he said, "Stop. Close down tonight. Do not work Friday, Saturday, Sunday. In fact, don't do anything until we let you know." He walked out. He didn't ask for a dime. He just came and brought that information to me. So I finished Thursday night. Friday morning I got up, took my box of dope, left whatever clothes—didn't even say nothing to the girls—and I went up to the Bronx to my mother's house. I just changed my clothes and I went down to 15 Pine Street and signed up to go to Lexington, Kentucky.

I stayed there about five or six days, then I signed out. I was afraid to come back here to New York. When the cop came to tell me to stop selling dope and stop the girls working, which is what I was doing, I knew he's telling me what comes from headquarters. So I went up to Chicago and stayed there for about a month.

Prostitution (handwritten annotation)

7.

Hooking

Among female addicts the most common form of hustling was prostitution, or hooking. (The word "hooking"—not to be confused with "hooked," in the sense of addicted—derives from the large number of brothels once found in the Corlear's Hook section of New York; sailors called the prostitutes from that area "hookers."[1]*) Hooking was a logical choice for many female addicts because it was easy to get into, always in demand, and, above all, produced lots of cash—far more than most addicts could earn in a legitimate calling.*

The relationship between addiction and prostitution was not one-directional, however. Just as many male addicts hustled before they began using narcotics, many women were prostitutes before they were turned on. This was largely a matter of exposure. The hookers' world was full of drugs and drug users—their customers, their pimps, their prostitute friends. Not only were drugs freely available, they also helped to alleviate the prostitutes' various physical and emotional problems, such as pain or fatigue or guilt. Narcotics, in a sense, made it possible for women to go on prostituting themselves. And, once they were addicted, prostitution made it possible for them to go on using narcotics.

The involvement of prostitutes with drugs antedated the classic era: late nineteenth-century surveys of urban addicts consistently showed them to be among the heaviest users of opiates, as well as alcohol and cocaine. This is still the case. According to one study, anywhere from 40 to 85 percent of prostitutes avail themselves of drugs.[2] *Although cash payment remains the norm, there is also a class of prostitutes called "barterers," who exchange sexual services directly for drugs or other commodities.*[3] *This appears to be a recent development, as it was not mentioned by the older women we interviewed. (The only exception, and a partial one at that, was a former prostitute who swore that she had been blackmailed into*

Narcotics = enabler ?? (handwritten annotation)

---

1. Eric Partridge, *A Dictionary of the Underworld* (London: Routledge and Kegan Paul, 1961 reprint ed.), 342.

2. Ira J. Silverman, "Women, Crime, and Drugs," *Journal of Drug Issues* 12 (1982), 175.

3. Paul J. Goldstein, *Prostitution and Drugs* (Lexington, Mass.: Lexington Books, 1979), 45–51.

*having sex with a policeman in his patrol car.) These women often lived with
men who supported their habits, but this was more in the nature of a long-term
relationship than an exchange for a one-time sexual act.*

MAY

*Born in Lynchburg, Virginia, in 1920, May was the youngest of three children
in a poor black family. Her parents separated shortly after her birth, and her
mother died when May was only five years old. She stayed with her grandmother,
but then her grandmother died in 1933, leaving May and her sister alone in the
world.*

Me and my sister got together and decided that we would leave town. We
didn't have nobody there. We were the only children—my brother had
left home about three or four years earlier. He just upped one night and
left. He came north.

People in those days kept iceboxes on their back porches. So we went
up and raided their iceboxes. We put the food in a sack. We went down
into a couple of basements and got some dungarees and sneakers and
things the white kids' mothers had put on the line. We put them on and
walked to Monroe, Virginia—seven miles, I think it was—and caught us
a freight train. We rode to Washington, D.C.

On the way we met this man, a colored man. He showed us how to
keep out of the way of the brakeman, and showed us how to get up on
the trestles to catch the train, and everything. But by the time we got to
Washington all our food was gone. So we went into a store and asked this
man, we told him we were hungry. He gave us a loaf a bread. That loaf of
bread tasted like cake.

Then we walked, and we walked, and we walked, and we came to the
precinct. We asked the sergeant if we could have a place to stay. He said,
"You haven't done anything, we can't throw you in jail. I'll tell you what
you do: you and your sister go to the house right down the street. There's
an old black lady who lives there. You tell her that I told her to put you
kids up." So we did, and she put us up. But she was poor too; they didn't
have nothing. The Potomac River was right near their house, and they
used to go fishing every day. I never ate so much fish in all my life. We ate
fish for breakfast, for supper.

We stayed there for a while. Meantime, my sister got a job working for
this white lady that owned a restaurant. I used to go over there and she'd
throw me some food out the window in a brown paper bag. Until one day
the lady caught her and told me, "Don't come around no more."

My sister was taking care of this lady's little girl. She didn't like the job
because the little girl was very fresh—she called her names and every-

thing. This lady had a son; he was also working in the restaurant. One day he changed his clothes and left about thirty dollars in his pants pocket. So my sister took it. I was out in the lady's yard playing with her grandchildren. I heard somebody calling me. I looked up and it was my sister. She said, "Just don't say nothing to nobody. Just come on." I said, "Where you going?" She said, "Come on." She had her suitcase. We went down to the bus depot and got on the bus. First place we stopped, I got out with my sister and went into the bathroom and washed up—'cause I had been in the yard playing. So I washed up, and she gave me a clean dress to put on. Then we got back on the bus.

We rode to Hartford, Connecticut, 'cause we had an aunt in Connecticut. We got off the bus and asked people where my aunt lived. They told us. We went there and knocked on the door. She opened the door —she hadn't seen us in years—and she grabbed us and hugged us and everything.

Now, I'm thirteen years old. What she should have done was put me in school. But she didn't. She had a son of her own. He was two years younger than me. She told us that she didn't know if we could stay with her or not because she was on the welfare, and if the welfare found out that she had two more children, that she might get cut off. Years later I learned that she didn't have to have done that. She could have went down to the welfare and explained to them that her two nieces was up here and didn't have no mother or father, and they would have put us on welfare with her. But she didn't.

I didn't know that my sister was pregnant. She was going on fifteen. The father was in Virginia. She didn't tell me, but she started, you know, showing. My aunt got very angry and told us we'd have to leave. So my sister got her a little job and worked until she got too big. Meantime my aunt let me stay there cause I was so small—but she didn't want me there.

My sister had the baby. It was a girl. We thought things would be better then after she had the baby. But my aunt got very, very mean. She would go downstairs in the basement and take the fuse out of the box so we wouldn't have no lights. She wouldn't send me to school. She'd sit down and eat, her and her son, and wouldn't offer us anything. So I made friends with some kids, and I would stay with them, one night at this one's house and then at that one's house. That went on until I started getting into teenage. Just shifting for myself.

My sister stayed there until the baby got about a year. She met a lady, and the lady told her she was going to New York. My sister asked this lady if she could go along with her, and she told her how things were. And the lady took her, and the baby, to New York.

I stayed in Connecticut, just from house to house and like that. I met a man who worked in a bar. He kind of liked me, although he was about forty-some years old. He used to give me three or four dollars when he'd see me, and I'd save it up. I saved up my fare and left Connecticut and came to New York.

I came to the same house where my sister was. I come to find out that it wasn't a nice house—you know what I mean. This lady was having girls come in with men and everything. It was a house of prostitution, almost. I wasn't used to nothing like that. So I got me a little job in Brooklyn, along Benson Avenue. I stayed with this lady—I worked for her for about a year, taking care of her little girl and boy. It was a sleep-in job. I'd come home on Thursday and every other Saturday.

In the meantime I made some friends in New York. I also found where my brother lived, in Brooklyn. I met a fellow and I started seeing him. One thing led to another and we started living together. I was about sixteen. We lived together for about ten years. I had two children by him. For the first time things were pretty all right for me. He made a pretty good salary. He worked as a handyman at the Franconia Hotel.

But he drank quite a bit. And there were other things. We broke up— I think my daughter was a year old. And, oh yes, my first son was born retarded. So, when we broke up, I couldn't handle him. I couldn't take care of him. So I put him in Willowbrook. That's the state school on Staten Island.

Things started getting kind of bad again. I had my daughter with me. I met another fella, but he was no good at all. He used to fight me. Him and I broke up because he hit me and broke my nose.

I started living together with my sister again. When my husband and I broke up, I had a little apartment over atop of hers. By him leaving, I couldn't keep the apartment, 'cause it took so long for me to get on the welfare. So I moved in with her. My sister wasn't an addict then. She was something like a madam; she'd let the girls come in with their fellas and charge a dollar. And she was doing it too.

Now she had some friends that were prostitutes. After work at night these girls would come in and sit down and smoke reefer. One night I walked in the bathroom and I saw this girl sitting on the edge of the tub with this rubber band around her arm and the needle. It scared me to death because I'd never seen nothing like that before. She said, "Oh, this is something. Try this." I said no, I wouldn't try it. She said, "Well, take a little puff of this." So I took a little puff of the reefer. But that was as far as I'd go for quite a while.

Anyway, things looked bad for me. My sister would say, "You might as well go on ahead and do it because you can make yourself some money, and for your child." So I started to hustle. I was twenty-six.

One night I took a little cocaine. Instead of snorting it, I let the girl wrap my arm up and shoot it in. It was a terrific feeling. I'd never felt like that before in my life. The only thing though, with cocaine, the more you get that sensation, the more you want it. But you never get the same sensation more than once. You understand? So then all our money was going for cocaine.

This girl said, "You're not going to get so high off of this cocaine, but if you take some horse and put in there and mix it, you'll get a nice, long high." So we all wanted this nice, long high; we all went for it, about seven of us. We all let her shoot us up. That was the first time.

One night, about two months later, one girl had just come out of jail, and she was sitting there telling us about how she'd kicked her habit cold turkey, and the things she'd went through. It scared me *so bad*. I said, "I'll never use another needle," and I actually meant it. I went to bed. The next day my back seemed like somebody was pressing on it, just terrible pain in my back. I couldn't understand why. I just laid in bed all day. I didn't have my appetite, or nothing. That's when I was getting hooked and didn't realize it. So the same girl come in. She said, "All you need is a little bit of something," and she gave me a little fix. The pain went out of my back—snap!—just like that. From then on I started using it regularly.

Buying the heroin was the easiest thing in the world. I was living at 111th Street, between Fifth and Lenox. All you had to do was walk out the door on Fifth Avenue. The Spanish boys and the black boys had nothing but drugs. You'd buy from anybody that had good stuff. You would ask around, and then they would say, "So-and-so's got some good stuff." You'd say, "Who else?" They'd say, "Well, so-and-so, but so-and-so's stuff is better." And you'd go get the best.

When I started, bags were three dollars, and seven people could get high off of it—it was that strong. I used maybe two bags a day. I could survive off of one bag—half of it then and half of it the next time. But it was hard to get three dollars if you don't have three dollars. I was hustling for my money. I had been cut off the welfare because I had moved downstairs. The check came to the old apartment and the super sent it back. In those days they were very strict, you know. They said, "You don't live there no more."

We hustled on 111th Street, between Fifth and Lenox. My God, it was like a parade. The white guys would come every morning, every evening, and on Saturday and Sunday. They came from all over. There were about twenty to twenty-five girls working, and they'd just take their pick. There were about two or three houses in the block; the girls would take them into these houses. Me and my sister worked in her apartment, and she let some of the girls work in there also.

I don't know how much I made a week hustling. When you're an addict you can't tell about how much you make, because as fast as you get it you're spending it on drugs. My habit wasn't bad when we first started out. But it wasn't very long before I was up to four or five bags a day. An addict gets greedy, you know: the more stuff they get, the more they want. And then prices went up too, to about five dollars a bag. That happened in the sixties, and the heroin wasn't like it was in the fifties. The price was higher, and the stuff was worse.

I wasn't hustling *all* the time. It was off and on, off and on. In between I'd have a nice guy, and I wouldn't do it. They'd support my habit. They all knew I was addicted. I never once lived with a man that had a habit, that was addicted to the stuff. But they helped me, they gave me money. I'd try to control my habit when I was living with somebody, because I'd know they couldn't afford it.

I married my second husband about three years ago—we'd lived together for about eleven years. He's a good husband. I met him when I was on methadone. I went into my first methadone program around 1968. Methadone has been a godsend to me, believe me. I don't know what I'd have done without it. You know, before, when I was using drugs and couldn't get it and was sick, I'd say, "God, why don't they have something to help us?" 'Cause nobody really wants to be an addict. Nobody wants to be tormented. When this doctor told me that there was a methadone clinic—oh!—he gave me a new life. He actually did.

Whatever happened to my sister? You wouldn't believe it, but she's a Jehovah's Witness. Yep. She straightened out too and got to be a Jehovah's Witness. Her daughter got sick with leukemia. She straightened up because she had to be taking care of her daughter's three children.

I don't know how she just stopped. One time, years ago, she went down to Kentucky and tried to straighten up. She came back and got back on the drugs. She used them again for years. Then, when her daughter got sick, she just stopped smoking, stopped everything. I mean without going anyplace, without any doctor. And she was addicted to heroin worse than I was.

She's very religious now. Uh-huh. She don't even want me to mention what we did years ago. She doesn't know I'm on methadone. Because she's a Jehovah's Witness now, she doesn't want me to mention nothing like that. So I don't tell her anything.

SOPHIA

Sophia was born into a working-class Italian family in Newark, New Jersey, in 1915. Her mother bore thirteen children: only three survived. In school she went as far as the eighth grade, although she later earned a high school equivalency diploma while in prison.

When I was seventeen I came to New York by myself. I ran away from home for no apparent reason, no reason whatsoever, other than that I wanted to go on my own. I just wanted to spread my wings.

Believe it or not, the first man I ever met in New York was a pimp. This was at Cortlandt Street. In them days the train used to stop at Cortlandt Street; there was no Port Authority.[4] I guess this man had me spotted as a runaway. He approached me and asked me if I wanted something to eat. I can't exactly remember what line he pulled on me, but I went for it. I stayed with him for about a week and a half, and then he started to work on me about going out into the streets. And, first thing I knew, I was in a whorehouse.

I'll never forget it: it was on Delancey Street on the East Side, in an old Jewish neighborhood. The madam was an old Jewish woman with a big belly. She always had something in her hand: she was always eating. She used to sit on the stoop with some of the neighborhood johns. She had three girls, all of different ethnic backgrounds. We all had lounging robes and lounging pajamas and what have you. We were dressed. But the joint itself was atrocious. It was an apartment in a tenement house.

I was living with Gino, the pimp, at the same time I was working in the house on the Lower East Side. He was Italian like myself. That's probably the reason why I stayed with him, because I didn't know nobody. He was young, a very nice-looking man. He was very good to me. I stayed with him a few years. I used to give him my money, and he'd dress me real nice. I gave him the money because I liked him, you know. A lot of pimps beat their women and get the money out of them that way. This man never threatened me. He was very good to me, really. He kept me well-dressed. I didn't want for anything: he kept me well-fed and in a nice hotel. I worked in good houses and made good money. He gave me plenty of money to spend, to buy anything I wanted. A lot of pimps didn't do that.

Just one time I got beat up by him. I used to watch him go to the bathroom—I'll never forget, I was living in the Piccadilly Hotel—and I used to wonder, "What the hell is he going to that bathroom for?" He had a big brown bottle; it looked like a cocoa drink, you know, chocolaty. And every time he'd cough, he'd go in and take two spoonfuls. He always told me, "Sophie, don't ever go take any medicine out of that bottle, because that bottle is made up especially for me." So I never paid no attention. Then one day, I got a terrific cough, and I said, "Oh, he always drinks that medicine and it stops his cough." So I went in and I did the same thing he did. I took two spoonfuls of that medicine. And then what did I do but put water back in it.

There was opium in the bottle, pure opium, that was cooked down and mixed with a Chinese medicine called *wom-poo*. After I drank it—oh!—I felt so high. I felt good. I was in a different world.

---

4. Port Authority Bus Terminal, a notorious hunting ground for pimps looking to entice newly arrived runaways.

Every now and then, whenever I felt bad, I would go to the bottle. But he found out. His medicine was getting more watery. It wasn't taking care of him the way it usually did. I happened to be in the bathroom one day and he came in and caught me taking medicine out of that bottle. Well, that's all she wrote. I hit every wall in the place. To this day I never got a beating like that man beat me.

He used this medicine because he was an addict. He didn't tell *me* he was an addict; he told me he had a chest condition. He had a slight condition, but that isn't the reason why he used it. He used it because he was hooked on it. The way he started was popping *yen-poks*. The kids in his neighborhood would cook them up and pop them in their mouths. But he didn't want me to get hooked. He was protecting me. So the story he gave me was that he had a chest condition and that the medicine was made specially for him.

I was eighteen years old when this happened. I was just using this medicine now and then. I wasn't hooked. I got hooked later in a whorehouse, honey.

A lot of the girls were drug addicts. A lot of them used the needle— I never bothered with them. They were prostitutes when they started to use drugs. Always. Prostitutes used to take junk just to forget what they were doing. I felt guilty. I had a very guilty conscience—I never wanted my people to find out. The drugs helped: it made me forget.

I started smoking opium when I was eighteen, nineteen, around that age. It was during the Seabury investigation,[5] if you remember them days. I had already graduated from the Lower East Side to a high-class house on upper Fifth Avenue. I smoked opium every time I got a chance. I would always look for people that were smoking opium. I loved it, I loved it. From the first time I ever smoked the first pill I was hooked—not in a physical way, but I really wanted it. I wanted that high, that feeling, because it really made you forget.

Lots of times I used to smoke with the Chinese. I used to go to one of them places down there and smoke. Yeah, the Chinese men were suspicious of me, but this was a Chinese girl I smoked with. That was unusual: she was the only Chinese woman that I knew of who smoked. She was very closemouthed. A beautiful girl. She worked for the syndicate, just like I did.

The syndicate? When Luciano was in power, he had a syndicate. You used to have to call in and pay a percentage of your earnings to the madam for the bookie every week, or you couldn't work in the joint. Every

5. A probe of municipal corruption, led by the anti-Tammany Democrat Samuel Seabury. Begun in September 1930, it culminated with the resignation of Mayor Jimmy Walker on September 1, 1932.

weekend the collector would come to the madam's door and collect his fee, oh yes. And if she didn't pay up, honey, that joint was demolished. The girls were beat up and abused: I seen that happen one time. It was pretty bad.[6]

No, I don't think that Luciano made sure that his girls had plenty of heroin to keep them quiet. I don't think so, because if they knew you were an addict in some of them joints, they wouldn't have you. The minute the madam would find out you were an addict, she would call up the bookie and say, "Get this dope fiend out of my joint." Needle users, any kind of users. But the opium smokers stayed, because they never knew us, you understand. When you went to work in a whorehouse and you were a smoker, you used to take *yen-poks* to work with you, or a small bottle of medicine. The time that you were working, you'd sip on your medicine; you'd go to the crapper, take you a little swig, and that was it for the day, until you got through work, then you'd go home and smoke. And they never found out who the opium smokers were—unless the madam was an opium smoker herself and she knew. The opium smoker was more tolerated. Needle marks were bad news. No needle marks. Flo and a couple of other of these madams, they weren't needle users themselves, and they wouldn't tolerate a girl being a needle user.

I got married in 1939. I used to go to a lay-down joint—that's where I met my first husband. He was a con man, a lemon hustler. In them days they were big. They used to swindle people out of thousands, their life savings. They'd take them to the bank and let them draw everything out. He used to come in from out of town, from Des Moines, Iowa, into this little place on Fifty-second and Broadway, the old Alvin Hotel. It's still standing, by the way. There were lay-down joints all throughout the building. I used to love to go there. And, it seemed every time I happened to go to a different lay-down joint, he happened to be there. I went this particular night and I laid on his hip. He said, "My God, every joint I go to, it seems like you follow me or I follow you." It was coincidence, you know. He asked me, "Why don't you come up to my hotel. I got a joint of my own. You can smoke with me." And I said, "Well, what are you coming to these places for?" "Because I got nobody to smoke with," he said. So, every time I wanted somebody to smoke with I used to call him up, you know, and I used to go up and smoke with him regularly. Gino and I got to fighting, and I finally left him. I started to live with Abe—his

6. Today Luciano is remembered primarily for his involvement in narcotics, but in the 1920s and 1930s he also systematically extorted money from the madams, call girls, and common prostitutes of New York City. Luciano's operation is described in Alan Block, *East Side—West Side: Organizing [sic] Crime in New York, 1930–1950* (New Brunswick, N.J.: Transaction Books, 1983), 142–48.

name was Abe—and we finally got married in 1939. We bought a home out in South Jersey, and we smoked out there with the doors wide open, with impunity.

When I married him I quit hustling. Before that, I earned about eight hundred, nine hundred a week. But you had to work. You worked—you were constantly busy. When you come out of them joints, you were dead. That was knockdown money too. You know what I mean by "knockdown money"? Tips men would give you—you wouldn't turn them in. In the thirties you would earn, oh, in the better joints, twenty dollars a trick. Ten, twenty—some higher than that. They used to pay by check. But you never really got what they gave you, what they wrote the check out for. You got a little portion of it—the madam got all of it really. Writing a check wasn't so indiscreet in them days. Or hundred-dollar bills, thousand-dollar bills . . . there were some fabulous joints.

My husband used to go in and out of town. I told you what he did—he conned people. I didn't have to work until he got caught and had to go to jail. That was during the panic, about '40, '41, '42. I was by myself. I had to hustle. I was back on the street again, back in the same old business. I worked on the streets because I was older and there were no bookies around, no booking joints. You didn't have a man to call up and make arrangements.

I was still making pretty good money working on the streets. In them days the cheapest date was ten dollars. During the war it cost me about sixty, seventy dollars a day to support my habit. Prices were that bad. Doctors would charge you twenty-five a scrip. Don't forget, they'd only write for so many: they'd want you to come back. Sometimes what he'd write for would just be a shot or two. You'd go have a prescription filled and you'd shoot it all up at one sitting. But ten dollars a trick was enough to keep me going until the next day. Then you had to get out and make some more money. I always made enough to look after myself, but on a day-to-day basis—like everybody else. If they told you any different, they were lying, believe me. Ain't nobody saved any money in them days, because every nickel they made they spent on stuff.

When my husband got out of jail, around 1946, he got himself a job as a bellhop. He went back to using, oh yes. He started to smoke and then it got too damn expensive; he couldn't smoke opium on a hop's salary. So he started to pop. After awhile he began to push stuff out of the hotel too. Junkies used to check in—that hotel was at Thirty-second Street and Broadway. It's down now. He worked there for many a year as night bell captain. He made a lot of money in that hotel: he was dealing at the same time he held down the job. Then in the latter part of '48 he got popped for selling junk. He did a year up at Riker's. He got out of jail in 1950, two weeks before he died. He died of one heart attack—he was never sick a day in his life. He was older than me. He was forty-seven when he died. I was thirty-four. Anytime he was around me, I was off the street. He wouldn't tolerate that. The only time I went into the street was when he was busted. Whatever money I had I used up, and I had to resort to working to maintain myself.

After my husband died, I went back on the street—a little. Then I started shoplifting. I shifted from prostitution to shoplifting because I didn't want to hustle no more. I never did like it; it rubbed me the wrong way. It's a quick way to make a buck, you know. What the hell, you can close your eyes and pretend. That's all it is anyhow. Anyone that says different, they're hung up on sex.

I shoplifted all along Fifth Avenue—Lord and Taylor, Franklin Simon, Bergdorf Goodman—all them fancy places. I used to carry one of these long handbags, nobody ever suspected. Oh yes, I was caught. The first place I was ever arrested was in *Bloomingdale's*! I stole a coat—I went to jail for that.

In '51 I started to sell some of my junk. I used to make up five-dollar bags and sell them to girls on the street. This person I used to buy my stuff from, I started buying ounces from him. Nigger Jim—I'll never forget—he's dead now. He was white. And his wife, Ethel, she was white, too. He was Italian, but they called him "Nigger" because his complexion was very dark. Very, very olive, you know, real olive complected.

I did five years when they caught me. In 1952 I was arrested for possession. The law had just come out: seventeen-fifty-one, that new law.[7] They stuck it up my backside, if you know what I mean. I was in Bedford Hills. And I did every blessed day. Every day. No parole, no nothing.[8]

First I was placed in the Women's House of Detention. I didn't get any help to reduce my habit. I had to go cold turkey. The cells were little cubby holes; all you could see were roaches and mice. At night you'd see nothing but . . . if you had a BB gun, you could shoot about ten mice. There was a sink and toilet—that was it. I was vomiting in the cell. They gave you nothing. They gave you a little old rotten cup.

Bedford Hills was different, though. You had your own room. The only thing you didn't have was a private bathroom. You could open your window and look down on the road—girls had escaped out of there and everything. The food was all right. I used to work in the cafeteria, cleaning the tables, stacking the dirty dishes and stuff. I did that for five years. They didn't try to teach me a trade.

I didn't have any problems with brutality or anything like that. But I

---

7. Sec. 1751, amended April 4, 1951, stipulated a minimum five-year sentence for "any person who shall barter or exchange with or sell, give or offer to give to another any narcotic drug." Apparently the police had more on Sophia than mere possession (*Laws of New York*, 1951, p. 1293).

8. Bedford Hills Correctional Facility in Westchester County, New York.

wouldn't say I was a model prisoner. I got into trouble: I was in segregation for thirty days because somebody told the supervisor I was getting narcotics. I wasn't, but I had someone else get it for me. They put the finger on me.

I didn't get narcotics continuously. Every once in a while I'd want some stuff. I'd have somebody pick some up for me. There was a girl, a lesbian, she loved me very much. She'd do anything I said. Her mother used to bring it in to her, and she used to give it to me. The girl would send her mother to another girlfriend of mine; the girlfriend would fix her up a package with a needle, a hypodermic—you know, a gun—and stuff. She'd roll it up real small so she wouldn't be caught with it: they used to search you. Sometimes she would put it in a cocoa can—they'd never go in and mess around with your food—and she used to bring it in.

The lesbian was an addict too. So we both used to take off. In the summertime they used to have baseball games up there; different prisons had baseball teams. We used to laugh at them, high as a kite. But this was only once every five or six months. Shoot, I didn't want to have no habit in there, man. Who wants to have a habit in jail? How do I know I'm going to be able to get it every day? It's ridiculous. No, I didn't want no monkey on my back in jail.

But the first day I came out of jail I put a needle in my arm. I couldn't get into New York fast enough. And, believe me, there was a girl there waiting for me with a hypodermic full of narcotics, to give me my shot. That wouldn't happen if I was hooked and needed a shot. You understand what I'm trying to say? There wouldn't be no shot there for me. But, being I was clean and everything, they drove up with a shot. This girl was also a shoplifter and a dealer. "Come back and join the team." So I started to use stuff all over again.

I started hustling again. This went on for a couple of years, until I married this man in 1959. This man never used a drop of stuff in his life. I met him as a trick, a twenty-dollar john. I used to see him all the time, every weekend he'd come up. He was a parolee from doing twenty years. He paid his hookers anything they wanted. He was very good in gambling joints: he always knew how to shoot craps. He loved them dice games—and he was always a winner too.

After 1959 I started to steal meat in a grocery. I stole a lot of meat. I used to hit one store four or five times, and I used to get nothing but pot roasts and porterhouse steaks. I had a certain type of a bag I used to be able to get it in. I had somebody outside—my husband used to be outside, a block away. I used to give the meat to him to put it in the shopping bag; then I'd go back into the store again. We didn't sell it on the street; we'd sell it to private parties. We used to clear about sixty, seventy, eighty dollars a day, just on the meat.

At the end of the week we had enough money to cover all our expenses.

The heroin used to cost me thirty, forty dollars some days. I would also shoot up coke, about sixty, seventy dollars worth every two days. So let's say I had a sixty-, seventy-dollar-a-day habit. The coke I bought from Harlem; the heroin I bought from friends.

This went on for a little while until I got tired of it and started to go to the department stores again. This time I latched on to nothing but bags —these things, pocketbooks. You'd go in without a bag and come out with a bag. I made some money with them bags, brother. I used to steal a-hundred-and-fifty-dollar bags . . . Saks Fifth Avenue, that used to be my favorite. I got busted out of there too. I paid a hundred-dollar fine.

I sold these bags in the Times Square area. I had a fellow that would buy it, and he had somebody that he was selling to. I made quite a bit. I used to take off a third, and I used to get nothing but expensive bags, seventy-five dollars up. I would make over five hundred, a thousand some weeks. What would I do with all the money? I'd gamble. I always liked to gamble.

I had only three convictions for shoplifting: two in the sixties and once in 1937. I was arrested about twenty-eight times for prostitution. Sure, I spent time in jail for those raps. They let me go lots of times, but most always I did time, from thirty to sixty days. I did six months one time. Altogether, I spent about ten years of my life in jail.

LOTTY

The prostitutes' subculture, like that of the larger world, was stratified. The lumpenproles were the streetwalkers like May; above them were the women who labored in the brothels; and above them were the high-priced call girls. At the very top of the heap were the "kepties"—mistresses of extraordinary beauty or charm who were supported by wealthy men. But even for these fortunate few, the tendency was always to drift downward.

I had big eyes and high cheekbones, rosy cheeks and platinum blonde hair, and I always had a very small figure. I had *women* turn around in the street and say, "Isn't she gorgeous?" Things like that would spoil you. When I went anywhere it had to be first class, or I wouldn't go.

I had beautiful clothes; I had one man give me seven hundred a week. He took me to Texas, bought me a house and a car. He was a cotton and wheat man. He lost three hundred and fifty thousand a day in the crash. So he told me, "Why should I waste my money that way when I can have a beautiful gal?" He had a ranch and all kinds of money besides the wheat and cotton. So I was his companion. I stayed with him for two years. I first met him at a cocktail party in New York City. He was very scared because I was still a minor, under twenty-one. The man that I met him through really wanted to ruin him by getting him a little bad publicity—he was a married man, see.

He got me this little five-room house. It was his, but he deeded it over to me. Then he bought me a little car, becuse you needed a car to get around, you know. He gave me two charge accounts. He never could understand why I always had children's clothes on there. He said, "Have you got kids?" I said, "No, those are my brothers and sisters. I'm bringing them up." He said, "I didn't take on the whole damn family! I took you on. You're my girl, not them."

At the time I was with him I wasn't using—he didn't even know about it. But, anyway, after two years I started thinking about that beautiful opium and I wanted to get back to New York. Even after you overcame the physical withdrawal symptoms, there's still a craving. You miss it. That was the reason I gave up a man that had millions.

Once I went into the hospital for treatment. A man I knew wanted me to get off. I knew him twenty years. He gave me all sorts of jewelry —he was in gold melting. He'd come every time on a Saturday night, bringing me a pin or earrings or a bracelet, and a hundred-dollar bill. I'd just stay all night. Nothing happened. He was an old man. He just wanted company, you know. We'd go to theaters and dinner. There was nothing there.

He wanted me to go to the hospital; he paid five hundred a week. It was called the Towns. It was on Central Park West. I don't think it exists any more.[9] As soon as you started getting sick, they would give you a shot. Then, when you got down real low, they'd call it "going over the hill," and they'd give you sedatives, sedatives, sedatives. And you were okay. But I never went to any other hospitals. I never went to any place like Lexington, Kentucky, or down on Eighteenth Street and Second Avenue.[10] That was sort of a bum line. In other words, I was more high-class than those type of people.

I started using heroin around 1933. For fourteen dollars I got what they called "Green Dragon." It came in a box, all tissued up. Fourteen dollars. Today you'd pay a couple thousand for it, or more. The seller even slipped me the needle and everything. I was all set. I didn't particularly want to do it, because they've got a bad reputation, the people who use white stuff. So I was a little afraid. But I put the needle where I could

9. The Towns Hospital was operated by Charles B. Towns, a former insurance sales-man who claimed to have a sure cure for addiction. At first the medical world was im-pressed, but gradually evidence accumulated that Towns's formula was ineffective, and he was discredited.

10. The address of Manhattan General, later known as the Morris J. Bernstein Institute of Beth Israel Medical Center, which once provided free detoxification for addicts.

get a job. I always shot in my upper arm, or back here where I could hide it with my bikini. We wore bikinis when we kicked our heels—I was still working in a chorus line. I always sterilized my own works; that's why I never got marked up so.

It was pretty tough sending my mother money every week—and I had to send that first. I had a trunk full of receipts because, if I was late, I would wire it to her. Then, during this time, I was going with an Italian boy and I got pregnant. I had a little girl by him. She was born in 1937. I was late having her—I was twenty-seven. My being addicted to heroin made it bad for her. I cured her myself, or she'd be dead. I used paregoric. Paregoric is wonderful for babies. Most of these hospitals didn't know it, but they could have saved many a baby if they knew about paregoric. You just give it a wee drop more, a little teeny bit more than you would originally give another baby. I went home to have my baby. The first time I gave her paregoric she slept eighteen hours and my mother said, "She'll wake up, and she'll be hungry." Sure enough, the first thing she wanted was her milk.

This Italian man I had my baby by was wealthy. He didn't support my habit, but we'd go to the El Morocco every night for dinner, and he'd buy me big orchids and all kinds of clothes. He paid my rent—I was a mistress, you know. I never had any problem with money. And I was able to buy my heroin. I had one man, the same connection for nine years.

I brought my daughter up until she was eight. But I had a wonderful girl who took care of her, because at that time I had a man who had a yacht, and we used to leave on Friday night and we wouldn't come back until late Sunday night. We'd have a hell of a good time: we'd take beer and roast turkey, and we'd dock and catch fish and cook them.

I took my daughter away when she started pounding on the door while I was doing it, and I saw that she was getting too hip. I got a family and I paid them to take care of her. They begged me to let them adopt her, but I wouldn't do it, because I knew I'd never have any access to her. But she came up beautifully—they were a lovely family, owned their own home and everything.

Just before the war I married this guy who had a liquor and a heroin problem. To tell you the truth, I met him at a heroin party—like it was ten or twelve of us. They were selling capsules then for two dollars apiece, and three people could get fixed up with it. I would shoot up alone if I was sick, but I liked a big party, I liked to see something going on. Some of them drank and shot heroin, but I never drank with it, I never liked booze. I carried my own works, because you never can tell what you can pick up. I didn't let other people at the party use my works. I'd tell them, "Look, for all I know you might have leprosy." [Laughs.]

They were a different class of people from the opium smokers. They weren't rich, but they were thieves, most of them. My husband was a thief. I went on a party and that's how I met him. Right away he started making a play for me. He was six-foot-four and very beautiful, very handsome, with blond-gold hair. He ducked the army—he did all sorts of things to get out of going in the war. That's the reason he married me.

I didn't have to act as a mistress to other men, because my husband made enough money. When you're stealing jewelry, you're making a lot of money. He once stole a forty-thousand-dollar necklace. He couldn't sell it that way; he had the jeweler break it up, and he would sell two or three stones at a time. He was good to me; he gave me two emeralds, he'd give me stuff that he stole. But he'd tell me, "Don't wear it right away." He'd be afraid they'd find it, you know.

He was very good to me, but I used to lose a lot of sleep. He was drunk all the time, and he'd shoot heroin—he was addicted to heroin. And, not only that, he'd take any kind of pill he could get his hands on. I don't like pills, I guess because I saw my husband take so many of them. The condition he'd get in. He'd put his head down and nod, and you'd have to watch him every minute. Otherwise you could be burned to pieces or anything could happen.[11]

I stayed twenty years with him. Then he met a girl, a floosie. It was one of those things. He took her to San Francisco. And that was my chance to get rid of him, because I had been trying to get rid of him for a long time.

I met my second husband in 1956. He said he'd had his eye on me for years. I met him in a doctor's office—this doctor's office sold Dilaudid, which is pure heroin, in the pure form.[12] All you do is mix it up and cook it up in water. It was during a panic: we couldn't get the heroin any more; it wasn't any good. You'd have to take a teaspoonful to even feel it.

My second husband was a Dilaudid addict. He could make any doctor in the city—both of my husbands could. The doctor who gave us the Dilaudid, we used to have to wake her up to get her to write, she was so full of it herself. She was in Germany during the war. She had two little girls, and one of them went crazy from the bombs, and sleeping out in the cold in the forest, and all that. She had to put her in institutions. When she came to this country she had practically nothing. She didn't know

11. Because of the cigarette dangling from the nodding user's mouth. One of the symptoms of narcotic addiction that experienced physicians look for is a rosette of cigarette burns on the patient's chest.

12. This is a fairly common misconception. Dilaudid is the trademark for preparations of dihydromorphinone; heroin (from the German *heroisch,* large or powerful) was the name given to diacetylmorphine, another and earlier semisynthetic derivative of morphine. Both drugs, however, are powerful analgesics and both are highly addictive.

what to do. One day a girl came in, and she wanted Dilaudid. So she gave it to her.

She was very reasonable. She only charged us twenty-five dollars. That was for each of us; she didn't even know we knew each other. And the drugstore charged us about twenty-five for filling the scrip. I went to her for about ten years. She's dead now, with hepatitis.

My second husband owned a pornography store. He sold film. He had a room, a suite in the Dixie—his store was right across the street. He'd take them upstairs and show them the film; if they liked it, they bought it. He made a mint of money—he had forty thousand dollars when I met him. I never had to go out and steal. The men in my life were very good to me, and my second husband was marvelous. Whether things were good or bad, he'd always put a hundred-dollar bill on the dresser. All I had to do was look at something and he'd say, "Do you want that?" I'd say, "Well, it's all right," and he'd walk right in and buy it. One night I said something about Paris, and the next day he comes by with the tickets on the SS *France*.

My second husband died eight years ago. He liked coke, in fact that's what killed him. The coroner took only one look at him and he said, "My God! His heart is so enlarged, he's choked to death!" Choked to death on his own heart. I had only one second to dial 911. I took him in my arms and said, "They'll be here right away." He just smiled, and that was it.

Before he died that night, he came in and he gave me a bank book. He said, "Tear this up." I said, "Why? What are you tearing it up for? You want me to put it in our joint account?" He says, "No, just throw it away. Tear it up and throw it away." It had eight hundred and fifty dollars in it —otherwise the cops would have gotten it. Now, I didn't know cops were such thieves. So when they start going through his pockets, what do they find but the store's money, four hundred and eighty-nine dollars. They put it in their pockets; they split it up between four of them. The next day they told the other man who was in it with him that *I* stole it.

Then I met a Jewish man, he was very sick. But he took me to Las Vegas twice. I was like a nurse to him—I'd take him to the doctor. There was nothing between us; it was platonic. He was selling drugs and using them, for the pain. His brother said he gave me too much money; he'd give me a hundred a day to shoot the dice and pull the machines and play when we went gambling. So, the second time we went, he told me *after* we got on the plane, "I'm not going to give you that much money to play with." So I hollered, "Hostess!" and I moved my seat way in the back. He begged me to come and sit with him and all, and I wouldn't do it. He finally came around and gave me the hundred bucks to play. And he bought me shoes and different things.

Then he got tight with his money. He said I used too much. So I said,

"This cheap son-of-a-B; I better get on a program before I'm caught without any money in the bank at all." I've been on methadone six years now. I don't like it. It's like poison. It does all kinds of things to you—like I got nauseous before. Methadone's something I don't know how to get out of. I just don't seem to know what to do. I'm an old lady now and I figure, "Oh, to hell with it." I'd rather have heroin: the heroin puts you to sleep right away. With methadone I sometimes don't sleep all night. But heroin's so hard to get these days; I think I would rather stay on something I could get. And methadone does keep me from getting sick.

My dose is very low now, because I went on a cruise two years ago. I only use forty milligrams now, and when I went on the cruise it was thirty —I had been using ninety. I went from ninety to thirty in four months' time. That's very fast. The methadone can do terrible things to you if you don't get it for two or three days. Like, when I went on the cruise, if I'd get busy playing bridge or doing something and couldn't get away, I'd get all kinds of aches and pains.

I went on the cruise by myself. I spent a lot of money, I spent twenty-five hundred, besides all the evening gowns. I wanted to look just as good as anyone. I figured, when I was told that I had liver trouble, that I may as well have a good time, that that might be the last good time I would have. But an old man hooked onto me and spoiled all my chances. I thought he was very repulsive. All he wanted to do was drink beer and tell dirty jokes —and I hate dirty jokes. I had the second dinner and he had the first; and when I'd come out he'd be sitting there waiting for me. I couldn't get away from him for a minute. He said I was his "doll." Even after I came to New York—I didn't know he had my address. He took it off the Customs. If he'd have left me alone, I might have met somebody nice. I might have gotten married again. [Laughs.]

If I had my life to live over again, I'd run like heck from drugs. Because I've met so many nice people that it ruined. If I stayed with that man in Texas, I'd be a millionaire today. He had a ranch, and he told me that when his sons grew up—they were big boys then—that he would give me the house. He and his wife weren't on good terms. His last son was a cripple, he had multiple sclerosis. He blamed it on his wife, and she blamed it on him—you know how wives are. She said if he hadn't have run away with so many prostitutes that it wouldn't have happened. But that's not true, that's from something else.

I've got a few hundred dollars saved. It costs me so much to live now, and no money coming in. I'm not living with anybody. I'm on the SSI. My check comes all right, but my stamps and my Medicaid sometimes don't come for three months. I'm living in this flea bag now on the West Side. The room isn't so bad since I've cleaned it up. It must have cost me twenty or thirty dollars to get the roaches out of it. Then I had a mouse, so I put glass in all the holes. They didn't come back, so it's pretty good.

But I'd lived in such gorgeous places; I lived in places that were furnished with French furniture.

I feel very depressed about this, yes I do. And now they want to take a biopsy of my liver. They think I might have cancer. I refused, for the simple reason I have lived my life, and it's been very beautiful, even with the drugs.

8.

Dealing

One of the more lucrative hustles open to narcotic users was dealing. It was highly dangerous, but it assured a steady supply of drugs for personal use and generated large profits on a regular basis. Astonishing amounts of money—in uninflated, pre-1965 currency—passed through the hands of the former dealers we interviewed. They also enjoyed prestige within the addict subculture: the more they handled, the larger the prestige.

In one sense dealing was a less serious offense than the various property crimes committed by addicts, since it involved a financial transaction between two willing parties. (If there really were sinister dealers in trenchcoats, lurking around schoolyards to corrupt children, we did not find any.) But, even though dealing was consensual, it was nevertheless responsible for a great deal of indirect harm. Making drugs available to users encouraged them to continue hustling rather than seek out treatment; it also made possible the further spread of addiction (usually through intermediaries) to people who could not or would not have obtained narcotics through licit, medical channels.

This is why Anslinger and other narcotic officials stressed the prosecution of dealers: if they were eliminated then existing addicts would be cut off and fewer new ones created. In practice, however, arrested dealers were quickly replaced, because selling drugs was such an attractive opportunity for cash-short addicts. What the police sweeps really amounted to was an imperfect, informal tax on an illegal industry; real price, measured in dollars and adulteration, was at least partly a function of the suppliers' risk. The higher the price, however, the more likely addicts were to hustle—and dealing, as we have said, was one of the best hustles going. The more one thinks about the social and economic dynamics of classic-era narcotic addiction, the more circular they become.

Continuous replacement of arrested dealers was not the only obstacle to effective law enforcement. The illicit market they sought to penetrate was complex and hierarchical in nature. Since there was no domestic poppy production to speak of, the heroin had to be imported. The importers, who dealt in bulk, sold to the kilo connections, who in turn sold to smaller dealers, and so on down the line. The distribution system, as it had evolved by the early 1960s, is shown in Figure 3.

Once the heroin reached the United States it was cut practically every time it changed hands. The result was that a kilo costing $3,500 in Europe ultimately retailed for $225,000, a markup of well over 6000 percent.

The multiple layers of the traffic made it difficult to prosecute the importers and wholesalers, who were generally not addicted to the narcotics they sold. When a low-level or middle-level dealer was arrested, he could only implicate the person above him—an uncommon occurrence, since dealers who informed or testified against higher-level suppliers risked sanctions far worse than those provided by the law. If dealers informed on anyone, it was more likely to be rivals on the same level of the traffic; by feeding information to the police they could take competitors out of circulation and temporarily increase their share of the market.

The upshot was that, while the police could never penetrate and smash the entire distribution network, they could pick off the small-fry dealers, and occasionally (with the accompaniment of much publicity) arrest a "ring" of higher-ups. Arrest represented a potential catastrophe for an individual dealer: federal sentences were averaging over five years in 1957.[1] There was consequently a strong incentive to divert some of the profits to purchase protection, i.e., to buy off police, judges, prosecutors, and politicians. Because there was so much money in narcotics, corruption reached the highest levels. In fact, one of the reasons Anslinger came to power in 1930 was that his Treasury Department predecessor, Levi Nutt, was touched by scandal. Both Nutt's son and son-in-law were in the employ of gangster Arnold Rothstein, who was posthumously revealed to be the country's largest narcotic trafficker. Although Anslinger himself ran a reasonably tight ship, his administrative powers were confined to the federal level. There was little he could do about police pay-offs in New York and other large cities, where both corruption and narcotic use were well entrenched by the 1960s.

CHARLIE

Charlie, born of Italian immigrant parents in 1908, was raised with his two brothers in Greenwich Village. When he was about three, his father abandoned the family and ran off with Charlie's godmother. Charlie did poorly in school, dropped out, and went to work in a chandelier factory in 1923. He began sniffing heroin regularly with another worker, became addicted, and lost his job. Sick and desperate, he learned from friends how to smoke opium to prevent withdrawal. This proved to be his entrée into a new and classier world.

When you got a habit, right away you didn't want to be a junkie. People used to look at the pipe smokers more as, you know, not too bad. Because

---

1. Isidor Chein, "The Status of Sociological and Social Psychological Knowledge Concerning Narcotics," in Robert B. Livingston, ed., *Narcotic Drug Addiction Problems*, Public Health Service Publication No. 1050 (Washington, D.C.: G.P.O., 1963), 165.

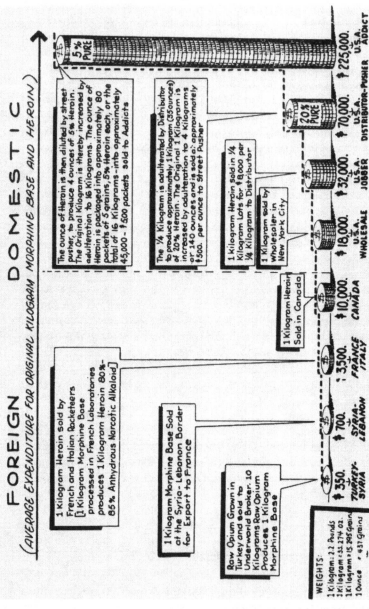

FOREIGN AND DOMESTIC PRICES FOR OPIUM AND HEROIN

FOREIGN   DOMESTIC
(AVERAGE EXPENDITURE FOR ORIGINAL KILOGRAM MORPHINE BASE AND HEROIN)

Raw Opium Grown in Turkey and sold to Underworld Broker. 10 Kilograms Raw Opium Produces 1 Kilogram Morphine Base

1 Kilogram Morphine Base Sold at the Syria-Lebanon Border for Export to France

1 Kilogram Heroin sold by French and Italian Racketeers [1 Kilogram Morphine Base processed in French Laboratories produces 1 Kilogram Heroin 80%-85% Anhydrous Narcotic Alkaloid]

The ounce of Heroin is then diluted by street pusher, to produce 4 ounces of 5% Heroin. The Original Kilogram is thereby increased by adulteration to 16 Kilograms. The ounce of Heroin is packaged into approximately 80 packets of 5 grains, 5% Heroin each, or the total of 16 Kilograms into approximately 45,000 - 1,500 packets sold to Addicts

The 1/4 Kilogram is adulterated by Distributor of 20% Heroin. The Original 1 Kilogram (35 ounces) is increased by adulteration to 4 Kilograms or 140 ounces and is sold approximately 500. per ounce to Street Pusher

1 Kilogram Heroin sold in 1/4 Kilogram Lots for 8,000 per 1/4 Kilogram to Distributor

1 Kilogram sold by wholesaler in New York City

1 Kilogram Heroin Sold in Canada

WEIGHTS:
1 Kilogram: 2.2 Pounds
1 Kilogram: 33.274 oz.
1 Kilogram: 15.295 Grains
1 ounce = 437 Grains

$350. $700. $3,500. $10,000. $18,000. $32,000. $70,000. $225,000.
TURKEY-   SYRIA-   FRANCE   CANADA   U.S.A.   U.S.A.   U.S.A.   U.S.A.
SYRIA   LEBANON   ITALY   WHOLESALE   JOBBER   DISTRIBUTOR-PUSHER   ADDICT

5% PURE   20% PURE

FIGURE 3   From kilo to five-dollar bag: the structure of the illicit narcotic market in the early 1960s.

Source: U.S. Senate, *Organized Crime and Illicit Traffic in Narcotics: Hearings before the Permanent Subcommittee on Investigations of the Committee on Government Operations,* Part 3 (Washington, D.C.: G.P.O., 1964), 753.

when you smoked a pipe you kept yourself clean, you was meticulous
pipe smoker was meticulous: he was neat about his clothes and everythi
Your better class of user was a pipe smoker. You went with women m
When you smoked a pipe, oh my God, you got on top of a woman, ___
Christ, she had to kick you off. It held you back, but a woman loved that.
With heroin, it ain't. With heroin, it dries you out. Half of the time you
don't even want a woman.

I was dealing heroin at the same time I was smoking. That's how I
was paying for my hop. In those days, I remember you could have got a
vial of H for two dollars. It was about what we would call a "sixteenth"
today. You know, we learned so much about it from this guy, Cago, that
we went in business. We bought an ounce of H—and this is H that's a
hundred percent, that came from Germany in a little square box with gold
rims. This Jack Diamond[2] had gone to Germany, and they had made a
big connection with a drug firm. At that time they claimed—I don't know
how true it is, because it never happened to me—they claimed that people
had a certain license that they could buy opium. But they can't sell it
directly to the United States; some way or other, they used to get it on
this ship that used to bring Scotch here. You understand, this is during
the bootlegging days.

We would take an ounce of H, at that time you would make two out
of it. Today they make [laughs]—I hear it's 1 percent out on the street. I
don't know because I don't go for it. Back then I paid thirteen dollars an
ounce for it. After we made two ounces out of it, it come to cost me seven
dollars—all right, a dollar for the little bags that I had to put it in. We
got on a corner, and I'd see the floosies come down—we used to sell it to
the prostitutes. And then, when we got through, we'd go to Chinatown,
to Cago's flat. And then, when we got to know the business, we got big:
we got our own flat, our own room, we rented a room in Chinatown. And
we had a chink cheffing for us. If you let him smoke with you, he'd chef
for you.

When I was starting out, I experimented. I went to Grand and Forsyth,
on the East Side, where I was. Hymie Rothman, he was one of the biggest
over there.[3] I talked to him and I got a couple of ounces on credit. I

2. Jack "Legs" Diamond, bootlegger and narcotics distributor, worked for Jacob "Little
Augie" Orgen and Arnold Rothstein in the 1920s. He was celebrated for having survived
several assassination attempts; "the bullet hasn't been made that can kill me," he once
boasted. On December 18, 1931, he was found dead in his bed with five rounds in his head
and torso.

3. Hyman "Hymie" Rothman, his brother Herman Rothman, and another man, Harry
Rubenstein, were arrested by customs agents on September 6, 1923. Found in their possession were ninety pounds of smoking opium, allegedly destined for Newark's Chinatown.

said, "Hymie, I want to go into business. I ain't doing nothing." He said,
"Yeah, all right." They liked me because I was a crazy kid—I had a
reputation already. I shot a guy one time in a poolroom. One day I had a
little argument with some kid, a fish. He was a little bigger than me, and
I wasn't going to let him punch me, so I had a little twenty-two gun and
I shot him. No, he didn't die. But that made you, you know, the dopes
started talking, "Oh, Charlie, he's a good kid." You know how the Jewish
people talked: they said, "That little guinea, he's a tough little guinea, he
shot a guy."

So Hymie said, "All right, Charlie, you want a couple of ounces? Sure.
Pay me when you got it." So I said, "What am I going to do?" He said,
"Go in the drugstore, buy two ounces of milk sugar. Go to your house
and get a flour sifter, like when your mother makes cake. Does she bake?"
I said, "Yeah." He said, "Well, get the flour sifter and sift it about five, six
times. Then put it up in packages. Do you know how to weigh?" I said,
"No." He said, "Well, you go in a stationery store and you buy a post
office scale. On there its got quarter ounce, sixteenth ounce, you know.
Then, whatever you want to make, you weigh it, and you get glassine
envelopes, and you put it in there." So I did that, and I was in business.

I went up around Times Square. At that time, you know *how many*
theaters were in Times Square? Legitimate theaters? For crying out loud.
Every theater up there had vaudeville too. So you had people that wanted
something, you know? Anybody that wanted it, I would sell to them.
Anybody that had the money. I didn't sell openly on the street, nothing
like that. Somebody would recommend you, like somebody that knew
somebody that was using or wanted some. They'd say, "Go see Charlie.
Tell him I sent you."

There were all kinds. Working people, everybody was a worker. You
never had what you've got today, muggers and thieves. Everybody had
something, a frankfurter stand, a newspaper stand. In the thirties a guy
could have a stand selling newspapers on the corner; he made ten dollars
a day and spent a deuce to get himself fixed up. You understand? It didn't
cost much. For five dollars I used to get three tins of hop and, if I wanted
to be conservative, I could have gone for a month. Three tins of hop—
five dollars! Well, no, not everyone was as conservative as me. Guys that
wanted to show off, that wanted a broad alongside of them, they smoked
a couple of tins a night.

But today, these kids that get habits, they're nothing but thieves.
They're snatching pocketbooks, they're snatching jewelry, because
they've got to get a tremendous amount of money. Do you know what
you had in the thirties? In those days you had sneak thieves that used to
jump on trucks and steal boxes of woolens, suits. They didn't hurt the
little people, like you see today. I never heard of anybody in my day steal

from an old man or an old woman, like you hear today. Do you know why? From the different methadone programs that I went to, I've met kids that don't know how to do *nothing*. Just that they've got to steal from their mothers! their sisters! There was one kid in that Bernstein Institute, he gave his sister eight stitches on the head to take her pay when she came home from work.

There were more men than women among the people I sold H to. On the average they were from, say, twenty-five to about forty. Most of them had jobs in the Times Square area. Guys were elevator drivers. . . . I used to go to what you call the garment district. One day I go to deliver an eight-dollar package of dope. The guy is a starter in a big building on Thirty-eighth Street between Sixth and Fifth Avenue. He's in the lobby, and it's one of those lobbies that goes from Thirty-eighth to Thirty-ninth Street, you know? It's a beautiful building. Do you know what a lobby is?—all marble, and he's got five elevators there, five elevators here. And here's this guy in this uniform with brass buttons. So he sees me and gives a sign that meant "I'll be right out." All of a sudden he changed his hat and put on his cap and came out. He said, "Could you come up tomorrow, bring me another package?" I said, "All right." He gave me the eight bucks and I gave him the package.

As I'm walking out of there a fucking bull grabs me. This is how I got away from him. In my hat, I had all the glassine bags. He searches me— what he was looking for was a numbers runner. So I said to him, "I'm no numbers runner. What are you looking for?" He said, "I seen you go in there and you took something." I said, "No, I had an address."

When he took the hat and looked in it three or four of the glassine bags fell in. He said, "What's that?" I said, "Oh, uh, I get asthmatic fits. I put them in a glass of water and I take them." He said, "All right, put them away." So I put them back in the hat and I put the hat on. So he said, "You ain't got no evidence on you for numbers. But I'll get you." And I walked away from him. [Laughs.] A bull, a first-grade bull.

I sold to a nurse, would you believe it? Her father and her mother used morphine and they lived on Eightieth Street between Columbus and Amsterdam, on the downtown side. The father was in a wheelchair and the mother used to take care of him. The daughter had a drug habit, her mother had a drug habit—they were from the South. Down in the South they all use morph. She got a habit from the father. The father was some kind of—what do they call them?—paralytic.

She came down there and somebody said, "Charlie, that woman is waiting for Joe and he's not around." He knew that I knew people on Grand and Forsyth. So I said, "What does she want? A couple of tins? Some H?" He said, "No, she wants morph." So I said, "I don't know if I could get any, but tell her to give me the money and I'll go see." She gave him the money, but when he came back with the money, she turned around and said, "Oh, I'll have to go with you." So I said, "Will you pay for the taxi cab?" And she said, "Yeah."

So I hired a cab, somebody from the neighborhood, you know. No strangers. We got in the cab, both of us, and we went to Grand and Forsyth. But I didn't go straight to where I wanted to go. I made the cab stop at Grand and the Bowery. I told her, "Sit in the cab and I'll be back."

I went to the restaurant where everybody hung out. I walked over to Hymie Rothman and I said, "Hymie, I never bought morph before, but I got a woman . . ." He said, "You didn't bring her here?" I said, "No, I got her three blocks away in a cab, a cab from the neighborhood." He said, "All right, what does she want? Cubes or . . ." I said, "What do I know?" He said, "Well, get cubes."

So I gave him the money, I gave him thirty-five dollars, see, and I kept twenty dollars. He went away and in about ten minutes he came back and he gave me this square tin box wrapped in cellophane. It must have come from Germany because it had German lettering—"*Drogen: Morphium.*" So I knew it was morph. I put it back in the paper bag and I went to the cab and I gave it to her. She said, "Will you ride uptown with me? I want to try it to see that you didn't give me no cubes of sugar." So I rode up with her.

When we got to Eightieth Street, we stopped in front of her house. She paid the cab driver, and I went inside. They lived in these brownstones. I went in with her and I saw this old man in a wheelchair. The daughter introduced me. The daughter had a white uniform on and she started talking to me while the mother and the father went into the back kitchen. She started telling me that she's a nurse, because I see the white uniform, I see the cap, you know. She said, "I'm going to work. I work for a doctor on Fifth Avenue. You're sure that's good morph? Because there's a lot of stuff in the market." I said, "As far as I know. I don't know much about morph, but the people that I got it from—it's good."

So, about five, ten minutes, the old man came out with the mother pushing him in the wheelchair. He said, "It was good morph. Good. Pure. Very good." It dissolved in the spoon. She took the hype, she fixed him up, and she fixed herself up. Then she told the daughter, "You want to go in? It's on the table. Go fix yourself." They were all using. I supplied them for about a year or two. Then something happened to me, and they must have got it somewhere else. I sold morphine to one or two different people, but I mainly dealt H.

The people I sold drugs to were just users. They didn't deal to others, nah. Guys that had jobs, that were working, they wouldn't go out and sell junk too. You had to be up against the wall to do it—you had no other way of making an income, you understand?

The customer had to be somebody that knew what they were buying and how to use it. I didn't deliberately recruit anyone. Somebody that might have done that was somebody that wanted a girl, like to put her out for prostitution. I've heard of that, a guy wanted a broad—but that would be a pimp. It wouldn't be nobody like us.

I heard about it from prostitutes themselves. Like I would say to her, "How the hell does a nice girl like you get into this racket?" She says, "Well, you know, I loved a guy so much, and he had a habit, and he made me get a habit in Philadelphia"—that was the most place they came out of. You had whorehouses in Easton, Scranton, Reading that was like illegalized [sic] because we used to go there on a Sunday. Like five, six guys would get in a car: "Where you going?" "Let's go bar hunt. Let's go to Easton." And you went there. And it was a big, big road house, had a big bar in it. Twenty-two, twenty-four, twenty-five girls on the side— Chinese, white, black, any color, any nationality. They'd come over and say, "You wanna go up, Johnny? Around the world? Come on, I'll give you a trip around the world." That meant that she took you and licked you from your toes to your head, "around the world."

The federal government's full of shit when they claim there were fewer addicts after the clinics closed. They got *more* because that's when the money went into it. See, that's where the profit came in. Now, you take a kid like me. If I could have went to the clinic, I would have been better off, because I would get it legitimately. Then, when I couldn't go to the clinic that they shut down, then I had to go to the mob. Then there was money for the mob, and the mob made millions. And they can buy, I don't care who it is—even if it's Jesus Christ—they can buy him, he's got his price.

There was still plenty of junk on the street. Plenty. They made it better, because they made profit. I'll tell you two of the famous narcotics men that we had: Primrose and Meyer, the bosses of Chinatown. They murdered and killed more Chinese and white people for drugs than anybody else. But they were on the take all the time. There were certain people, certain dealers, that got to them.

Then there was another guy that was famous, Two Gun Murphy, a little short Polack that come out of the army and made the narcotics division. He was Polish. They wrote a story on him—Brodski, Polowski, something like that—and he changed his name to "Two Gun Murphy." He came into Harlem with two big thirty-eights. He shot up Harlem. On a roof he shot two drug sellers, boom, bang. Oh, they called him "Two Gun Murphy." It's true. You could go to the narcotic people—he worked for them.

I'll tell you about that son of a bitch. There was a guy that got sixty years —Chewy, from Houston and Norfolk—in the little Hungarian restaurant. He had a young girl, a blonde, Eva; she was about eighteen years old. This son of a bitch Murphy was looking to fuck her in the worst way. What did he do? He used to make Chewy have a clear sail to sell junk, hop. This Eva one time told us stories about Two Gun, how he came down to the little Hungarian restaurant, took her to Broadway shows, and all that. Took her to hotels. And that's why he gave Chewy the protection.

I never paid off a policeman myself. But my sources did. Sure, Tammany Hall was bought off. They had to give the OKs. You see, you take like on Fourth Street and the Bowery, Harry Perry had that club. He was a big leader, that Harry Perry; he was one of the strong arms of the Tammany cat. Well, he had that club and, in the nighttime, that club used to run the most powerful card game. Two men got killed up there, Pat Russo, and the other guy was Griffin.[4] They were bodyguards for Harry Perry. They ran one of the biggest games up there. And you know who went up there? All the detectives, narcotic men, went to shoot craps.

One time I went with these three detective sons of bitches that picked me up to the Huron Club. Do you know what the Huron Club was? The Huron Club was Mayor Walker's home. He lived on St. Luke's Place with his wife and little dogs. We used to fight to walk those dogs when we come out of school. Well, about four blocks down was the club, the Huron Club. Upstairs were bedrooms where Jimmy Walker, when he was too drunk, his chauffeur and bodyguard would bring him up there. Downstairs they had a bar. All the federal men used to come in there and drink and everything. The biggest connection—the Mayor! What are you talking about? In New York, money made money.

I was pushed out by the Italians about '38, '39, before the war. Then I had to start getting anything I could get to keep my habit up. See, around about '36, '37—no, just a little before that—the Jews had the drugs. They had everything, the hop and the H. Who were the big dealers? Hymie Rothman, one of the biggest. Murray Marks, the guy that got killed on Pelham Bay Parkway, he was a big one. Murray Marks, Hymie Rothman, Waxey Gordon—oh, you could go on naming them till the cows come home.[5]

4. On January 31, 1926, an embittered gunman known only as "the Kibitzer" shot and killed Red Russo (Vincenzo Montalvo) and Patsy Griffo (Pasquale Cuoco), and wounded another man as they were playing at rummy. The incident took place on the second floor of Harry C. Perry's Second Assembly District Democratic Club. "Cat" refers to the Tammany tiger. The tiger became the emblem of the New York City Tammany organization after the Civil War, presumably because it was the emblem on Boss Tweed's fire engine.

5. Murray Marks, who was gunned down June 29, 1933, was an aide to Waxey Gordon (Irving Wexler). The investigation into Marks's murder netted several caches of opium. Gordon himself became involved in narcotics as early as 1917, when his cocaine distributing activities came to the attention of the New York Kehillah's Bureau of Social Morals. During the 1920s he specialized in bootleg beer, which he reportedly ran through sewers in pressure hoses. He was set up in the business by Arnold Rothstein, one of the pioneers of rum-running in New York. Another Rothstein associate who eventually became involved

The Jews were satisfied to make a dollar on you. See, the Jews were businessmen: they gave it to you the way they got it. They knew you were going to hit it; but they figured you'll be in business, and they'll get you, you understand. He knows you'll come back tomorrow, and he'll make another dollar on you, and another dollar, and another dollar.

Then the wops started to get in it, and they started to knock off the Jews, they started to clip them. This was in '26, '28, around there, and the wops took over. They'd find the Jews in the East River if they kept selling it. We had a lot of kids on the East Side killed—Allie Wagner and his brother, they killed them.[6] Soon as the wops found out that they were selling against their orders not to sell—bingo! bingo! bingo!

First it was the Italian guys with the handlebars: Don Pepe, all the mustache guys, you know, Don Pasquale, Francesco. Then the Americanized guys came in, the Mafia guys. Charley Lucky got in it, Frankie White got in it, they all started to get in it. Then Tony Bender got in it, Vito Genovese got in it—that Vito Genovese got convicted. I think he did ten years.[7]

The Italians were selling shit, chemical, acid. You bought one, and if you made three out of it, it wasn't worth a nickel, because they were already cutting it. These sons of bitches were so hungry for money that they cut it half a dozen times—then he sold it to his brother-in-law and his nephew, and by the time *you* got it, if you touched it, it was ruined.

The Jews, they would take the hop that was smuggled in and keep it as hop, as opium. And sell it as opium. But then, when it went to the other sons of bitches' hands, they didn't make it come here any more as hop. Because hop is too bulky—do you know how big a pound is? A pound of opium is this big [indicates a fair-sized lump with hands]. And there's no way you're going to make it any smaller. Now, do you know how much a pound like that in heroin is? Holy mackerel! For Christ's sake, you could make a hundred ounces, or more.

It got to be that there was no more money in it. You couldn't do nothing

---

in narcotics was Jacob "Yashe" Katzenberg, "who undoubtedly knew more about procuring heroin in Asia and smuggling it into the United States than anyone else in the world" (Alan A. Block, "The Snowman Cometh: Coke in Progressive New York," *Criminology*, 17 [1979], 91–93; Hank Messick, *The Silent Syndicate* [New York: Macmillan, 1967], 95, 100, 122; Albert Fried, *The Rise and Fall of the Jewish Gangster in America* [New York: Holt, Rinehart, and Winston, 1980], 94–102, 214 [quotation], 215).

6. In the early morning hours of February 21, 1931, gunmen ambushed the Wagner gang in a hotel suite. Al and Abe Wagner, bootleggers and suspected narcotic dealers, had been feuding over turf with the John "Aces" Mazza gang. Al Wagner was killed outright in the attack; Abe was wounded but escaped. He was murdered a year later in St. Paul, Minnesota.

7. In early 1959 Vito Genovese, a powerful Mafia don who was formerly a lieutenant of Charles "Lucky" Luciano, was sentenced to fifteen years on a federal narcotics charge.

no more. Then you had to go out and steal, because you couldn't make a living at it, because, the way they gave it to you, you was going to starve to death.

Not only that, it got to be that they came around, like to the neighborhood I was in. There was a guy there by the name of Inky. This Johnny Spotelli came around and gave him an awful beating.[8] "You ain't selling junk in this neighborhood no more," he said. They took it over.

They put you out. They wanted their man there. See, they had their man. You had to be a button guy, you had to kill three, four people and be somebody that they look up to. They took your customer away. To get him, they'd say, "What does he charge you? Ten? Here, we'll give it to you for five." You lost him. But the dopey bastard don't know that, soon as *I'm* out of business, they'll charge him twenty for what I'd give him for ten.

The Jews were wonderful; they were businessmen. They wanted to make a buck on you today and a buck on you every day. The fucking wops, they wanted *ten*, and tomorrow maybe choke you for fifty.

CURTIS

Curtis was born in Wilmington, North Carolina, in 1904, the second of six black children. His father was a barber and itinerant musician, his mother a washwoman.

I smoked reefers and used a little cocaine when I was nine years old. I got it where I worked as a delivery boy in a drugstore. They used to sell

---

He died of a heart attack in his Leavenworth cell ten years later. Tony Bender (Anthony Strollo) was one of Genovese's lieutenants. He was improvident enough to help put Joseph Valachi in the narcotic business; Valachi later turned government informer.

There were Italian dealers in the 1910s and early 1920s, but they were mainly small-time operators. Most written accounts agree that Italian criminals did not begin to dominate the wholesale traffic until the 1930s (*New York Times*, April 6, 1924, Sec. 9, p. 13; Humbert S. Nelli, *The Business of Crime: Italians and Syndicate Crime in the United States* [New York: Oxford University Press, 1976], 123; Louis Vyhnanek, "'Muggles,' 'Inchy,' and 'Mud': Illegal Drugs in New Orleans During the 1920s," *Louisiana History* 22 [1981], 261–62, 278; U.S. Senate, *Organized Crime and Illicit Traffic in Narcotics: Hearings before the Permanent Subcommittee on Investigations of the Committee on Government Operations*, Part 3 [1964], 630–40; Part 4 [1964], 913, 918).

8. Probably Innocenzio Stopelli, alias John Stoppelli or "Johnny the Bug." According to FBI and New York City Police summaries, Stopelli's record dated from 1924 to 1948 and included arrests for possession of a gun, robbery, bribery, and violation of federal narcotic laws. By the early 1960s he was said to be "one of the most active large-scale wholesale narcotic traffickers in the United States" (*Organized Crime and Illicit Traffic*, 1056).

reefers. It was legal at that time. Marijuana, they called it; they had it in cigarette boxes. No, it didn't have any medicinal use: they used to make ropes of it.[9] I never cared for this reefer, but I smoked it. On Sundays, this fellow I was hanging out with, he'd smoke cigarettes and reefer. On Sunday, that's all. Just for the devil of it you'd smoke it. I didn't know, really, that it was a drug, or that it would make you feel funny.

There were a few older fellows that were addicts in this town. They knew I worked at this drugstore. They told me if I would see a bottle with a cross and a skeleton on it to get them some and they would give me a little change. I used to get it for these fellows, but I didn't know what it was—I just got it for the money. I'm sure they were also using morphine. They used to be around a poolroom where I would go, and play pool and things. See, even kids could go to poolrooms there, as long as they had on long pants.

The cocaine I sniffed only a few times. But I didn't care for it then. And I quit the cocaine and reefer. I only worked at this drugstore for five months or something like that—a short time. I didn't start using cocaine again until I was about twenty, until after I had come to live in New York. I had gotten into trouble in Wilmington. I always liked money. I burglarized the same place twice, but I got caught the second time. After that I lived up here with my aunt.

One day I met this fellow from my home town. He said to me, "Come on, let's go over here and get some of this cocaine and sniff it." So I went with him. He took me to this apartment on Lenox Avenue where this girl was selling cocaine and heroin. She was a black woman, a nurse in Harlem Hospital. I don't know why she quit, but she had stopped nursing and started selling drugs.

For two years I used to go there, but I wouldn't use no heroin. I just sniffed cocaine. But I used to have pretty good money for my age. And if you have money, these women would try to get you hooked so you'd spend money. So one night this nurse sneaked heroin in my cocaine. And this like to kill me. I fell on the floor and I vomited a lot.

This place was a house of prostitution. There were a lot of women there using heroin. They were old addicts, they were all older than me. They got angry at the nurse—that's how I knew. I didn't know she had done it, but they knew because they were all of them dope addicts. They bawled her out for sneaking it on me—you know, I was a kid then. But I continued to use drugs. I wasn't having no habit, but I was using. See,

---

9. Marijuana was an important cash crop in the Midwest and Upper South in the nineteenth and early twentieth centuries. The hemp fibers were used mainly in the manufacture of twine.

Takes a long time to become dependent

you can use a little heroin, like today, and don't use nothing for two days; you can do that for two or three or four years and not get a habit. Well, I did that for a couple of years.

I went to see this nurse one night to get some heroin. But the police were bringing everybody out of the house, including her. She was the madam of the house and was selling heroin. She got two years. She got locked up that night by the police, who were bringing them all down to Jefferson Market.[10] She tried to escape. But she was well built: she was too heavy for the sheets, which must have been rotten. The sheets broke and she killed herself.

There was a fellow who lived with me at 128th Street. He had a habit, but he didn't tell me. We were using cocaine mostly. But cocaine, if there are two or three of us in a party, we can sniff or shoot up a thousand dollars a night. Now, that's a lot of money—but maybe we're selling, that's how we can shoot it. But the other people who came to this house, they had habits. They were elderly people. So he said to me, "Gee, we're spending two or three hundred dollars a night, and those people are taking one shot, and it lasts them all day." You see, with heroin you only shoot up two or three times a day. At that time it only cost fifty cents a shot—now it costs ten dollars. That's the difference. So he told me, "Why should we spend three hundred dollars when we can get a habit and only spend a dollar and a half, maybe, for the whole day?" Now, that's a lot of difference, and it made sense to me. So then I said, "We might as well get a habit." So I just went on and got a habit, and then I only had to spend a dollar and a half, maybe two dollars a day. I was twenty-two when the two of us decided to get a habit. But he had had a habit before, and I didn't know this. [Laughs.] He really talked me into it.

There was plenty of drugs then, more than there are now. I sold drugs for a few years. In my house I sold it, on 133rd Street. I started selling after I got out of the reformatory, after '26, maybe around '29. The people I sold to were real drug addicts—you know, some musicians, some thieves. I used to sell to Billie Holiday. Those addicts didn't go dirty. They were mostly all musicians and people that could do something. They were professional people mostly: if they weren't professional on the stage, they were professional in the street. They were, ah, what you would call professional thieves.

I was stationed up in Harlem the whole time I sold drugs. I sold to black people, whites, too, and Chinamen. I had all that Chinaman trade

---

10. A famous prison and courthouse at the intersection of West Tenth and Sixth Streets and Greenwich Avenue, built in 1878. An imposing brick edifice with unlit, dungeon-like cells, it was used to process the hundreds of addicts picked up in police sweeps and to detain them until they were sent to Blackwell's Island or some other institution. Jefferson Market was razed in 1929 to make way for the Women's House of Detention.

down there—I used to go to the laundry down on 116th Street. When the Chinamen buy stuff, they all buy it together. They'd buy a couple hundred dollars worth, there'd be ten of them. They bought in a group —they are together, the Chinese, you know that.

So I had a mixed trade: white, Chinese, black. I didn't deal with too many Spanish. I used to buy from them Spanish fellows down at Fifth Avenue; there were quite a few of them selling down there in them days. But there weren't too many Spanish people here until the United States bought Puerto Rico.

The addicts of that day weren't like the addicts today, because the pressure was not like it is now. We got real drugs, good drugs—not like the 1 percent they get now. We were using 35 percent drugs then. Strong. It would kill these people now, but we were built up to it. It's a different class now than it was then. There's just as much difference between them as between cheese and ice cream. The people in the thirties had more respect for other people; they had more respect for themselves. You would hardly know an addict when you saw him. You didn't see people nodding out on the street, like you see today. If they got in that predicament, they'd go home. In the 1920s it was mostly adults that used drugs. Not too many kids, because they wouldn't sell to them. When I started, I used to have to get someone to go buy mine, until the man got to know me. There was a fellow who came here to New York from Detroit; they called him Detroit Jimmy. The old people know him: he used to live at 128th Street and Lenox Avenue. He is the one who started this selling kids drugs in New York. That was in '33, '32, somewhere around in there.

Most of the drugs we bought in quantity. We'd buy like an ounce, or, if we were short, we'd buy half an ounce. They had two kinds of drugs in them days. One was called Green Dragon—it had a large dragon on the box—and they had White Horse, with a stallion, a white stallion, on the box. Pictures, you know: it was made up in factories, in a box.

At that time, in the 1920s, a whole ounce only cost you from twelve dollars up to twenty-five dollars—the only thing is that the twelve-dollar was not quite as strong as the twenty-five-dollar ounce. Today that twenty-five-dollar ounce would cost you five hundred dollars. If you got the same quality of stuff. But they don't get that kind of stuff now.

Before I'd buy the ounce, I'd get my place set up so I can mix it and so forth. And then, if I'm in shape, I'd get scales and things. I'd go to the drugstore and get stuff to mix it with. You'd get bonita—there's two or three things you can cut it with. In the twenties you were cutting it with milk sugar. How I would package it would depend on what the man's buying. In the twenties and the thirties we didn't use bags; we put it up in little paper packets—then it was only fifty cents. Now, if you were buying a quarter or a half an ounce, we had envelopes, you know, like you buy a thousand in a stationery store.

There were also capsules. They have had different prices: some for two dollars and, some, we had them as cheap as a dollar and a half. Number five caps. I don't know if you know them, but they're little small caps. You can buy them right there in the drugstore. Well, those were made after Detroit Jimmy started selling to youngsters. He didn't put drugs in caps, but other people that were selling small quantities started making up caps so these youngsters would have enough money to buy dope. That was in the thirties; you had caps after World War II, too. The last time I saw any caps was maybe fifteen or eighteen years ago. Around in the sixties they kind of started weaning off. Some of the grown people would buy caps if they didn't have any more money, you know, but mostly the kids would buy them. I know, definitely, because I made up something special for that purpose myself. I didn't start kids to using it, but after they were using it, then I'd make them up.

Now, when I was selling, I used to put up the packages for the adults, which is the quarter- and the half-ounce. We'd never sell them an ounce —only the larger dealer would. I'll only sell them (because I'll make more money) the half-ounce—but mostly not that much. I'll sell them in the quarters, eighths, and sixteenths, and in the little small caps, and the fifty-cent packages.

I sold out of my apartment. I had a couple of fellows working for me who used to go into the street. But I wasn't no big seller: I had to buy my drugs from somebody else, a black man. Who really controlled it was the bigger people on the East Side, the Sicilians. In the twenties too—no, in the twenties the Jewish people had it.

Now, *that's* a story. The Jewish people don't mess with anything that's not profitable. They saw that it wouldn't pay, that it was too much time for the money. Any time is too much time for them people. And they're too smart to sell it; they gave it up because they saw it was too hot. They gave it over to the Italians—they're more gangsters.

The black people handled the largest quantity of drugs after it left the big connections, when it came to the country. I used to live on the East Side where they live, those Sicilians. The police would go around there; and that's why they took it [to the blacks], because if they handled it they got killed. Do you understand? So the Italians took it; now, when they get it, they take it and deliver it to, like, the San Juan Hill, which is the biggest stop after it comes in. There were more drugs sold in the San Juan Hill than anywhere in the world. It was called "the jungle." Have you ever been down there? It's only one block, Sixty-third Street, down on the West Side, between Tenth and Eleventh Avenues. This was a black neighborhood, all black. No white people lived down there at all. They used to come down there though—some of the biggies—I've seen them come there in a Rolls Royce, with chauffeurs and things.

In 1939 they busted everybody that was dealing drugs there. They had a stool pigeon—I worked with him over on Riker's Island. He was doing a hundred days. He came out and he made buys and things off of different people. Then he left. But if you work for the government as a stool pigeon, they don't let you go. They either catch you or have you killed, if you play with the government. When he left for New York they had circulars out for somebody, anybody to find him. They don't quit, once you're a stool pigeon. Even if he leaves the country, they'll find him.

When they busted the San Juan Hill, they changed the drugs, the price —they changed everything. It happened suddenly, overnight. Just like Prohibition—it happened doggone near overnight. When the government stepped in, the Jews would have nothing else to do with it. The price? The night they busted the San Juan Hill, the next morning the drugs jumped from fifty cents to ten dollars, five dollars—that's the cheapest you could buy a bag, five dollars. There wasn't even no three-dollar bags. It was five dollars after they busted that Hill. It changed just like that. That's how hot it was when the government stepped in.[11]

When the Italians came in, I didn't have any problems making connections with them. I lived with Italians. I used to work for the biggest guy in New York. I knew the big connections at that time. But it was better when the Jews had it. The Italians, they started to cutting it. They got so good that they discovered all kinds of chemicals that they'd mix it with. Now we don't know what they're cutting it with.

World War II, that's another story altogether. There was no heroin— that's why don't tell me they can't stop it. They can stop it if they want to: there's too much money. In World War II they stopped the heroin. I mean you couldn't buy one bag nowhere. This went on for over a year, longer than a year.

But you don't stop no addict from getting no drugs—he'll get it one way or another. Then they started using morphine, everybody had morphine habits. They'd get it from the doctors, and some from the drugstores. We'd take it. We'd write scrips. Everybody was writing them that could write. I couldn't do it, but I had two girls that I knew who could

---

11. There were actually two raids on San Juan Hill. The first, on February 1, 1939, netted twelve arrests and ten ounces of heroin; the second, on the night of February 4, 1939, netted four arrests and twenty-six ounces of heroin. The first raid was spectacular, even by New York City standards: an armada of forty Treasury Department agents, sharpshooters, and radio cruisers descended on the Hill. West End (Eleventh) and Amsterdam (Tenth) Avenues were blocked off by cars to prevent any escape. These raids were part of a city-wide crackdown on heroin and marijuana dealers (*New York Times*, February 2, 1939, p. 2, and February 6, 1939, p. 3).

At first Curtis stated that the Italian involvement in the narcotic traffic coincided with the San Juan Hill bust, but, as the interview unfolded, it became apparent that he knew of Italian wholesalers before 1939. This is consistent with the recollections of other dealers, such as Charlie, and the fact that the heroin seized on the Hill was highly adulterated.

write Latin; they had no trouble. And they had other ways to get to the morphine.

It very seldom happened that we couldn't get the morphine. It might happen for an hour, two hours—but in less than two hours somebody is going to get something from somewhere, even if they have to stick them up. I sold morphine during the war. I used to get it and sell it, just like everybody else was getting it and selling it: scrips.

Then heroin came back. Who controlled it? Whoa, now that's a question. Big people controlled that drug—you would be surprised. Maybe in the White House. Even on the street here it's a problem. I mean, you only get to know to a certain extent. You *think* you know, but that won't be the head. You don't get to know the head man, most likely, until he gets busted or something.

I reestablished my connections after World War II. I was the first one to get heroin when the first load came in—the man I was dealing with was the first one. He was a black man, but he was getting it from—all of it was coming from—them Italians. The black man don't have no ships. The white man brings all the drugs here. Everybody knows that. The black man may get some if he's working on the ship and smuggles a little bit in, but the white people control the drugs. And a lot of it's controlled by the law. Yeah.

In the first of the fifties they had what you called a "seventeen-fifty" package. To survive, I used to get, say, two of those packages, which would cost me thirty-five dollars. We'd get twenty-two number five caps out of each package, which is forty-four caps out of the two. I could take and sell those for two dollars a cap. Twice twenty-two times two is eighty-eight, and it cost me thirty-five, so I'd make—how much?—fifty-three dollars. That's over double your money.

Heroin has been getting worse and worse right along because of greedy people who don't care what's the outcome. Money, they don't care how they get it. They're even killing people, they're selling poison, anything, to obtain a dollar. Today it's dangerous using dope out there on that street. It's very dangerous. Before it wasn't like that; I know the time when a person would not sell you a bad bag of dope. Maybe you got *one*, but—they just didn't do it. Times have changed.

The price of heroin has stayed the same, but it's not the same because you don't get the quality for your money. You get less heroin in a five-dollar bag, and worse heroin, but the price is the same as it was when it went up. It's been quite awhile since I sold any. The last dope I sold was around '57, '58. I was living over at 125th Street and St. Nicholas Avenue. My friend had a bootblack stand, with papers, sandwiches, and things, and we were selling there. I stopped selling because too many stool pigeons started stoolin'. I couldn't last three months before the police knew my name and they were coming to get me. They'd know how much I've got, they'd know me as good as my mother, because the stool pigeons talked.

I never was a real big dealer. I could have averaged a thousand dollars a week clear profit, but I didn't care for too big a traffic. But I was making maybe five or six hundred dollars, that's all. What did I do with the money? Spend it. I have money in the bank, but most of it I just spent, oh, on so many things. You had cabs, taxicabs. And, back in those days, dope fiends used to *dress.*

RALPH SALERNO

The allegation that the Jewish dealers had been driven out of business by the Italians, who then adulterated drugs to unheard-of levels, surfaced repeatedly in the interviews. Charlie, Curtis, and several others made this complaint. However, Arthur had good relations with his Italian suppliers (see chapter 6), as did Jerry, whose narrative appears later. Jerry, in fact, denied that the Jews had been cut out. "There was no such thing as control," he said. "I was getting it from the Jews, the Italians in the thirties and forties. I don't think there were any combinations; they were somehow able to get it as individuals."

Faced with contradictory testimony, and curious about the role of organized crime in the narcotic traffic, we interviewed Ralph Salerno, an intelligence specialist who spent over twenty years with the New York City Police Department. Following his retirement as Supervisor of Detectives in 1967, he co-authored a book, The Crime Confederation *(1969), and served as a consultant to several investigative groups, including the House Select Committee on Assassinations. The last of eleven children in an Italian immigrant family, he graduated from high school and then joined the navy in 1943. He served in the Pacific theater, was wounded in a PT-boat action, and was discharged in December 1945. He considered going to college on the GI Bill, but felt handicapped by the commercial courses he had taken in high school. So instead he joined the police department.*

I had a rather unusual police career—I'm terribly overspecialized. My wife teases me about it by saying I'm a "police academy dropout." I never completed the three-month police academy course. I joined the police department on September 16, 1946. It was the first group of recruits following World War II. The prescribed training course at the academy was three months, which meant that I would not have graduated until mid-December. But on election day, November 1946, there was a murder in East Harlem. A Republican precinct worker had gotten up early to go to the polling places, and he was set upon by three young men who beat him savagely. I don't think it was their intent to kill him, because they had not used any weapons, but evidently he struck his head against the sidewalk as he fell from the blows; his head was fractured and he died a few days later. His name was Joseph Scottoriggio. It was quite an infamous case in its time. The headlines were "ELECTION DAY MURDER." Some of the earliest leads indicated that the motive for this terrible crime was some minor political double-cross involving Scottoriggio and the congressman in that area, Vito Marcantonio.[12] The indications were that people in organized crime had ordered the beating of Joseph Scottoriggio as a favor to the congressman, to teach Mr. Scottoriggio a lesson.

At that time we had two thousand recruits in the police academy. Today, 1982, fifteen hundred personnel is a sizable police department. It's hard for people to grasp that we actually had two thousand recruits in the police academy, because of the limited hiring that had taken place during the Depression and then during the war years. Well, they came through the academy and were going to interview everyone who was of Italian background, who could speak or understand a little Italian. The original plan was that those selected would work undercover in East Harlem to try to pick up what the community was saying about this crime. East Harlem had been an Italian ghetto—every member of my family, other than myself, was born there.

I was fortunate enough to be one of twenty-five young men that they finally selected from the number they interviewed. And so, without ever having completed my training at the police academy, I now found myself involved in an investigation that had political and organized crime overtones to it. The twenty-five of us worked on that case for about eight months. I learned to have a little bit of resentment for the journalistic phrase "unsolved gangland homicide," because, to our own satisfaction and to a moral certainty, we solved that case. We knew what had caused it; we had an idea who had ordered the young men to beat up Mr. Scottoriggio. We didn't have that proof in the form of legal evidence that could be

12. A protégé of Fiorello LaGuardia, Vito "Marc" Marcantonio was a shrewd machine politician who happened also to be a staunch leftist—an improbable cross between Richard Daley and Henry Wallace. First elected to Congress in 1934, he seemed to have a lock on his district; in 1942 and 1944 he even managed to secure triple nominations from the Republican, Democratic, and American Labor parties. But in 1946 he lost the Republican primary to a former Air Force intelligence officer named Frederick Van Pelt Bryan, who benefitted from the postwar backlash (*Time*: "Veto Vito?"; *Newsweek*: "The Red Darling") against Marcantonio's style of radical politics. Marcantonio hung on to win the general election, a no-holds-barred struggle culminating in Scottoriggio's beating, which was witnessed by his wife from their apartment window. A routine, desultory investigation of Scottoriggio's death caused a public outcry (led by Republican presidential hopeful Thomas Dewey) and a major shake-up in the city's police department. Damaged by the scandal and assailed as a Communist, Marcantonio was finally defeated in 1950. He died four years later, August 9, 1954 ("New York Police Shake-up," *Life* 21 [December 30,

presented in the courtroom, so no one was ever successfully prosecuted for that crime. But I always felt that we had solved it.[13]

That case was a tremendous education, it influenced me in many ways. I realized, even though I was only twenty-one, that we were really doing two things in our investigation. Number one, we were trying to solve that homicide. Number two, we were being used in a way that was going to be very, very helpful to the Mayor of the City of New York, William O'Dwyer, in winning his next election, because we were learning a lot about his political enemies and those who were pretending to be his friends but who were really his enemies. So I realized that there could be some abuse of police assignments for some political motive or gain by people in the political structure above the department. And O'Dwyer was reelected in 1949; then in 1950 he sought and obtained an appointment by President Truman as Ambassador to Mexico, and resigned the mayoralty. There were investigations which showed corruption in various parts of the police department, also the fire department. Many people felt that Mr. O'Dwyer had left "one step ahead of the sheriff," before the scandals totally exploded.[14]

Following our assignment in the Scottoriggio murder case, we were thanked for our services and told, "OK, now you can go out in uniform and be policemen." I went to a precinct. I was there two weeks in uniform when the man who had been our supervisor called me and said, "I want you to come back to work for us." There had been some interest by another high-ranking officer in police headquarters in these "young rookies who had done such a good job." He had some additional assignments for us in the area of organized crime. Our assignment was heavily oriented toward electronic surveillance—surveillance that was proper, lawful, legal. We did a great deal of wire-tapping and bugging.

We did that for about three years. Then in 1950 we were made detectives and that little group of young men was broken up, assigned to

---

1946], 13–16; Annette T. Rubenstein et al., eds., *I Vote My Conscience: Debates, Speeches and Writings of Vito Marcantonio, 1935–1950* [New York: Vito Marcantonio Memorial, 1956]).

13. Michael "Trigger Mike" Coppola and Joseph "Joey" Rao were held as material witnesses in the case, but finally released. One by-product of the investigation was the indictment of six Mafia drug dealers, including Charles "Little Bullets" Albero, an associate of both Rao and Coppola. The narcotic probe even spread to "Boss of Bosses" Frank Costello, who took the unprecedented step of calling a news conference and denying any connection with the traffic. "I detest the narcotic racket," he announced, "and anyone connected with it. To my mind there is no one lower than a person dealing in human misery." According to some accounts, Costello tried to get the syndicate out of narcotics in 1948. He did not succeed (*New York Times*, December 19, 1946, pp. 1, 5; December 21, 1946, p. 20; *The Valachi Papers* [New York: Putnam, 1968], 231–32).

14. The investigations centered on police protection of gamblers, especially Harry Gross, who operated a large bookmaking ring in Brooklyn and who later testified that he

different detective commands. Some men went to the pickpocket squad; some men went elsewhere. Three men went to the narcotic squad, which was being expanded from fifteen detectives to eighteen. Even though we had a police department of twenty-three thousand people, the narcotics squad had fifteen people in it, which was less than one one-thousandth of our total personnel. There was not a big priority for narcotics work at that time.

I was added to a group of ten experienced detectives who had been borrowed from other commands to form a new unit because in 1950 Senator Estes Kefauver from Tennessee was embarking on a national look at the problems of syndicated crime. We knew that he would be coming to New York City, and we wanted to have some material for his consideration. So one supervisor and ten men were assigned to take a look at major crime figures. We found out where it was they were living, what automobiles they were driving, and who they associated with, where they spent their time. Senator Kefauver's staff was very complimentary of the work we had done, so it was decided that this work should be continued. At first we were kind of buried in office space that had somebody else's name on the door, but it eventually became a formalized unit under Police Commissioner Stephen Kennedy in July of 1957. Everyone thought it was just another one of Commissioner Steve Kennedy's brainstorms, which would probably not last much beyond his own tenure. Yet, within five months, he looked like a brilliant genius. In November of 1957 state police discovered a meeting at Apalachin, a tiny village of a thousand people in upstate New York. The sixty-odd people identified there showed clearly that this was a national crime meeting. People had come from California, New England, Colorado, Texas, Florida. That we could immediately tell the police commissioner something about the twenty-three New Yorkers who had attended that meeting showed that the work of this unit was important and should be lasting. So I stayed in what then became the Police Intelligence Unit, and the Intelligence Division of the New York City Police Department, for the rest of my career.

By the early 1960s I had come to be considered something of an authority on organized crime. I think the fact that I was Italian was a big contribution to my success: maybe I could understand Italian criminals a little bit better than other detectives might. See, I believe that a policeman is a people-watcher. Some policemen limit themselves by watching people only to see what they do, until such time as they have openly violated

had made massive pay-offs up and down the line. Subsequent inquiries by the Kefauver Committee in 1951 revealed that O'Dwyer had connections to Frank Costello and other syndicate figures.

the law, and then they want to capture them. I think that you should go deeper than that in being a people-watcher. I think that you should try to understand the person that you're watching, what he does and *why* he does it. If you do that well, you approach becoming the ultimate detective, who can almost sense or guess, in an educated way, what someone's going to do *before* he does it. And then you can be there first with the most.

I was not involved in narcotics enforcement per se when I served with the intelligence unit. Our primary interest was syndicated or organized crime groups. But, if you were going to pursue that primary goal, you naturally were going to see the importance of narcotics—it was a big moneymaker for them. When we came across leads close to the narcotics area, we would give them over either to the New York City narcotic squad or the Federal Bureau of Narcotics. They would actually do the field investigations leading to prosecutions. Ours was more of an intelligence unit—we weren't on the street with the smaller dealers. The same thing would be true if the person we were interested in seemed to be a major figure in gambling operations. Once we got close to, say, the actual location of the bookmaker's wire room, where he takes bets on the phone, or the place where the policy betting slips are delivered, that information would be turned over to an operational unit—they would actually go out and try to effect the arrests and testify in the prosecutions. It reduced our down time. When you make a case, there's a great deal of time that must be spent in preparation with the prosecutor. Testifying in court reveals your identity—we didn't want to have to give away our identities or methods of operation. So the strategy was to give the information, after we had developed it to a certain extent, to an operational unit which would face all of those problems while we went on to bigger and better things.

The syndicate figures we were interested in were made up of many nationalities, backgrounds, and religious affiliations, but were dominated perhaps by two groups, Italians and Jews. I once described it to *Time* magazine in this way: the success of organized crime results from the happy marriage between Italians and Jews, in which they produce together the "three m's"—moxie, muscle, and money. "Moxie" is a Yiddish word which means brain power; it seemed to me that the Jewish people made a big contribution of the moxie. The Italians had kind of taken over the violence. The shooting gangs of Jewish young men, from the thirties and forties and Murder, Inc., had disappeared. The only young shooting gangs we had were Italians. So the Italians took over the muscle, Jews put up the moxie, and they split the money.

The impression we got is that the murder of Rothstein was like a signal for Italian dominance in the narcotics field, that by the end of the thirties the Jews were out of narcotics and it was basically an Italian-run endeavor. Is this true? You seem to say it was a marriage. But people who lived in the Lower East Side, who worked and sold drugs, told us that a lot of Jewish gangsters were killed by the Italians, in terms of gaining territorial control over the narcotics.

I believe you've correctly identified the key figure as Arnold Rothstein. He was murdered in what is now the New York Sheraton, just south of Central Park. His heirs were a mixed group, some Italians and some Jews. These were the people who, while working with, for, and around Rothstein, had formed partnerships: Frank Costello, Charles "Lucky" Luciano, Meyer Lansky. Murder, Inc., was headed by two men: Lepke, whose name was Buchalter, and Albert Anastasia—an Italian and a Jew, in a marriage controlling tough guys and hit men. When Walter Winchell, a famous columnist, arranged the surrender of Louie Lepke Buchalter to John Edgar Hoover, he was actually a federal fugitive on a narcotics case. In the late thirties going right up to the early forties, just prior to his surrender, he was very big in narcotics. So you did have Jews in narcotics. You had Italians in narcotics. And *these* Italians and Jews were not fighting each other.[15]

In fact, they did nothing but work very, very well together since they formed their relationships during the Prohibition era. Meyer Lansky shook hands with Frank Costello and Lucky Luciano in New York in the 1920s. The same thing was happening in Chicago when Al Capone met a fellow named Jake Guzik. In Boston it was "King" Solomon, prominent Jewish gangster, shaking hands with Frank Cucchiara. In Philadelphia it was one of four Italian brothers shaking hands with "Boo Boo" Hoff and "Nig" Rosen, two Jewish fellows. Amicable. Amicable because the Italians' and Jews' immigrant experiences came within ten years of each other: they ran into each other in the 1890s and 1900s coming to the United States. Their sons were young men in their twenties in the late 1920s. That's when Louie Lepke met Albert Anastasia, and they got along very well. There's no record, on that level of important crime, of Italians and Jews fighting.

Let me point out something to you: if you're talking about New York City in this era you have got to forget the nonsense of the Fourth-of-July speeches about America being a great melting pot. If you take a look at the map of New York City up to World War II—and I'll draw the map for you—it is a mosaic, not a melting pot. You can be a big gangster on

---

15. Lepke was certainly involved in narcotics, but other versions of his fall indicate that it was his erstwhile Cosa Nostra allies, rather than Winchell, who induced him to surrender. Before he went to the electric chair for murder, March 4, 1944, Lepke himself charged Frank Costello with betrayal (George Wolf with Joseph DiMona, *Frank Costello: Prime Minister of the Underworld* [New York: Morrow, 1974], 120–22; Maas, *The Valachi Papers*, 171–72; Fried, *Rise and Fall of the Jewish Gangster*, 212–14).

Mulberry Street, and if you cross the Bowery onto Delancey Street and Essex Street, you're in foreign territory and you better watch your step, because that's a Jewish community. An Italian gangster can't be a big shot in crime in the Jewish community because he's not in the politics of that community. So, for Italian drug pushers to invade the Lower East Side, they wouldn't last two weeks, because the Irish cops will be told by the Jewish politicians, "Get rid of those guys!"

What your people might have seen was a low-level street peddler who was a usurper—that might have ended as a violent scene. I think you have to do some analysis of the people you are talking to. Someone growing up on the Lower East Side who says, "Oh, he was a big guy in narcotics" or "He was a big gangster," can be talking about a local criminal whose sphere of control went beyond no more than four blocks, from Rivington to Stanton Street, from Essex to Allen. Describing someone as a big gangster is a very relative thing.[16]

After World War II, following Louie Lepke's arrest and conviction, you did begin to see a rapid withdrawal of the Jews on the importation level. They saw that there was a lot of money to be made in organized crime but thought, "Narcotics is generally looked at as a dirty business, it best behooves us to make our money elsewhere." It was a voluntary withdrawal on their part, in exactly the same way the more successful Italian gangsters voluntarily withdrew by the early 1960s. They said, "Too much attention brings a bad image to our legitimate businesses that we're running illegally, to our gambling businesses that nobody seems to resent. Too much heat on narcotics—let us withdraw."

The Italian domination really set in with the old French connection, when the predominance of heroin came from Turkey, Lebanon, through Italy to Marseilles, following World War II. Outside the United States the control fell to six literal Corsican *families*, people actually related to each other. Almost all of the heroin the United States wanted, they could supply it. Who had the bona fides to sit down with these six Corsican families? Only the Italians, and a few Jews who lingered after Lepke passed from the scene—and they were in the field largely through their

16. The generation of the criminals referred to is also important. Albert Fried and other crime historians make the point that it was the rising young Italian and Jewish gangsters who were most willing to join together and rationalize crime. But their less assimilated elders, such as Joseph Masseria, were openly contemptuous of outsiders. The passing, natural or otherwise, of the old guard during the early 1930s paved the way for greater Italian-Jewish cooperation. When someone like Charlie (ch. 8) insists that there was conflict in the late 1920s, it is not necessarily inconsistent with collaboration later in the 1930s when Young Turks like Luciano and Lansky seized power (Fried, *Rise and Fall*, 119–28; see also Peter A. Lupsha, "Organized Crime in the United States," in Robert J. Kelly, ed., *Organized Crime: A Global Perspective* [Totowa, N.J.: Rowman and Littlefield, 1986], 45–52).

affiliation with some Italian. You could have had 40 million dollars and, if you were a black man, you couldn't even get to sit down with that Corsican. He didn't want to know you; he didn't trust you; he didn't know if you were working undercover for the narcs. All that he had to sell—and all that could be sold—he sold to Italians that he knew very, very well.

Joe Valachi gave a pretty good indication of how the traffic was organized. You'd make a deal with the Corsicans in Marseilles or Paris. You would pay X number of dollars for the actual narcotic, and then you had an option: did you want to pay for it delivered in the U.S., or would you pick it up in Europe and arrange for its delivery? If you wanted it delivered in the U.S., there was an additional charge to cover the costs of the courier and the risk involved.

During the 1950s the Federal Bureau of Narcotics had a small book; I think it was labeled "Known and Suspected Major Dealers." These were people who could bring in two kilos or more. I don't believe there were more than 125 bios in that book. It was a very limited number of people, dominated by Italian criminals. There were still Jewish dealers at that level, but in the overall representing no more than perhaps 20 or 25 percent. The rest were Italians. I don't believe there was a black man who could bring two kilos of heroin into the United States up to 1960.

A big Italian dealer is going to sell it in one-kilo, two-kilo, half-kilo lots to people that he knows and trusts well. You're not going to get others in the picture until you get down to what we used to call the "ounce men": people who buy a quarter kilo, mix it a couple of times, and sell it in ounces. This could be anybody. But who is he going to sell it to? He is going to be required to sell it, really, in his own community. If a black ounce man has cut it down into decks, and he's selling a little package of forty glassine envelopes, he'll be selling to another black guy. If he happens to be Jewish, he'll be selling to somebody who's probably Jewish too.

The one area where you might see some difference is show business. That's a Jewish industry. Where does a black musician get his drugs from? He probably gets it from his agent. Who's who? Who's Jewish. In the 1970s and 1980s they're saying, "You want to book that rock group? You got to give them X number of dollars and their cocaine supply for the two weeks that they're playing for you." That's part of the deal, see. So if you want to be in the entertainment business today, you're in the cocaine business, whether you want to be or not.

I would say that the biggest change in narcotics trafficking since 1946 has been the expansion of the market. I tend to think of it in terms of a huge, illegal business, and the number of possible customers expanded tremendously in the fifties, certainly in the sixties and seventies. Drug abuse used to be regarded and treated as a very limited problem, engaged in by people in the entertainment world and by some people in the lower socioeconomic classes. That changed radically. It became recognized as a much wider problem that had invaded the middle class, and even the more affluent and better-educated people in our society.

Again, I look at it as an economic market. It is a market that cannot advertise on television and radio, or with billboards. But it goes through a form of expansion created by the people in it. A person who becomes addicted to, let's say, heroin will find some difficulty in meeting the costs of supporting his habit. Whether it's actually suggested to him by the person he's buying from, or whether he figures it out all by himself, one of the easiest ways for him to be able to support his own habit is to introduce the joys of heroin to three other people. He'll be their contact. They will be returning to him for additional heroin. He can then start purchasing in larger bulk, and he'll have his three friends actually covering his cost. In the process he has expanded the market 300 percent.

I didn't sense a deliberate attempt by the higher-ups to expand the market. They didn't conceive of it that way. They would become aware of the increased demand, and be very happy to satisfy it, without giving a great deal of thought to what created it. I think they were wise enough to see that it was expanding by itself, without any help from them, so they didn't actually exercise a conscious plan to further the market.

In the popular novel, The Godfather, *and in the motion-picture version, there is a deliberate conspiracy by Italian syndicate figures to sell narcotics, but to sell them to a very specific group: the blacks.*[17] *Is there anything to that at all? Because another thing we see in the fifties, in addition to larger numbers of users, is more and more minorities becoming involved with drugs.*

No, there was no conscious plan in that sense. But the more sophisticated Italian and Jewish criminals who were in syndicated crime have always relied, and to this day rely, upon a certain amount of community acceptance and support. During the 1950s on Mulberry Street, in the lower part of Manhattan, the Italian gangsters' image was: "We keep the drug pushers out of the neighborhood." And they did. They exercised the kind of control that anyone who tried to sell drugs to young people

17. In the famous conference scene the Detroit Don, "Joseph Zaluchi," explains that "There's more money in drugs. It's getting bigger all the time. There's no way to stop it so we have to control the business and keep it respectable. I don't want any of it near schools, I don't want any of it sold to children. That is an *infamita*. In my city I would try to keep the traffic in the dark people, the colored. They are the best customers, the least troublesome and they are animals anyway. They have no respect for their wives or their families or for themselves. Let them lose their souls with drugs. But something has to be done, we just can't let people do as they please and make trouble for everyone" (Mario Puzo, *The Godfather* [New York: Putnam, 1969], 288–89).

in the vicinity of a school would be physically assaulted and thrown out of the neighborhood. They earned community support for that. But it wouldn't stop them from selling a kilo of heroin to someone, as long as they knew he wasn't going to try to trickle it back into their neighborhood. As long as they're not selling it, or allowing it to be sold—by blacks or whoever—in their own community, they're not undermining their bases of power. It isn't that, "We're going to sell it to blacks and therefore. . . ." It's, "We will not allow it to be sold here."

I had mentioned that the Italians began pulling out of the traffic in the early sixties. What happened was that the federal government passed a bill, known as the Narcotic Control Act of 1956. Prior to enactment of that law, if there was a joint operation between federal officers and New York City policemen, the federal officers would be very happy for any prosecutions to be made in the state courts of New York—even though they may have put up more of the resources, put up the buy money, and paid the informant for information. They felt that the possibility of obtaining a conviction, and the penalties that would be given out in the state courts, were better than in the federal court. But everything changed a hundred and eighty degrees with the enactment of this law. One of its principal features was that it established a federal violation for a "narcotics conspiracy." It made it easier to convict a higher-up who had never seen, touched, or tasted the drug, but who had put up the money for it. And the penalty for being convicted of a narcotics conspiracy was as great as it would have been if you had been found carrying two kilos of heroin.

All of these advantages, from the law enforcement point of view, were recognized by the people in the drug traffic. When the statute became effective, July 1, 1957, a lot of them said, "Uh-oh, the ball game has changed. I can get hooked." I believe that was one of the important things to the people at the Apalachin meeting four months later, that it was on the agenda for discussion.

It has been mistakenly said by many people, including Joseph Valachi, that at that meeting they passed a law which said, "All people connected with our criminal organizations must get out of the drug traffic or be killed." That's not true. There were no dead bodies to indicate that it ever was true, and there was continuing involvement by Italians in the heroin traffic after that date, without their being killed. What actually was said, by the older and wiser heads, was, "We're getting out. We would *recommend* that everybody get out. The rule that we are making, which we do intend to enforce, is, if you are going to continue to deal in heroin, it is required of you to tell your friends and relatives, 'I'm doing something for the next three months, so don't come and visit me, and I'm not coming to visit you. I'll tell you when everything is OK.'" This was to avoid the possibility of inadvertently implicating a friend or a relative in a narcotics conspiracy. They understood that what could—and sometimes did—happen was that federal officers or detectives would follow a courier, who would sit down with the person who was going to pay him for taking the heroin from one point to another. That meeting might be finished at eight o'clock in the evening, but the officers would stay with him, and when he went to visit his brother-in-law or a friend at nine o'clock, that would be part of the surveillance report, and perhaps help implicate them. . . .

I had an electronic surveillance in that period of time. There were two young men, reading of the indictment of some fellows they knew. They said, "Oh, my God, look at that! They're indicted for drugs. They didn't tell anybody. They're in *real* trouble. They're gonna be lucky if they don't get hit"—meaning killed. Shortly thereafter their mentor in the criminal group came in. They said, "Hey, did you see that? These guys are in real trouble." He said, "No, they're not in trouble. Read the whole article. When you get all the way down, you'll see that this indictment, although it fell today, goes back two years. That was before they made the rule. So they are OK." Criminal confederations don't make *ex post facto* laws. Not only that, they don't make any laws they do not intend to enforce. If they had made a law to get out entirely, you would have seen a total absence of Italian-connected criminals in the heroin trade.

You have seen, over the years, I guess billions of dollars spent in an attempt to suppress narcotic traffic. Yet we've seen the narcotic traffic go from basically a bilateral French connection, which was a significant organized crime activity, to a multinational activity, which was even more significant in terms of overall organized crime revenue. Do you personally feel frustrated, do you sometimes wonder what the hell's the point? Do you see the drug situation as being basically a replay of Prohibition in the twenties?

When I read in the paper of a request for an additional 130 million dollars by the attorney general and the president for the diversion of two navy aircraft from Norfolk down to Florida, and increased personnel in the customs service, it is a repetition of something I have seen now a dozen times: "New increased effort." "This is going to be the answer." And so on. I saw the federal Bureau of Narcotics, which was making all those big cases in the late fifties and sixties, grow from an organization of two hundred and twenty-six persons to ten times that number—and more. I still think of myself as a law enforcement person. I see myself as a member of a profession that is saying, "This is how we have been attacking this problem for thirty years. It hasn't worked, but we are committed only to a further attempt to these same areas." I know that across the country there are twenty-seven thousand people, on all levels of government, in drug enforcement; I do not know of twenty-seven people who are being paid by the United States government to sit in a room and *think* about a better approach to this problem.

It's a very confused problem. We don't know what it is we want to do. Do we want to protect society at large from the crimes that addicts are committing? If that's our number-one priority, we would do certain things. Do we want to help the people who are abusing drugs? If that's our number-one priority, we would do other things. Let's establish our priorities, one, two, three, four, and then our master plan, which has got to be participated in, not just by drug agents and the customs service, but by the medical, social, and educational authorities. But we're not doing it that way, we're not doing it that way at all. The kinds of things I'm advocating are not as politically healthy-sounding as, "Oh, yeah, another 130 million for drug enforcement." It's always a heavy emphasis on the enforcement thing, which hasn't worked in thirty years, and won't work again.

Enforcement does not work.

9.

Working

The hustler-addict was an American phenomenon, by no means generalizable to all cultures and legal systems. In other times and places working people made up the bulk of regular users. Thomas De Quincey's celebrated 1821 Confessions *described opium eating among Manchester textile operatives as so prevalent "that on a Saturday afternoon the counters of druggists were strewed with pills of one, two, or three grains, in preparation for the known demand of the evening." Rural chemists and shopkeepers likewise piled high their counters, selling prodigious quantities of opium to agricultural laborers, especially to those in the unhealthful English Fens. Their customers dosed both themselves and their children; babies were routinely stupefied into silence so that their parents could go on working. Narcotics were a cheap form of day care for the nineteenth-century laboring poor.*[1]

Chinese coolies, who toiled as indentured immigrant workers in Southeast Asia and the United States, were notorious as opium smokers. How much they consumed will never be exactly known, but opium smoking was widespread among them and there were a large number of addicts. Some historians have gone so far as to argue that opium was the key to the coolie labor system. A coolie was not much better off than a chattel slave as long as he was in debt to whomever paid his ocean crossing. Although his wages were meager, it was theoretically possible for him to set aside money and eventually buy his freedom. Possible, that is, if his savings did not go up in smoke. Both imperial administrators and Chinese merchant-creditors were happy to keep the coolies supplied with opium; not only

1. Virginia Berridge and Griffith Edwards, *Opium and the People: Opiate Use in Nineteenth-Century England* (London and New York: Allen Lane and St. Martin's Press, 1981), 21–48, 97–109; Terry M. Parssinen, *Secret Passions, Secret Remedies: Narcotic Drugs in British Society, 1820–1930* (Philadelphia: Institute for the Study of Human Issues, 1983), 22–58.

was it a lucrative source of revenue, it made the workers quiescent and extended indefinitely their terms of servitude. Opium was the opiate of the masses.[2]

During the classic era, proletarian narcotic addiction largely disappeared from the United States. This was partly due to the fact that a growing number of addicts were recruited from the urban underclass, and hence were under- or unemployed. You cannot be a worker-addict if you cannot find work. Even if steady work were available, it was barely adequate to cover the cost of heroin, to say nothing of ordinary living expenses. Addicts, however tightly controlled their habits, were constantly tempted to hustle to make ends meet.

There were, however, an exceptional few who stuck it out, working at legitimate jobs and supporting their habits for years at a stretch. It is interesting that three of the five narrators in this chapter were immigrants, newcomers to the city who were used to long hours and hard work. It is also significant that four of the five had access to the New York City drug market. "I've never known a place where you score as well as in New York City" is the way one addict put it. "This is the master." As bad and as expensive as New York drugs would one day become, they were usually better than what was available elsewhere. That was of some help to addicts trying to lead conventional lives.

JANET

Janet was born in Virginia on Mulberry Island (now Fort Eustis) in 1916. Her father, a black oysterman who squandered his earnings on other women, died when Janet was six. "They almost had to hang me to get me to go to the funeral, that's how much I hated him." Janet learned to do domestic work from her mother, a housecleaner, and she eventually found work as a live-in maid for a wealthy family in Jersey City. She liked the arrangement but, when the family moved to California in the mid-1930s, she decided to stay on the East Coast, closer to her mother, who was still in Virginia. So she crossed the river to Manhattan, looking for work.

I was an expert at pressing shirts. I had never worked in no laundry, but I knew that because the man I worked for in Jersey used to always compliment me. He said, "Janet, you can't leave us, because I know I'm never going to get anybody to do my cuffs"—he used to wear those long sleeves with French cuffs.

2. Carl A. Trocki, "Opium and Social Control in Colonial Malaya," paper delivered at the Conference on the Historical Context of Opium Use, Philadelphia, June 1–5, 1981.

One day I was walking on 125th Street and I saw a Chinese laundry there, and I saw the girls doing shirts. So I went inside and asked them, did they need any help? One said, "Yeah, I think the boss is looking for someone. What do you do? Backs? Collars and cuffs?" Well, I didn't know what she was talking about because I thought, if you do a shirt, you do the whole thing. I had never used no pressers before. So I said, "Yeah, I can do all of it." But I didn't know they had two girls on a machine, one to do the seams and the bosom, and the other girl the backs. She said, "You see that little man? Go back there and talk to him. He'll probably hire you, because he needs a backer." She kept on saying "a backer," but it didn't get through to me what a backer was. But I thought it was easy: the girl on the front, she'd do the whole thing and I'd just do the back. So I went and asked him, did he need a girl to do shirts? He said, "Where's the last place you worked?" Well, I wasn't slick enough to lie then. I wasn't going to tell him that I had worked at such-and-such a place, 'cause I really had no address to give him, noway. I said, "I just left my job in Jersey." He didn't question me about that. He said, "Can you work nights?" I said, "I can work day or night." He said, "Well, you come in tomorrow at three o'clock." I thanked him all the way out the door: "Lord! Thank ya, thank ya, thank ya!"

The girls were very nice. They had to show me how to do the shirts: the machines in them days weren't as modern as they are now, you know. I caught on easy, but they could do it much faster, because they were doing piecework, a dollar twenty-five cents a hundred. Some days they would do a thousand shirts, some days they'd do eight hundred. These were girls that were really experienced. They're fast; they don't pick jobs that just pay a salary. And the Chinamen don't pay that bad: they have a lot of work, and they want their work out. But the girls wouldn't skip me, if you know what I mean. They said, "If your shirts pile up on you, we'll help you do them until you learn how to do the machine. But so far, for somebody who hasn't used the machine before, you're doing very good." I said, "Thank y'all for helping me out."

I worked for that man, off and on, for about eight years. I worked there during the fifties, sometimes. He always stayed in touch with me. If a girl was out sick, or on vacation, or had to go home on account of something, he always depended on me. When I started work I was paying eight dollars a week for a room. I used to take home at least sixty-five dollars, some weeks seventy dollars. That was a whole gob of bread at that time. I had a little bank account—I'd never had one before in my life.

I wasn't hooked when I got this job; I was just playing around. I started using drugs in 1936 or '37, one of those two years. First I was smoking reefers. I just met different people, and they'd say, "Let's go up to the pad, Janet!" All those places were wide open, like you're walking into

Grand Central. I used to go up and smoke all the time. I never got high off reefers, but I saw some people, they'd smoke and be on Cloud 12. [Laughs.]

My first habit was morphine. I can't say that no one really put me on drugs. I had a friend, she was a sporting girl, a top-notch booster. I used to see her using morphine. She asked me, did I want a little bit? I said, "Oh, no, I don't want that." She said, "Come on, I'm going to give ya a little skin"—I didn't know what she meant by "a little skin." Well, we were very close, and every day I used to be with her, and I would get that little skin. And I skinned up on a habit.

My habit didn't bother me at work, because I always had plenty of drugs. My girlfriend gave me morphine—she had doctors who wrote for her. So it didn't cost me anything, at least in the beginning. But then the feds cracked down on the doctors and they had to stop writing the prescriptions. So I started using heroin.

I got the heroin from a boyfriend. I think I met him . . . see, years ago, they used to have clubs, the majority of them were on Lenox Avenue. They had music, but they didn't have dancing or nothing. They sold drinks and food there. Well, I met him in one of those places, and we started going out. He had a habit, but you'd never know it. He was a cool cat, he thought. I used to see him snorting. He had a mayonnaise jar he kept full of heroin. When he would come by my apartment on Edgecomb Avenue, he would always go into this jar. I thought it was cocaine. He had taken me to one of those coke joints in Harlem. You could go up to a pad, an apartment, and sniff coke. You'd order it and they'd put it on a saucer. You'd put the stuff on a mirror, or on the saucer, and make these lines, you know. There were blacks and whites sniffing—the white people came up to Harlem in the thirties to connect. Some were show people, some were ordinary people.

Well, I'm thinking that what's in this jar is coke. [Laughs.] I'm a dummy; I don't know. One day I said, "I'm going to try this." I was in that jar every day. I wouldn't use too much, but I used enough to get hooked. I didn't know it. I used to keep an appointment every two weeks with a beautician. This one Friday morning I woke up and went out on Seventh Avenue, where my beautician lived. I said hello and then, ooooh, I started throwing up. You know, I had never had no symptoms of being sick; I had been using the morphine and heroin continuously. I went back home and said to my boyfriend, "I'm so sick, I don't know what to do. You know, I think I'm pregnant." He said, "Yeah, you pregnant, all right. You *heroin* pregnant." I said, "Oh, don't say that." He said, "You been in that jar, and I've known it for a long time." I had to admit it. So he said, "Come on, I'm gonna get rid of that baby for ya." [Laughs.] But he was real upset about it, because he didn't want me messing around.

I continued using heroin, although I liked the morphine better. The morphine was cleaner, and I knew what I was using. If morphine had been so that I could get it, I would never have known what heroin was. But I always tried to have one connection for heroin, so that I wouldn't have to be running around. If you have one connection, you know what you're getting. But if you go out on the streets, especially if you're sick, and somebody "recommends" somebody, you don't know what you're getting. Even in that day, you might get a bad bag. That's why I sniffed the heroin. I started shooting later, when my nose got sore. But that frightened me, because I never wanted to use the needle with the heroin.

I used to get my stuff, and I'd take off before I came to work in the afternoon. I could have taken it to work, but I wouldn't take that chance. When I'd go home I'd take off in bed. Once in a while I'd shoot up with other people, but mainly I was alone. I don't like a lot of people.

Let me see, how much was it in them days? Five dollars a bag, and you could get caps for two dollars. And that was the real thing—you could take half a bag. I think I once got half an ounce; I paid thirty-five dollars for it. That lasted me a good three weeks. I'll tell you something. Once, when I was going home to Virginia, I met some people I knew. One of them said, "Janet, what're you doing here?" I said, "I'm going to see my mammy." He said, "Yeah? I know you're straight." I said, "Yeah, I'm all right." He said, "If you're not, all you got to do is look me up." That shocked me, because I didn't even know people in Virginia knew anything about no dope—that's how green I was. But you never know what's going on: they were taking stuff from New York and going down there dealing, and getting five times as much as they got here. If it's five dollars in New York, they'd go down there and they may charge you fifteen dollars for a bag. I couldn't have made it with a habit in Virginia, not with a legitimate job. But, at least in the thirties, I could work in New York City and still pay the rent. My habit was about forty or fifty dollars a month, tops.

I don't think the drugs helped me with my work. In '42 or '43 I went down to Virginia to visit, but I stayed and worked at the Quartermaster Laundry, Ft. Eustis, the same place I was born. I was making big bucks, more than in New York, because I was working for the War Department. But I wasn't hooked. I had kicked in New York, before I went to Virginia. I kicked my habit cold turkey: just laid there and suffered for five days. I didn't want my family to know that I was on dope. And, after a while, you get tired of using, even though you need it. It's a rat race. You're not getting high anymore, you've just got to have it not to be sick. Well, when I got that job with the government, I wasn't hooked, but I was the best worker in the laundry—they had a billboard down there, and my name stayed on top. I did a thousand shirts a day, the whole shirt, by myself. The captain was so surprised, he said he'd never seen nothing like it.

When I filed my application, he said, "If I hadn't needed a girl, I would have taken you just to find out if it was true that you could do that many shirts."

I came back to New York after nine months. I wasn't here but a month when I started on drugs again. I didn't feel no yearning; I felt physically all right. I don't know why I went back . . . just foolish, nothing else to do. And then I didn't look for another job because I was using stuff. But I had money from my savings. I was able to reestablish my connection—he was a black man, his place was downtown in the Thirties, on the West Side. He dealt with choice people. I didn't know them personally, but they looked clean-cut. White and colored, dressed neatly. That's another thing about me: I can't stand to see a greasy, dirty woman. I want to cut her throat.

I got married June 23, 1943, here in New York City. My husband had known me a long time. He had been addicted for years, way before me. I'm still legally married to him, but we were separated in 1968. We never had any children. I don't think that had to do with drugs, because my period never stopped.[3]

He was a beautiful husband—I got everything he thought I wanted. He was a thief; he stole from the government in the yards, where they had those cars and packages. He made enough money that he could support both of our habits. And he was well dressed, wore choice clothes from the best of stores. I didn't have to work—I didn't have to do nothing with him but look good.

He was arrested, did some time. I was left pretty good: I had money set aside. But when I saw my money getting low, I . . . you know, I know how to get money too, but he just wouldn't allow me to. I would sometimes work for the laundry, but that didn't stop me from stealing, at least when he went away. I was a pickpocket—I learned myself. Man, I made so much money picking pockets, I don't know. I came home one day about three o'clock in the afternoon, I think I got to thirty-two hundred and stopped counting. I worked the streets, never the subway. If a guy stopped me and talked to me, I'd say, "Baby, come on over here." I would stand with him in the doorway, and I'd pat him—it took me a long time to learn to do this, to be perfect at it. After I hit his hide, I'd peel off it. I'd never take it off—if he had a wallet, I'd pick his wallet, clean it out, and put it back on his hip. You see, when you take a man's wallet, and you walk away from him, and he sees he ain't got no wallet, right away you're busted.

You got to work fast, sure. You can't mess around, but don't be running when you leave. Take your time and walk away. I repeated these same

3. Some, but not all, women addicts experience amenorrhea and cannot become pregnant. If they do become pregnant there are often serious complications for their infants, including narcotic dependence. Opiates can affect either the fetus or the nursing child.

tricks over and over and over again. I was using my looks, and I was good with my hands. I didn't do a thousand shirts a day for nothing.

L I

Li was born near Fu-chou, China, in 1917. He was the first of three sons born to young, landless laborers—his father was sixteen when Li was born. Fleeing poverty and Japanese invaders, Li left Fukien province for Singapore, then went to sea aboard a tanker in 1939. Li spoke some English, but several portions of the interview were in a Fukienese dialect and appear here in translation.

I came to this country in 1942. I was in Philadelphia, my ship was leaving, and I missed it by two hours. After that I got a job washing dishes some-place in New Jersey. I made only sixty dollars a month, and I worked sixteen and a half hours a day, with no day off. But I wouldn't go to sea no more. It was wartime; a lot of people were killed then. I was scared.

I came to New York City in 1946. That's when I started to use heroin. I bought it by myself, used it by myself. I lived alone in an apartment, 34 Mott Street. I owned my own works, bought needles in a drugstore, and boiled them every time I took a shot. I didn't have any opium-smoking Chinese friends. You see, my original tongue is Fukienese, which is a minority among the Chinese group. Even if I had wanted to smoke opium, language would have been a problem—the majority of Chinese in New York spoke Cantonese.

Most Chinese go to some secret place, some cellar in Chinatown, to buy drugs. But I went out of Chinatown to different groups, to blacks and Puerto Ricans selling on the street corner. That's how I started. I was sick. I had hemorrhoids, you know, big ones on my asshole. I was asked by a Puerto Rican who was selling heroin in the street if I wanted to buy some; he told me it would be good for the pain. I bought it, and it killed the pain. It also made me high and happy.

After World War II the heroin was very pure. I liked it. But year by year it was worse, sugar powder was mixed up with it. In the forties I had to use ten dollars' worth—two bags—a day. Sometimes it would go to fifteen, but not too often. I could pay for it because, by that time, I had become a cook in a Chinese restaurant. I had to work Saturday, Sunday, seven days a week. The job paid four-eighty a month, and I was spending three hundred a month on drugs. That left me a hundred and eighty dollars to live on. Eighteen dollars of that went for rent. The apartment I lived in had gas, but the toilet was outside and there was no hot or cold water. I had to go across the street for water. Then, about two years ago, the landlord abandoned the building.

I was able to work throughout my addiction. I didn't do anything illegal, only spend money from my salary on drugs. I was only arrested once, for possession. I was in the Tombs for a month. No medical treatment, nothing. Just cold turkey.

I tried before to get help for my addiction; I tried to detox six or seven times at the old Manhattan General Hospital. But when I came out I would stay off heroin only two or three days, because of the pain from the hemorrhoids. I eventually had two operations for the hemorrhoids, but these were in recent years, when I was already on methadone. I came onto the program around late '69 or early '70. I was getting old, and I felt I couldn't maintain my habit.

I kept a part-time job for a few years after I came on methadone, but physical problems forced me to give it up. I have an ulcer. I drink, but not that much: two bottles of beer a day. Right now I'm living in a Salvation Army furnished room on the Bowery. There are five other Chinese men there—three of them are on methadone. I support myself with Social Security. I get two checks: one from Social Security Benefits, the other from SSI. I really don't know what the total amount is, because the checks are mailed to the Salvation Army. They cash them and give me a hundred and eight from Social Security and thirty-something from SSI. They keep the rest.

AMPARO

Amparo was born in San Juan, Puerto Rico, in 1909. When asked whether she came from a large family, she said, "No, there were only eight of us." Her parents were poor and Amparo, the youngest child, only went as far as the third grade in school. She also spoke little English: this narrative is in translation.

I came to this country on July 12, 1947. I came here on board the *Marine Tiger*. It was a famous ship.[4] I came by myself, in the care of six nuns. I found myself lonely in Puerto Rico. Times were hard. There really wasn't that much work. But I found a job right away in Nostrand Avenue in Brooklyn in a shoe factory. I learned the trade here, I picked it up as I went along. I made a lot more money at this job than in Puerto Rico. But I didn't send money back to my relatives in Puerto Rico—there was nobody to send it to. By this time they were all dead. That's why I was lonely.

4. The *Marine Tiger* was a Liberty ship that made several trips between San Juan and New York after World War II, carrying many thousand Puerto Rican immigrants. "Marine Tigers" became the derisive nickname for these newcomers, who were looked down upon by Puerto Ricans born or long settled in New York.

In 1949 I took a job in the kitchen of the Long Island College Hospital in Brooklyn. I made friends with the black people who worked there. I had never used drugs in Puerto Rico, and I wasn't using anything there. But then, all of a sudden, after three years, they stuck this particular black lady in the kitchen. She used drugs. When we used to go on break, I would watch this lady digging in a little bag—she was snorting—and then she would fall asleep. Curiosity got the best of me. I wanted to know what was in the little bag. That's how it started. I knew nothing about heroin, nothing about the street, nothing about needles. It was just like a brand-new game.

The first three times she gave me the drug free. She told me, "You use this for three or four days, and you're really going to like it." After the fourth day she wanted money—ten dollars. I think she wanted me to become addicted so she could make money. There were a lot of other Spanish ladies, and her logic was to addict me so I would in turn addict the others—then she could make money dealing to us. The black woman worked on the day shift; her husband worked on the night shift. He used to steal syringes and Dolophine, which is now called methadone, out of the hospital pharmacy. So they had a little thing going: he would take care of the men at night, and she would take care of the women in the daytime. Language really wasn't a problem: the woman had a little box, with twenty-, ten-, and five-dollar packages. She knew enough Spanish to say, "This is twenty, this is ten, this is five."

When I first used heroin I threw up a lot. I kept throwing up and I was very dizzy. And then I just nodded out, I went to sleep. I tried it again because I like the sleeping part of it, the nodding. I had had problems sleeping before, but when I took heroin I slept well. In the morning when the alarm rang to go to work, I was well rested. Heroin relaxed me. It made me sleepy. And after awhile the throwing up subsided, and I felt very comfortable. Heroin also helped me at work: it gave me all this energy. After I sniffed, I would have energy to clean windows and do work that wasn't even my own. They liked me a lot—I'd do other people's work if they didn't come in. I had a real good record there.

The black woman turned on other people in the kitchen. She would sell to the other blacks. People would also whistle from the street and she would go down and serve them. So she was actually dealing out of the hospital, both to the workers there and to people who came by during the day. It got to the point where they called me on the carpet and asked me what I was doing with this black woman. I told them that she was selling this powder. I knew it was heroin—I was addicted by this time. The police were then called in, and the woman was taken upstairs. By this time she was herself fully addicted, she had a big habit. I never saw her again—they dismissed her from the hospital. But I had to go to court twice, because the woman's husband threatened to cut my face for telling on her.

I used heroin so I could straighten myself out, so I could go to work. It wasn't a matter of getting high, or wasted. I always injected myself at home—I started mainlining about a year after I became addicted. I never took a fix in a shooting gallery or at the hospital. I would take a fix in the morning before I went to work and at two o'clock, when I had a break and I came back home. They never became aware of my addiction, because I was always by myself. When I had done my work I grabbed a book and read. I never mingled with a lot of people there or bought drugs at the hospital. After the black woman was arrested, another guy who worked there told me about heroin up on 111th Street. He would cop for me, and I would give him a taste. So I didn't have to deal with the people on 111th Street, just with this particular guy. I was his fix.

Back then I used to buy twenty-dollar quarters. That quarter would last me the whole week, because I would only get off myself. I wasn't giving away any of the heroin, and I was taking small fixes. Heroin now is garbage, but at that time it was unbelievable. You could keep a reasonable habit for twenty dollars because the heroin was that good.

Eventually, after about two or three years, my habit became fifty dollars a week. It was the price going up, more than it was my habit increasing. When I went with my twenty dollars to cop the guy said, "Nah, it's not twenty dollars any more, it's fifty." I said, "Why? I always paid twenty." He said, "We're paying more, you pay more." I also noticed two things. When I mainlined it I suddenly started to itch a lot, which made me think it was being cut with something. And when I got to work, I didn't have the energy I used to have. Like, my energy would cut off quick.

I didn't hustle when the price went up, but I did try to cut down on the amount I used. When that didn't work, I got on methadone. What happened was that one day, around 1971, I was standing on a corner near the hospital. I had just come back from Delancey Street, where I had bought six packages of heroin. A girl asked me for some money. A cop was watching—nothing intended, but he looked a lot like one of you, with a suit and beard and glasses. He saw my bag and asked, "What do you have there?" I showed him the heroin. He said, "Do you know what you've got there?" I said, "Yeah, I know what I have; I use this so I won't get sick." I was arrested for possession and sent to Matteawan.[5] Prior to this I had put in my papers for Lexington, Kentucky, but I had backed out at the last moment. So when I went to court for this possession arrest, it was in the record that I had supposedly gone to Lexington for a year. But I had

5. Matteawan State Hospital for the Criminally Insane, Beacon, New York, a mental institution that functioned essentially as a prison.

reneged on that, so they gave me two and a half years up at Matteawan. No parole. I did go in front of the board, and they offered me parole, but I turned it down. I didn't want to owe them anything or report to anybody. So I maxed it out.

I didn't have a hard time there at all. I worked, minded my own business, and did my time. I didn't feel a yen for heroin, but I came directly to methadone when I got out—I feared that I might go back to heroin. A lady professor who was doing a research project at the prison took an interest in me and told me about methadone. She gave me a letter of referral. And when I came out of Matteawan, that was it. I never looked back again, never used heroin again. I got on methadone, and I've never had a dirty urine.

I don't have a private pension. When I left the hospital after eleven years they gave me a large sum of money, a kind of settlement. I used some of that to put stones on my mother's and father's graves. But they don't send me any more money now.

EMANON

"Emanon" was born in Washington, D.C., in 1923. He was the only child in a relatively prosperous black family. Both of his parents worked, and his father had a lucrative bootlegging business on the side. Although Emanon's mother was a disciplinarian who "thought ass-whipping was the answer," she was unable to keep him in school and off the streets.

I dropped out of the tenth grade. After I left school I did nothing. I hung out. I was a bum. Then I got pushed by my mother, who said, "If you're not going to school, you're going to have to go to work." So I got a job working at a homeopathic hospital in D.C., working as a porter. The job paid ten dollars a week. Some weeks I lied to my mother about what I got paid: I'd say, "I broke something on the job and had to pay for it, so I only have X number of dollars this week." She'd say, "Well, if that's all you got, keep it," and she'd give me a lecture about breaking things. All the time I had the money anyway. This was so I could go out with the fellows and ball.

My old man had bought me a car, a used Oldsmobile. I wasn't old enough to drive it myself. But I had a friend who drove—all my friends were older than me. This friend was my chauffeur. But I'd also drive myself: I'd wait until my old man was asleep, steal into the house, get the keys, and drive around. Having a car made me somebody special in the neighborhood. I'd pick up girls, you know, and screw them, even though I was only thirteen or fourteen. I was doing the same thing that guys in high school and older were doing. There used to be a taxi stand two blocks from my house. We'd sit down and listen to the older guys' conversations. Most of it was about numbers, horses, or screwing some broad. We'd get that information and we'd try to practice it.

This porter job was full-time employment. But, before Pearl Harbor, someone told me that they were giving examinations for apprentice machinists at the naval gun factory in Washington, D.C. If I took the exam, maybe I could get a better job. Well, I took the exam and I passed, and everybody was cheering and slapping me on the back. "Wow, man," they said. It made me think I was one of the luckiest people alive.

I went there and I stayed about a year. The prejudices were terrible. I was the only black in my section, and there were only about four black apprentices in the whole navy yard. The first day there I was introduced to the quarterman, and my immediate foreman, and the guys I was going to work with. There was a white machinist, a big guy with bib overalls who came over to me. He said, "Hey, what's your name." In my neighborhood I had a nickname, and everybody who knew me would call me by my nickname. Everybody I wanted to be friendly with, I would tell them my nickname. But the way he came to me, and his being white, I was apprehensive—I suspicioned something. So I told him my full name. He said, "Naw, I don't want to know that. I want to know what they call ya." That kind of fucked me up. Like, I'm black, I got to have a name other than my real name. He had a southern drawl too—he was a typical redneck. I said, "Well, I've got one of those nicknames," and I told him what it was.

Then he asked me if I could dance the jig. I told him no. He said, "You mean you can't dance the jig?" I said, "Naw, what is the jig?" I knew—in fact, I used to want to be a dancer—but I told him I didn't know what it was. He said, "You know, butt dancing." Now I figured I had him. I said, "No, I don't, but I tell you what, I'm pretty agile and pretty athletic. I believe I could if I wanted to, if I tried. How do you do it?" So he showed me. While he was showing me, I was clapping out the time, helping him along. There was a circle of white guys around us, and a couple of blacks. At first they were getting a kick out of it. Then they realized that I had switched roles on him, and the expressions on their faces started to change. I remember this very distinctly: their expressions were starting to change. So I said, "Naw, man, I don't think I could do that," and I turned and walked away. The redneck didn't know what he had done to himself. He didn't know what he had allowed me to do to him either. But the rest of the people seemed to be aware. I even heard a guy say, "Goddam it, he made him dance. He was the one supposed to be dancing. He's a dumb motherfucker." [Laughs.]

By the way, I grew to like this guy. I learned a lot from him. I was put to work alongside him. We started talking, and I found that he had done this out of ignorance. He wasn't vicious, didn't mean to be vicious. He said that in the part of Carolina he came from, this is what it was about. He said he thought blacks enjoyed doing this for white people. Then he told me how poor he was. He was far more poor than me, and he caught hell for being a poor white in his section of the country, just like blacks caught hell for being black, no matter what. He had wanted to be a professional football player, and he had wanted to go to school, and all these things, but he wasn't allowed to because he was poor white trash. I could relate to him, and we got to be very good friends. In fact, he was the only white person I worked with during this time, other than some youngsters, who invited me to his home to meet his wife and family. I thought that was quite a thing. The guy was for real.

I also hung out with some younger white guys. They were both Jewish. One had come down from Brooklyn; the other was a Washingtonian. We liked the same things as far as music was concerned: the Basie Band, and things like that. Zoot suits were in, and the guys were wearing their hair long—not so long as it is now, but then if you had hair on your neck it was supposed to be disgracefully long. The zoot suits had full pant legs that tapered around the knee. The pants were, say, thirty-something in the knee and maybe sixteen at the cuff. The coat was long, and some guys who really went for it had big lapels and big hats and chains that hung down below their coats. I think I had two zoot suits myself, although they were kind of moderate, not too zooty.

These two white guys I hung out with were trying to duck the draft. We had a little song:

I got a job on the fence, baby, not because I need the money,
I got a job on the fence, babe, not because I need the money,
I got a job on the fence because I want to duck the draft—and that ain't funny.

We used to sing that around. It turned out, though, that I later went into the service. I lost my job because I was fooling around. I was doing OK the first year. I passed. But the second year, I started drinking, smoking a little more pot, chasing a few more broads. I was coming to work after I'd been up till four o'clock in the morning. I couldn't keep up with my studies—and I was getting help, too, from my white friends. So I lost the job.

I went to work for a carpet company, washing and delivering carpets. Then I went and joined the army when I was about twenty. I knew that I was going to be drafted soon. I was also tired, and I saw myself going toward trouble. My mother was always on me about my behavior, and I knew that I needed discipline. I thought that I could get it in the army. My mother said, "For God's sake, when you go into the army behave yourself, because if you don't you're going to end up in a federal penitentiary." I promised her that I would do things right, and I was serious.

I liked the army except for the prejudices. I got my basic training at Aberdeen Proving Grounds in Maryland. I was working on guns, light artillery mounts from mortars to seventy-five millimeters. That came easy to me, because at the naval gun factory I had worked on antiaircraft gun mounts, so I knew some of the theory and principles involved. While I was there, this white instructor took a special interest in me. I was working hard. I had said to myself, "This time I'm really going to give it a try." The instructor called me aside one day, and said he wanted to know what school I had attended. I told him, and he said he'd never heard of it. I said, "Maybe not, it's just a high school." He said, "How much physics did you have?" I said, "Listen, man, I don't even know what physics is." He said, "You're right up there with these other guys who've gone to Rensselaer Polytech. I'm going to talk to your company commander and see if I can't get you to stay over and go to cadre school." I felt good about this: I was doing something. But they wouldn't allow it. They'd had a black cadre school, but they'd cut it out, and they wouldn't put me in a cadre school with white guys. That really fucked me up.

I had this buddy whose attitude was just about the same. He had been working at the arsenal in Springfield, Massachusetts, and they wouldn't let him into cadre school either. But we were made promises that we'd be made noncoms—that's noncommissioned officers—because we had been trained in Aberdeen, and we were qualified because of what we knew about maintaining and correcting the malfunctions of weapons. Then we were shipped to Kentucky, and they didn't have any black ordinance men—the ordinance companies were all white. We were given something manual to do, lifting boxes of ammunition. That just added fuel to what we already felt. We felt that we'd always be treated as niggers, no matter what kind of effort we made. So I went to war with the army. [Laughs.] I'd fuck 'em any time I could—if I got a weekend pass, I'd come in late, or I'd needle certain noncommissioned officers. I didn't get into too much trouble, just some extra duty.

It turned out that I was never shipped to Europe. I got out of the army because I had ligament problems with my left knee. I had this condition before, but I think it had gotten worse. So I was discharged medically: I was only in the army six months and ten days.

I went back to my old neighborhood in Washington and started to write numbers. I didn't work too hard at it; I only made about thirty dollars a day. I was afraid to take too much, because I had no bankroll. I had no way of paying anybody if they hit. I thought, "I'll write some numbers for a while, and back them. And if somebody hits, then I'll go and take a trip to my aunt in San Jose or my godfather in New York." As luck had it, nobody really hit in the three months I wrote numbers. I would take the money I collected and gamble with it at night, or maybe buy some pot and some coke. Then I just quit the numbers. I never was much on finishing anything—I don't care how good it was.

I took an examination and got a job in the Justice Department. It turned out that I worked there eighteen years: I started off as a messenger, and then became a clerk in the civil division. I began work in December of 1944. Six months later I got married, in June of 1945. My son was born in December of 1945. You see, I'd already made my wife pregnant before I married her.

By this time I was using heroin—I was about twenty-two years old when I first started. I was a weekend user for a couple of years. I had pretty good control—I thought I did anyway. The heroin was only a dollar and a half a cap. But then I found out that I couldn't function without it. It was always, like, feeling bad, or anticipating going to cop or to get a shot. By this time I was shooting the heroin. I was doing it more frequently, and I was told by the people I was using with, "Man, it's better to shoot it. It's better, it's cheaper, it won't take as much, and you get high quicker." These people were mostly working people, working for the federal government.

By this time my second child, a daughter, had been born. I had to account for the rent and the other necessities of a family. I was earning fourteen hundred and forty dollars a year, and I was spending about three dollars a day on heroin. I'd shoot up twice a day, morning and evening. I kept my works wrapped in paper, hidden in the house. I'd wash them out good with warm water after I used them. Sometimes I'd use alcohol, but very seldom, because it was a hurried thing with me. I was usually on the run, because I was trying to keep my habit from my family and I was trying to get to work.

If I didn't get my morning shot, I'd take a long lunch period, sometimes three hours. I'd be looking for heroin. I'd buy it up around Seventh and T Streets, and later Fourteenth Street, in North West; sometimes in North East. I knew from somebody else who was OK and who wasn't. I'd buy from guys with good reputations. Believe it or not, there was more honor among users then. If you were short of money in the morning, and if you were a regular, the guy would give you your shot and say, "Man, bring my money back tonight like you said."

But the price started going up: two dollars a cap, three dollars a cap. Then caps started getting scarce, and you had to buy bags. Let's see, it was in the sixties that the caps disappeared. To meet expenses I got a part-time job, doing janitorial work in buildings. Then I started subcontracting myself, as an individual, for janitorial work. I also turned my car into a taxi. I was hacking, doing janitorial work, and working at the Department of Justice—and just making ends meet.

There was one break in my use of heroin. At one point I stopped using for two years. I got into religion, into Islam. I was hooked up with a sect that came out of Pakistan. I attended a meeting of the Black Muslims, but I didn't like it because it reminded me of fascism turned backwards, of fascism in a different color. If we did as the Black Muslims taught us, the world wouldn't be any better. Maybe the blacks would be able to thrive for a certain length of time, but we'd be doing what the white people had already done, so what's the use? It would be the same condition with another kind of person in trouble, and I couldn't buy that.

I didn't make my family convert to Islam. My wife came in, but my children, I just exposed them to it and said I'd like them to be in it, but that they could go to other churches. "Go to Greek Orthodox," I said, "Go anywhere you want, but I want you to compare. You're supposed to be the one to select this kind of thing." But they went to services with me all of the time when I'd go to the mosque. They would participate in fasting periods on a small scale—for a day they'd fast for the hell of it. Things were good for that two years. I was abstaining from heroin. I was doing the things that were prescribed, but then I rebelled against the discipline. One day I just decided I wanted to shoot some drugs, and I started using again.

All the while I was using, I never went to the hospital for detox. I was afraid. You see, nobody in my family knew, and my employer didn't know. My wife didn't notice any needle marks because they never showed. Even now you can see that I'm hardly scarred at all. I was careful, I used sharp needles, and for some reason I didn't scar badly. I'd nod out sometimes, but I'd take a pint of whiskey or wine and gargle with it, to be sure she smelled the alcohol. It seemed like drinking to her. And I didn't lose interest in sex while I was on heroin. In fact, [laughs] I think maybe I was on my wife too much, you know. It wasn't until my forties that I lost interest in sex—and not completely then.

But she eventually found out. One day, my habit was really getting the best of me. This was in the early 1960s, when Kennedy was president. I was using maybe about twelve dollars a day. My wife was sick: she was worrying about how I had started getting sloppy with paying bills, and she got an ulcer. This was getting to me, so I took the day off from my job. I decided to do some painting in the house, and I had on my paint clothes. I saw some addicts, a girl and three guys. They didn't work, though I was on a friendly basis with them. There was a near-panic in the city at this time. I asked them, "Where is it?" They said they were looking for the guy now, and asked if I wanted to walk with them. I said, "Yeah." My wife was used to my saying, "I'm going to go get a pack of cigarettes," getting in the car, and then she wouldn't see me for four, six, seven hours, or maybe longer than that. So, to give her some comfort, I decided to leave the car at home. I'd go and catch the bus and then walk over to the part of town where I'd find the junkies hanging out.

I went with them. We were walking around, looking for this guy with the heroin. As we were crossing the street, a car stopped at the intersection and the driver called the group over to him. I suspected it was the police. I kept walking, as if I wasn't one of the group. I started thinking, "I'm dressed shabby enough to be one of them, but I'll ignore it." But the cop called me: "I'm talking to you too." I pretended that he was crazy, that I didn't know him. By this time I knew he was a cop, because of the conversation he was having with the other four, who were known addicts. He said, "What's your name?" I said, "Well, why do you want to know?" I tried to play it like I was indignant. He said, "I want to know because you're with them." I said, "No, I was just walking along with them on this block, and then I was going over to Fourteenth Street." He said, "No, we've been trailing you for about ten minutes, and you've been with them, and that by the way you were behaving, and your conversation, that you know them."

At that time they had a "narc-vag" law in Washington. If two or more addicts got together, they could arrest you. And we were together. The cop said to me, "I've never seen you before." Another cop said, "Ah, I think we've got a fresh one. C'mon you, roll up your sleeves." I rolled them up, and he saw tracks—even though my wife hadn't been able to see any there. Then he said, "Let's see some I.D." Well, the only I.D. I had was in my wallet, with my Department of Justice pass. They saw the pass. The cop said, "Well, Jesus Christ, look what we got here. This *is* an extraordinary one. This guy works for the Department of Justice, down there with Brother Hoover." They cracked up at this; it was funny to everybody but me. I said, "Hey, man, what does this mean? Are you guys going to have me lose my job? I got a wife, two kids. I haven't been using too long, I'm trying to get myself together. This won't help me any. Don't tell anybody." So they didn't arrest me. They didn't arrest the other guys either. But they said, "If we ever catch you again, we're going to bust you."

This happened on a Thursday. I was shook by it, but I went to work on Friday and nothing happened. Everything was cool. But on Monday, when I came back from lunch, there was a note on my typewriter saying that the administrative assistant and I were supposed to meet in the assistant attorney general's office. Now it was, like, "Wow, since when did the assistant attorney general want to see me? What is this all about?"

The time came. The administrative assistant, who was a very good friend of mine, had been called to another meeting, so she couldn't be there. I saw the assistant attorney general alone. He started talking to me about my being approached by narcotic agents who said that I was a user. He said, "I'm going to tell you that the administrative assistant told me this couldn't be true. She said the agents were lying, and that she knew you well enough that you couldn't be an addict or a user." I told the assistant attorney general, "I'm sorry to disappoint the administrative assistant, but this is true." I was tired and, in a way, I was glad that it had happened.

He talked to me for an hour and a half. I was amazed that he would spend so much time with me, holding all calls and everything. He said, "You know, you handle confidential mail and things like that. If you're addicted, we can't keep you working here. But the way the administrative assistant talks, she thinks you're a good person. Did you ever think of going for the cure?" I said, "Yeah." He wanted to know why I hadn't, and I told him, "I got these people dependent on me, and my wife doesn't know anything about it." He said, "I understand you have a taxicab too. How do you do it? You've got three jobs—how can you handle this one?" I said, "Well, I do it." He said, "Well, I'll tell you what, let me see what I can do."

He called up HEW and talked to someone he knew, who connected him with somebody else. They suggested I go to K.Y. I said, "No, man, I don't want to do that. Is there anyplace I can go into treatment in this area?" He talked some more and was told, "Yeah, there is a doctor who is very competent who has a program at D.C. General Hospital." I accepted that. I said, "Yeah, I'll go there." I came back to my office, gave away some things on my desk, and then I just left. I didn't tell anyone that I had resigned. The assistant attorney general told me, "You have to resign, but when you finish this treatment, you can come back and get your job back, if what the doctor has to say is favorable." I said OK—what else could I do?

Now I had to go home and tell my wife. She was fucked up, man. Boy, was she fucked up. She wanted to know how I could deceive her all those years. She threw things at me like, "I've been getting in bed with you every night. I had your children. You did this and didn't tell me about it! You kept it from me." I felt like a pile of shit naturally. She was crying, and the whole thing. I told the children too. They were broken up, because they never pictured me as an addict, you know. I told them what I knew about addiction and that a lot of what they'd heard about the behavior of addicts was old wives' tales. If drugs would have been accessible, this never would have happened. If I could have gone into a place and gotten the drug legally, I could have functioned on the job—because I was a functioner, in spite of my use. Very seldom did I nod out, because I didn't take that much. Like, if I bought more than I thought I could handle, I wouldn't shoot it all up.

I was in treatment for three months. They withdrew me with Dolophine. Then they had rap sessions in the hospital, and sessions with the psychologist and psychiatrist. We also helped keep the unit clean. I used smuggled drugs on occasion, about four times while I was in treatment. When I came out my wife was warned by the doctor in charge to watch out for me, because, if I could keep my habit from her for that number of years, I could do it again maybe. He told her what to watch for, the dilated pupils and other symptoms of being high.

I knew in my belly that I wasn't ready to stop using. But I went back to the Justice Department. The doctor there was very biased; he really didn't want me back anyway. He looked at my arm to see if there were any fresh needle marks. That he didn't see. He told me to come back, he wanted to follow up on me for a couple of weeks, to see how I was doing on the street. But I said, "Fuck it, I ain't going back." I could have gotten back though.

With the little money I had left I got back my cab from the taxi people. And I started shooting again, sometimes heroin, sometimes Dilaudid. The Dilaudid was cheaper. My wife didn't know right away, but she caught on because there wasn't any money. I had to lie about the money I was making from the hack. We could have lived off the money I made from the hack, if I didn't have to support a habit. And I'd given up on the subcontracting job. I wasn't motivated to that extent anymore. The last job of any substance I had was with the Washington Urban League, about '64 or '65, I guess. I was a community organizer. They didn't know I was addicted, but a co-worker told them I was. I was confronted by the director, and she told me she couldn't have it. So I was back into the street.

It was about this time that I was forced into stealing. I stole out of my own house; I sold just about everything in it that there was to sell. I tried to shoplift—"boost," they call it in the street. I was a terrible booster, but I made out, you know, for some years. I was arrested once for petty larceny and one time for burglary. And then I sold Dilaudid and heroin for a while, about five years.

My wife? She became my ex-wife in 1966. We separated and were divorced. I deserted her, you might say. In spite of everything, this woman was waiting for me to straighten up. She was still fixing my meals, and waiting for me to come home, and all that shit. I just got sick of myself, real sick, you know. I wasn't doing anything, but she was still going through these changes like I was doing something. So one day I just walked out of the house.

LOW

One way around the problem of bad and expensive heroin was to leave the United States and go directly to the source. Low had an occupation that permitted him to do just that. Born in San Juan, Puerto Rico, in 1922, he was brought to the United States at the age of five. Low was one of three children, each with a different father. He regarded his stepfather, a merchant seaman, as his real father. "He was very good to me . . . I used to call him 'Pop.' " Low went as far as the tenth grade in a vocational high school, then dropped out to look for work.

I was brought up in New York City, Spanish Harlem, 110th Street, 111th Street, and Fifth Avenue. The neighborhood was full of prostitutes; nothing but pimps, thieves, pickpockets, and a few bootleggers. Ninety-nine percent of the people who lived there were Puerto Rican. There were very few Cubans, they were on Lenox Avenue. We had gangs—mine was the Dukes, the Puerto Rican Dukes. We had the Devils, the Madison Flashers. . . . Anytime we had a fight with blacks, we used to send word to the other groups that we were in trouble, and they would come over with baseball bats and we'd go and beat up the blacks. Or the Jews— when I was very young, my neighborhood was predominantly Jewish, and we fought against them. Then the Jews started to move to the Bronx, they went away fast, around 1930, '31. Then the blacks started coming in and we fought them. We fought with the Italians too. We couldn't go across Lexington Avenue, we couldn't go to their Jefferson Park swimming pool because they'd knock our brains out. And they couldn't come over across Lexington because we'd beat them up. Nobody ever crossed over and made friends. Never. They didn't want nothing to do with us, and we didn't have nothing to do with them.

I started smoking marijuana when I was about seventeen. There was a lot of it in the area, and it was cheap. We used to get seven joints for a dollar. A package of twenty-five cost two dollars. We all used to smoke pot and drank a lot of white port wine—it cost a quarter. This wasn't accepted by the, uh, lower middle class. If you smoked marijuana, they'd stay away from you. They'd say, "Oh, that guy, he smokes marijuana! Don't mess around with him." We'd hide the marijuana from the police, anytime we'd see a policeman we'd throw it away or swallow it, so we wouldn't be caught with it in our possession. The people who distributed the marijuana were all Puerto Rican and colored. Guys who worked on boats brought it in from Mexico. Then it would go through the vine: one guy would buy a pound and he'd make joints out of it, a thousand joints. A pound used to cost about fifteen dollars, and he'd make about one hundred and fifty dollars on a pound. That's how it got around.

We feared heroin addicts. We'd tell them, "We don't want no junkies around here. Get out of here!" and we'd throw them off the block. These were mainly young boys, Spanish boys in the eighteen, nineteen bracket. I used to see them turning into bums, being all dirty. Guys who were pimps, dressing good—and all of a sudden they'd be raggedy.

I went into the merchant marine when I was nineteen, then the war broke out. We were carrying soldiers and supplies and ammunition to the battlefields, and for the invasion of Sicily. I'd smoke pot on the ships —lots of the crew smoked, I'd say about 40 percent. The ships were all integrated: I met a lot of southerners, white guys from Texas who smoked pot. It was common. I'd get it in Casablanca or I'd stock up right here in New York, an ounce for five dollars. And in Le Havre, during the invasion, the Moors sold us marijuana. Pot and champagne: a very good high.

I stayed in the merchant marine after the war. I made a living out of it. I got married in 1944—my wife is Puerto Rican, of Spanish stock. We moved up to the lower Bronx in 1945. It's all desolated now. This place they talk so much about, Fort Apache, that's where I was. But it was nice when I moved there. You slept on the fire escape, left your doors open, no dope. It was Spanish, Jewish—you know, integrated. People would be playing dominoes on the street, drinking beer on the stoops. Everybody would go to work, it was working-class people. Then it got flooded with dope. When the junkies started to invade the place, people started closing their doors, putting on three locks, buying dogs. I got robbed three times, right in the apartment where I lived. I knew they were junkies. One time a guy in the pawn shop pulled out a coat that was robbed from me. He wanted to sell it to me, but I said, "Hey, that's my coat!" [Laughs.] He gave it back to me.

I started using heroin in 1949 when I came off the ship. I used to go into this bar on 111th Street with lots of money—"Set 'em up," I'd say. This colored guy was watching me. He said, "Try this, try this. Man, this'll give you a high you'll never forget." He was giving samples away, five-dollar bags. He knew I had money. He wanted to get me hooked. He'd put an ashtray on the table, full, and say, "Here, here, getcha higher —that whiskey'll kill ya." So I sniffed it. I started to vomit, vomit. I said, "I'm not going to use that stuff, that stuff makes me vomit." But after the vomiting you feel a sensation that no other high like marijuana or liquor can give you. You just sit down. You'll be asleep, but you'll be hearing everything that's going on. You'll be noting what's going on, but you can be sitting there like a mummy.

I kept on using the heroin, but I kept on working too. I worked as a ship's waiter until I retired, in 1968. I used to make over five thousand a year, a lot of it in tips. My wife got an allotment from the company to keep up the house. She always worked too: factories, pots and pans, assembly lines. I was away at sea twenty-two days at a time. I would get heroin here in New York, an ounce would cost me three hundred dollars, and last till, say, Casablanca.

On the twelfth day, when we hit Genoa, I'd buy a fifty-dollar bag of *pure* heroin. I used to cut it ten times. It would last me until I got back to New York. I'd buy it in a Puerto Rican bar in Genoa—yeah, in Genoa. [Laughs.] The guy who ran it was Italian. He used to sell you square match boxes full, pressed down. I'd buy about five of them, for a hundred dollars. Then I'd spread it out on a mirror and get *manita*, a cutting agent: a spoon of the pure stuff and four spoons of *manita*. I had other connections too. I used to get it from a woman, an Italian prostitute, whose husband worked on a boat. He'd bring it in from the Middle East, and that's one of the three best heroins money can buy—Turkish, Hong Kong, and Vietnamese. And we'd buy heroin in Beirut, Lebanon, when we'd go there once a year on fifty-two-day cruises—we'd hit all of North Africa and then come back through the underbelly of Europe. When we hit Beirut, everybody'd be ready. The change in money was five for one; I'd say for a dollar, you'd get about a ten-dollar bag. Pure heroin. I'd speak in French to the guy, "*Vingt-cinq dollars donnes moi*"—give me a twenty-five-dollar bag. Then I'd cut it, and it would last me to New York, and back to Italy.

When we got back in New York we'd only stay twenty-four hours. The next day, twelve noon, we'd be pulling out, back to the same run: Gibraltar, Casablanca, Italy, Spain, the Azores . . . If I had enough heroin left, I wouldn't buy it in New York. If I needed something, I would. There was a panic in nineteen-fifty-something, but I never went through it, because I bought in Italy. But I kept very quiet about it, because if I said something about my heroin, everybody would know it. Everybody'd be running around New York—you should have seen the panic. [Laughs.] It was like the country was in chaos, you know? You'd see groups of people, twenty-five, fifty junkies running from one block to another, saying, "Oh, they've got some up on 125th Street!" Then people would run up to 125th; when they'd get there, it was already finished. "Hey, they've got some on 110th Street." People just running . . . I used to say, "What the hell's wrong with the police? Don't they see these things?"

When I'd buy it in New York, I'd go straight to a guy I knew, Moe. He was Jewish. He was from the Bronx, but he would come into 116th Street to sell. I'd call him on the phone, "Look, I want to see you." He knew what I wanted, and he'd have it ready for me. I'd have the money for him—sometimes I didn't even have to give him the money, he'd tell me, "Pay me later." He was a very good friend of mine. We grew up together in Spanish Harlem—his was one of the few Jewish families that stayed there. He used to speak Spanish. If you spoke to him you thought he was Puerto Rican instead of Jewish. He died of an overdose.

On ship I'd take the heroin and tie it up in a brown cellophane bag, put it inside a bottle, seal it with candle wax so air wouldn't get in, and stash it in my mattress. The mattress is the only place customs wouldn't look, because they couldn't break anything that would cost the company money to repair. They could unscrew things, search me, search my shoes, and that was it. You see, the thing was, if you got caught with heroin, they'd confiscate your seaman's papers. But I was never caught, never arrested. I didn't have marks. Anytime I was in a roundup, they'd check my arms. I'd say, "I'm not a junkie. I haven't got a mark. I never inject." So they let me go. My membranes they never checked. My membranes are okay, because I didn't cut with quinine. I didn't like it. One time I tried it with quinine and it stuffed my nose up. It used to kill me. Anytime anybody sold me anything with quinine, I'd take it right back. I'd put a gun at his head: "Give me back my money or I'll blow your brains out!" I used to get my money back. You had to be tough out there. You couldn't be a softie, especially when you were dealing with junkies. I wouldn't hang out with them. In the heroin business, they'll fuck you in a minute. A heroin addict will go and fuck his mother.

My habit cost me about three thousand dollars a year. I could have bought more dope, but I just used enough to get high and fixed, to get straight and work. You couldn't go into a dining room nodding. I'd take a sniff in the morning, twelve o'clock, six, and a sniff before I went to bed. The reason I didn't nod out is that I cut the heroin with sugar milk, and I knew how much to take. I'd put a little on a toothpick that I walked around with and—bing! bing!—that's it, go to work. When I worked I felt nice, I felt fine. After I finished, nine or ten o'clock at night, I would go and take a shower, lay down in my bunk. [Laughs.] This is funny: I used to put a soup plate full of water on top of my chest. I'd be smoking and reading in my bunk. When I nodded, the ashes or the cigarette would fall into the water, so I wouldn't set the goddam place on fire. You smoke a lot when you use heroin—I don't know why.

I would generally snort by myself. I'd go in my room, lock myself up, and do my business. Nobody would be with me. The only guys that used with me were my friends, tight friends that I knew were all right. They were Puerto Rican. Like, we would be going ashore, dressing up, and I'd walk into my best friend's room. I'd say, "C'mon, they're waiting for us outside." He'd say, "Hey, take a couple of snorts before you leave." So I'd take a couple of snorts.

There was a lot of heroin going around. Whoo! I'd say 60 percent of the guys in this company I was working for were junkies. There were lots of alcoholics too; it was about even. I can't say how many of the junkies used the needle, because we had a segregation system. See, if a guy was on the needle, we stayed away from him. We'd say, "Oh, that guy uses the needle! If he gets caught, he'll rat on everybody!" So I only associated with sniffers. But I skin popped one time. I had chipped in to make a buy with some guys who were mainliners. They were on the needle and I wasn't. They took the same needle, burned it with a match, cleaned it with alcohol, and then passed it to the next guy. I just took a little skin pop, but I still contracted something. I looked in the mirror and said, "Hey, I'm yellow." I went to the hospital. They said, "You've got jaundice."

The other seamen who were using like I was all died. One died from a heart attack, another one died from cirrhosis—he got on methadone and turned into a wino. He drank when he took heroin too. His belly popped up like he was nine months pregnant. But I knew of some guys who were addicted who said, "I'm not taking no more stuff," and they stopped completely. They even kicked the methadone habit—they went onto methadone and they detoxified slowly. Now they're leading completely new lives. I envy them. I've never tried to get off methadone.

10.

Creating

Creativity (handwritten)

The relationship between psychoactive substances and creativity is an often-discussed topic, and one that has given rise to a number of theories. Sociologist Charles Winick, for example, has speculated that the progressive cooling of American jazz from Dixieland to swing to bop was related to the musicians' changing preferences for drugs, which moved from alcohol to marijuana to heroin.[1] In the field of American literature, Julie Irwin has reinterpreted F. Scott Fitzgerald's fiction in the light of his deepening alcoholism during the 1920s and 1930s.[2] Although there is no consensus on the extent to which drugs and alcohol shape an artistic work or performance, the question is nevertheless an important one, given the increasingly heavy use by artists and performers during the last hundred years. As early as the 1880s there were reports of spreading opium and morphine use among actors and actresses. During the classic era, narcotic use flourished among both stage and screen stars. Almost from the beginning, Hollywood acquired a reputation as a drug mecca, with scandals marring the careers of such popular entertainers as Wallace Reid, Mabel Normand, Juanita Hansen, Barbara La Marr, Alma Rubens, and, later, Bela Lugosi.[3]

We did not set out to explore the connection between drugs and the performing or literary arts, but it happened that we encountered two individuals, a saxophonist and a dancer, who were professional entertainers of some note. We then spoke with a semiprofessional trumpeter who had played with jazz combos in Harlem in the late 1930s, before dropping out of the music scene to become a full-time hustler. We asked these three men if and how the drugs they used

1. "The Use of Drugs by Jazz Musicians," *Social Problems* 7 (1959–60), 252.

2. "F. Scott Fitzgerald's Little Drinking Problem," *American Scholar* 56 (1987), 415, 418–20, 422–24, 426–27.

3. Kenneth Anger, *Hollywood Babylon* (San Francisco: Straight Arrow Books, 1975), 9–12, 39–40, 49–54, 60, 63–68; Michael Starks, *Cocaine Fiends and Reefer Madness: An Illustrated History of Drugs in the Movies* (New York: Cornwall Books, 1982), 137.

affected their performances, and why they thought entertainers, especially black musicians, became so deeply involved with narcotics. We also met and interviewed a remarkable woman, a jazz afficionada who had been married to a serious jazz collector and later to a world-famous jazz musician. She spoke about the role of drugs in the arts from a different perspective, that of an individual listening to and interpreting a performance. Finally, we asked William S. Burroughs, unquestionably the preeminent drug novelist of the classic era, if he would talk about his life and work. He agreed, and offered several insights, particularly in relation to his first, autobiographical book, Junkie, *published in 1953.*

RED

Red was born into a middle-class black family in Newark, New Jersey, in 1916. In 1939, after a year of college, he dropped out to join a band.

My feature instrument was the tenor saxophone. I play all the saxophones and most reed instruments, but the tenor was my feature. I haven't had an extensive musical education. For instance, I never went to a university or to a musical college or had anything big like that in the way of musical education. But I was thoroughly tutored. I got this right around the corner from where I used to live in Newark, New Jersey. There was a gentleman there, a wonderful man. In fact, he was a Jewish man. He was one of the best saxophonists that I've ever encountered. He was a virtuoso. For many years I had the instrument and was doing things by ear, until somebody said, "Gee, you're doing so much with that, why don't you really go and learn what you're doing?" So I went to him and he took me on for two dollars a lesson. Two dollars a lesson—it meant nothing to him: he just liked doing it. He passed it off to me, one of those kinds of things. He also taught me the rudiments of music. He taught me other instruments —the clarinet, and a little bit of flute—but mostly he acquainted me with the saxophone. It was his instrument, and he said I had a thing for it. I could just pick it up and run over it.

I was fourteen when I started taking lessons. I didn't start when I was a kid. I didn't even know that I wanted to be a musician that early, when I was seven or eight. My parents didn't start me into music. My parents wanted me to be a doctor, a lawyer. My mother and father had higher aspirations for me. And I would have gone into something like that—I was all right in school. But I was gifted with music. It just took me over. I would learn right away. I have a perfect ear: I can pick out a C when you make it and all like that. I can identify any instrument playing. I can go further than that. Like, if I write an arrangement and I'm rehearsing the band and somebody makes a wrong note, I can tell when it was made and who made it, or what instrument.

I took lessons from him for four or five years. By the time I was out of high school, I was actually ready to play, but my mother and father wouldn't let me. Every now and then I used to get to play a job when some of the musicians who wanted me would come by and ask my mother, beg her actually: "I'm going to look out for him tonight." "I'll see that he doesn't get with any women or drink anything." That kind of thing. I got to see a little bit of professionalism that way. That's how I got out into doing it.

In the big bands whole arrangements were put together in an ad lib idiom, little by little, until everybody in that orchestra, fifteen or sixteen, knew an arrangement that wasn't on paper. We could play it. Just knock the time off, and we could play it. People would say, "What are they playing? We're looking at you playing." That became a style of different bands that I went with, to be able to do that. And if you couldn't do that, you had to take the arrangements home and learn them, memorize them, so that we could do that.

I was introduced to heroin in 1955. We were doing what you call a broken engagement. We weren't working steady. We were using San Francisco as a home base. We would go to, like, Oakland and play a date and come back, or go to some other town in California and come back. So, one of the off nights, there were a few fellows up in my hotel room, and we were having a few drinks, and had a few girls, and we were sitting around, and, you know, one thing led to another. Somebody else came in, another friend of a friend, and was introduced to everybody, and he introduced the heroin. Nobody held any handcuffs or any gun on me to force me to take anything—I tried it. I sniffed it and it made me sick as a dog. I was high, but I was so high it made me vomit all over the place. It passed from euphoria, into ecstasy, into something beyond that I couldn't control. It was powerful stuff.

That same evening, after I was left alone in my room, I writhed in the bed. Sleep was out. I could forget about going to sleep—I was miserable! It was twenty times worse than a headache, the worst headache you ever had. I had to hit the air. I had to get out. So I went out of the hotel. I put my key in my pocket, locked my door, went out. I don't know where I walked. I just walked around, down by the waterfront and everywhere. I walked around, trying to get myself back to normal, trying to work it off. I even drank hot coffee. I became so miserable that I just sat down on the curb. The water ran right behind the heels of my shoes. I just sat there, I was so miserable, just praying to God, you know, like you've done something, and you know it's wrong. "Just let me get through this, I'll never do it again"—one of those things. I was sick that whole night and the next day too.

But as soon as I got over that, I wanted to see what it was really like. Everyone had said, "You vomit and everything because your stomach has to get used to it. That happened to most of us the first time. Your second time out is when you really get to know what it's all about." So I wanted to try it again, and the next time I tried it its effects were as everyone had told me it would be. I was immediately hanging in a nod from the sniff. This was very good heroin. In fact it hadn't been cut but two or three times, they said.

I'll try to describe the feeling. I'll give you an example. Say you wake up and you don't feel too well, you're not too spunky—it's just a dry day. You have no desire to do anything or go anywhere. Then you turn on, you sniff a little heroin. Do you know what that does for you? I'll say within twenty minutes you get a *crawling* feeling that comes over you until it enhances your whole body. And then you feel different, you feel good. That's what makes people become subjects of it. If something is hurting you, or you're troubled with something, it makes you feel good: your pain is lessened, your troubles practically leave you—at least the thought of them momentarily leaves you. But I don't have the excuse that "I did it because I was troubled." I just did it, and I liked it.

Heroin didn't change my musical style, though. It had no impact on my playing or my style or anything, except for one major fact. And that was . . . how can I put this, the *desire* to play or to perform. You see, up till this time, when it was time for me to go on, I had to psych myself up to it. I was nervous. "The curtain's getting ready to open now; we're getting ready to do it now"—I had to psych myself up to it. Sometimes, even while on, I was nervous a little because I was aware the public was out there listening to me. Even my solos, my solo work and stuff like that, I would be . . . I had to psych myself up, more or less, to do it. But if you had some heroin in you, you were ready. At all times. You just went on. The heroin took away the stage fright. In fact, it was almost a must to have some.

I think that was the major inducement for so many jazz musicians to use it; that, and the fact of the particular euphoria that it gives you. You know, the fact that you're just overwhelmed at all times. But very coolly and calmly, because it's not an exciting thing like pot would be. I've seen youngsters, and old people too, smoke some pot, and they're all giddy. Scratching themselves, or whatever they're doing: they're racing, and they're talking, and what not. They're pepped up. But heroin is not as spontaneous. It's a quietening thing. Nobody would even know you were in the room, unless they wanted to find you. You conceal yourself.

Marijuana was also very common among musicians in the big bands.

In all bands, in all categories. Marijuana to me is just like a next-door neighbor. I've been aware of marijuana, known all about it, most of my life. I was introduced to it, I guess, my first job out with a little hometown band. If somebody had some and would offer me some, I'd smoke it. Fine. I'd get high, have a good time. When it was over, that's all. There was no more. I might not have it again for two months.

Alcohol was also common. But drinking with musicians is mostly sociable. In fact, I don't think I've ever known an alcoholic musician. You know, an alcoholic: what I know alcoholism to be.

Cocaine? Oh, yes. Along the way with heroin, I've been introduced to cocaine. But cocaine you can put in the same classification—at least I always did—as marijuana. It's not habit-forming; it's not addictive. When you have some cocaine, fine. Beautiful. But it's a short-lived euphoria. It doesn't last long. I used cocaine lots of times when I was performing. Even speedballs. I used to mix it with the heroin and snort it. I learned to do that from other addicts I saw mix it with their speedballs when they shot themselves. Cocaine is a lot more expensive than heroin. So when you mixed some cocaine with heroin, it was done sparingly.

All I ever did was snort. I never did skin pop, or never did spike—shoot it into my vein. I've always been deathly afraid of needles. So that kept me away—it almost kept me away from the heroin, because at first I thought you had to put it in you through a needle. That night when I was introduced to it, my friends said, "No, you don't have to use a needle. You sniff it up through your nose. Just sniff it like this." Somebody did and I said, "Yeah?" That's when I tried it. Sniffing served as the answer for me.

But it absolutely ate my membranes out. As many years as I've been unaddicted, I have no membrane between the two sides of my nose. They're absolutely eaten out, and I would like to say this to anybody that ever thinks about sniffing: do not do that! Do not put it in your nose and think that you're beating it, because it will eat your membranes out. And not only that, if you're not fortunate enough to get off it fast enough, it will eat your nose up. It will eat it off your face.

OTHA

The youngest of thirteen children, Otha was born into a black family in Memphis, Tennessee, in 1918. He was a precocious dancer at a time when dancing still commanded a wide popular audience. Although he began injecting heroin in 1935, he did not become addicted until 1946. He used only semi-regularly during the 1930s, and not at all between 1941 and 1945, when he was on tour for the U.S.O.

My mother taught me how to dance. Steps had names in those days. In 1922, when I was four, she taught me how to do the Black Bottom.[4] That's the first step I ever learned. She danced too. She was five-three, and weighted a hundred and fifteen. I used to take her to dances—she was the only one I could waltz with. The average kid don't like waltzes, but I did.

When I was a child, I always had a dream of seeing my name in lights on Broadway. And it happened. We had a theater in Memphis called the Palace Theater, on Beale Street. Butterbeans and Susie[5] had a show that week and on Wednesday, amateur night, I won first prize. I was eleven years old. That was 1929. My mother hollered out in the theater, "That's my boy." Then Susie said, "Who's that hollering out there, kid?" I said, "That's my mother." She said, "Call her backstage. I want to talk to her." Butterbeans and Susie got permission from my mother to take me with them. They had a tutor that was teaching their daughter. Their daughter was a contortionist—she was in my age bracket: she was eleven herself. Her name was Margaret. I learned along with her. I got as far as the eleventh grade. So I had my schooling; my mother found that out before I left. She said, "Will he still get his schooling?" They said yes. I grew up in Chicago. I lived with them in a home on the South Side.

I was in Chicago until 1939. I met another kid; he was a dancer too. We did an amateur program at the Regal Theater in Chicago. That's on the South Side. First prize was fifty dollars. The m.c. at that amateur program was also a booking agent, which I didn't know. After the show, he held his hands over the contestants' heads, and the audience applauded. The other kid's name was Johnny. Johnny and I got the same amount of applause. So he gave Johnny the fifty dollars and he said, "I'm going in my pocket and give Otha fifty dollars too. And I want both of you boys to come down to my office Monday morning and I'm going to put you together." That's what he did. We called ourselves Otha 'n' Johnny.[6]

Now I envisioned that after we got together, Otha 'n' Johnny would be in New York. But they needed a dance team in Detroit. They had a new club opening in Detroit called the Club Zombie, on the North End. So this booking agent sent us there—this was in '39. Midwestern dancers don't dance like eastern boys. A midwest dancer, he attacks a step. An eastern boy, he just slides—like Fred Astaire, he caresses a step. A midwest boy like myself, he'll *hit* it, he'll *get* it, like he's fighting. That's

4. A popular 1920s dance featuring sinuous hip movements and rocking steps. The term "black bottom" originally referred to the low-lying black residential district common to many southern towns.

5. A husband and wife comedy act popular on the black vaudeville circuit.

6. "Johnny" is an alias. Johnny died in 1946 of an overdose.

the difference: people like that aggressive style. We went to Detroit with a two-week option and we stayed two years.

I started messing with drugs in 1935 with five or six other dancers. They were mostly addicted. I mainlined the first time. It made me sick, very ill. I thought I'd be through with it after that, but I wasn't. In the theatrical world you cannot drink and dance. Your balance is thrown off. Alcohol . . . it don't mix. But you can shoot stuff, smoke pot, use coke, and you can still dance right.

The heroin was just something to stay in with the in-crowd. Either you did it, or you were out. These were top musicians. One band leader was very famous. There was a male vocalist who was very famous—still is —and another female vocalist, she's very famous too. All of these people were using H at the time. Why do I think so many black musicians used heroin? Escape. They tried to escape.

As a matter of fact, we interviewed another person who was a very well-known jazz musician, who played in a big band. He said to us that the thing about heroin was that he did not feel nervous. Before he started using heroin, he always had butterflies in his stomach when the curtain went up. After he started using heroin, they weren't there. Do you buy that?

Yes, I buy that description. When you're dancing when you're high, you're more relaxed. You can feel your audience. I mean, there's a certain vibration that comes from the audience to you across the footlights; you're more relaxed and you work harder for them. I'd break a leg for an audience like that.

During this period I'd always speedball, unless you couldn't get the coke. If you couldn't get the coke then you'd use the heroin by itself, and you'd smoke you a joint. It's almost the same reaction, although the speedball is better, because both products are going through the bloodstream. It's very relaxing. I speedballed before I performed, definitely. In the dressing room, just fifteen or seventeen minutes before you were going on stage, that's when you'd take off. When the band played your introduction, the product got a hold of you then. You were ready to go on, yes indeedy.

WEST INDIAN TOM

Born in Trinidad in 1925, West Indian Tom came with his family to Harlem in 1929. Although his father died when he was four, he was well provided for.

Most kids in the street come from broken homes. But West Indian people are like Jews and Italians: they're very firm on their family, they keep them together. I never missed a plate of food or went with holes in my shoes. I come from a very good, spiritual home.

I don't think there was a better place in the world for people to live than Harlem when I was a child. Harlem was known as "the place of gay feet." You had speakeasies, one on every corner; you had all sorts of nightclubs. All your rich white people used to come from downtown to uptown. They had the Cotton Club, the Savoy Ballroom—oh, God, they had so many different places where people could come and enjoy themselves. What really turned Harlem out bad was, as soon as the war started and they started letting the men and women from the southern states come for better jobs and for more advantages, they began to bring their bad elements with them. Like, the crimes they committed down South and the way they lived down South, they brought all that back up here with them.

But before the war Harlem was a beautiful place. You didn't have too much of that, uh—I want to find the correct word, because this is my first time talking to you—you didn't find that *prejudice* thing that you have now. You see, now you can actually feel it in the air, you can sense it. You could be walking down the street and see me and another man standing on the corner, and the first thing that will come to the average white man's mind is, "Oh, let me be careful, they might want to rob me." This is the thing that's in the air. Everybody can sense it. But there wasn't that much hostility back then, definitely not. That hostility came after the war.

I started using heroin when I was about thirteen or fourteen. I was hanging out with a bunch of musicians at the time, because I played a trumpet. Started when I was ten or eleven. You couldn't say I play it now, but I can hit the notes. Anyway, I was hanging out with a bunch of musicians. Everybody wanted to be Charlie Parker or somebody. I got heroin from one of the musicians in the combo I was playing with. It was very strong. At the time there was no such thing as heroin being white. The heroin was the color of my skin, very dark brown. It came in a number five capsule, the smallest capsule they have. It was only a quarter, or fifty cents.

At that time, to be a real solid jazz musician, you had to be into *something*, and whiskey wasn't it. And reefer was secondary, reefer was like for kids. The heavy guys that really knew their music didn't mess with no reefer. Half of them didn't even mess with morphine. They messed with coke, or heroin. They thought that was the thing to give them more of a drive. Most people did it for the drive that they would get out of it. They would be able to play more way-out music.

You take this guy that died, John Lennon. When they questioned him several years back, he told them he got a feeling from the stuff that he was using that gave him a different sensation, that the crowd didn't bother him. In other words, like he could wrap himself up in his music so deeply that he didn't even pay any mind to the people who were out there hollerin' and screamin' at him. This was a reason why he used drugs. You see, everybody you ask might have a different opinion on why they do certain things.

Do you think that getting away from the crowd was a reason applicable to the people that you knew, or to you yourself?

They used it to be, I guess, more noticeable. Their playing? It was good. They played very good—to me, because I guess I was on the same kick. Look at Billie Holiday: she went out there and sang her heart out. And on a lot of Billie Holiday's records, if you listen to them, you can tell that that woman was high. She missed notes, her voice got flat in certain parts. You've heard her records: you know yourself that on some parts you can tell that she's high, because she'd just go out of the pitch altogether —it seems like somebody's touching her—and then she'd come back in again.

Those were her late records, not the early ones.

Yes. On the early records she was, well, more of a lady. They should have called her "Lady Day" then, not later.

ANN

Ann was introduced to opium in 1942 by her second husband, a repatriated black musician who had smoked with Jean Cocteau in Paris. Like everyone else, they eventually had to give up opium for heroin. "I can't tell you how ashamed we felt when we first snorted," she said. "Like we couldn't even look at each other. It was so ingrained in us by the people we'd been in contact with, by everything we'd ever heard, that the worst thing you could be in life was a heroin addict." Before using opiates, however, Ann was strictly a marijuana smoker. She and her first husband made of marijuana a ritual—a ritual that was always accompanied by music.

I was born on March 9, 1919. We lived in what is now called the South Bronx. My parents were Jewish immigrants from Russia. They came from Orthodox families but they were hardly religious. My father was a housepainter. My mother worked in a dress factory; she was a member of the ILGWU. I had one sister. Ours was not a happy childhood. My parents were poor, and they were not happy together. They fought constantly, and they separated constantly. My sister and I never really had a home.

When my mother and father finally divorced, I was about sixteen, my sister about ten. I graduated from high school when I was seventeen and I got a job. It paid fifteen dollars a week, [laughs] the most money I had ever seen at one time. I did an awful lot with that fifteen dollars: I saved money, gave my mother money, bought my sister clothes so she wouldn't have to wear the kind of clothes I'd had to wear to school, *and* bought myself clothes. All for fifteen dollars. It's amazing.

My mother was very dependent on me. It was like I took my father's place. I married the first young man who asked me, just to get away. I was nineteen. My mother never forgave me, and it took my sister twenty years to forgive me for leaving them. But I guess I was a survivor, and I knew I would never survive there.

My first husband was also Russian, but not Jewish. When I met him in '37 he was smoking marijuana. We went to a movie once and he lit up a joint. No one even was aware of it. They thought maybe something was burning. People were so unfamiliar with it.

My husband had a white friend in show business who was a tap dancer. It was through this young man that he was able to make a contact in Harlem to get marijuana. Harlem was the only place you could get it. It was very difficult, at least in the middle thirties. But it was very cheap. It was already rolled, and it was like five for a dollar. If you bargained, you got six.

I didn't know marijuana was considered a drug; the people I knew never talked about it as a "drug." In those days it was called "gage," "weed," or "tea." So there was no connection to drugs—although I would say eventually it led to drugs, because in that era you had to meet different people even to get the marijuana, so that occasionally you might meet a drug user, although you weren't aware of it.

My husband opened a neighborhood bar and grill in the South Bronx the year after we were married. We had decided that we didn't want children, so I kept working as a secretary. By that time I was making twenty dollars a week. He also kept his job with Con Edison, so that he was working two jobs in order for us to, you know, make it. We had a very lovely apartment that we gradually furnished. But we could only do it by his keeping the job at Con Edison and working in the bar at night. We would smoke marijuana in the apartment with two other couples. We would gather on the weekend, on a Friday or a Saturday night. We were the only ones who had our own apartment, so it was natural for them to come there. The big thing about smoking was listening to jazz records. My husband and his friends loved jazz music. He had a tremendous collection. He had been collecting records ever since he was seventeen, back in '31 or '32. He explained to me that I could enjoy it better, and understand the music better, if I smoked pot.

The atmosphere was very important. It was very important to have a blue or a red light, and no one *dared* to speak while the record was playing. I remember that, if someone spoke, the word was, "He's a bring-down." Like, he just brought the whole atmosphere down, from everybody being tuned in to whatever we were listening to. And it was always black jazz. Benny Goodman, forget it—he couldn't really make it. [Laughs.]

We listened to *real* jazz: Teddy Wilson, Billie Holiday, Louie Armstrong. Did you know that when I married my second husband, the musician, that I became friends with all of them? I never dreamed when I was listening to their records that I would ever know these people. And, interestingly, not all of them used drugs. Teddy Wilson, for instance, never, never smoked marijuana or used any drugs. There were a great many black musicians who knew that others did it, but were not interested in it.

The music was *so* beautiful in those days. I can understand marijuana —it really went with music. It was a serious way to enjoy jazz, and a very "in" thing, you know. It was important to keep it in: you never let anyone know you smoked marijuana. You wouldn't even let them listen to these artists. If they wanted to hear music, you'd play Benny Goodman for them. You wouldn't let them hear Billie Holiday.

In the beginning our jazz group was like a weekend thing. We'd meet on Saturday night, spend the whole night sitting around, playing records, and smoking. Someone would light up a joint and pass it around. Before that one was finished, another person would start another joint, depending on how many people were there. We would sometimes have as many as ten people, all white, all working class. Definitely no underworld or show business people.

When the record was over everyone would discuss passionately whose solo was better. Or they would say, "On the other record, Herschel Evans played this, and on this record . . ." The discussion was always about music. I remember one young man who was paranoid, though. For a while he would be right in with all the rest of us, but then he would get very paranoid under the influence of marijuana. He was the first one I ever saw like that, and it didn't start until maybe the second year he was smoking with us. I don't think that anyone ever put the two together; we never understood that the marijuana could affect some people that way. We would just think that he was very funny, because his reactions were odd. He would sort of accuse some of us of making fun of him. When you smoke marijuana, you know, things will strike you as funny for no reason, or for a reason you couldn't ever explain.

As I say, we smoked just once a week. But I liked it, and I started to ask my husband during the week if he had any tea. I'd want to light up because it gave me a good feeling. It made bearable feelings that were coming up within me: things that were happening in my family, things with my husband that were kind of hard for me to deal with in my head.

Weed of wicked ale [handwritten margin note]

I didn't understand my own feelings about things but I found that, gee, if I lit up a joint, it didn't bother me any more. I wasn't upset. So, after a while, it wasn't just to listen to music.

In the beginning my husband would never smoke except when he was at home. But then he too started to run into the kitchen of the bar to smoke some marijuana. There were a lot of problems running a bar, even a neighborhood bar where you didn't have to deal with tough people. The marijuana made him feel better able to cope, 'cause he didn't drink. Never did. There wasn't any drinking while we listened to the jazz either. As a matter of fact, the big thing was making a pot of coffee. Even though my husband owned a bar, nobody even thought of asking for a drink, and we never thought of offering one. It just didn't seem to go with pot.

I don't know what's happening now with marijuana, whether you drink with it or not. But then it was just pure marijuana with the jazz. I don't know if it was different marijuana then, or what, but it was very pleasant. I have smoked marijuana at different times of my life, and I have never, ever enjoyed it again the way I did in that period.

Do you think the context, listening to this exciting music with your friends in your living room, had anything to do with the effect of the marijuana?

I would say so, yes. I would say that it helped a great deal, because you felt you were doing something very hip that other people were not enlightened to. They didn't even know this wonderful music existed. You felt very privileged that you knew about marijuana and knew about this music.

Eventually we changed the weekend marijuana sessions to Friday, because my husband started hiring musicians to play in the bar on Saturday night. He would hire three-piece groups. He always wanted music he'd enjoy, so he'd hire three black musicians to come up and play. We found that it was very good for business, because there was no place else in that area to dance, and young men could bring their girlfriends there. Previously, it was a bar that no one would come into but the drunkards in the neighborhood. But with the Saturday night dances, young people started to come in. They didn't have to drink a lot; whatever they spent, it was just that much better for business. At first the regulars grumbled, "What's going on here?" They wanted to play the jukebox and hear "Melancholy Baby," or whatever. But, after a while, hearing it every Saturday, you'd catch one or two of them trying to get the beat. [Laughs.] They began to like it, and it became a regular thing.

That's how I met my second husband. I was in Manhattan one day, coming from work, when one of the musicians who'd played in the bar said hello to me. He was with another man, the man who would become my husband. When I looked at him, that was it. I just fell in love with him like that [claps hands]. I spent that whole night with him. I met him at six in the evening and didn't come home until eight in the morning. I told my husband that I'd fallen in love with someone else and that I'd have to leave him. He was stunned. Three weeks later I left.

WILLIAM S. BURROUGHS

This interview is different from most of the others in this book in two important respects. No alias was used, since details of Burrough's career are widely known and his identity would quickly have become apparent. The other difference is that we abandoned our usual step-by-step, life-history line of questioning, since Burroughs had already written and pseudonymously published Junkie,[7] *an autobiographical account of his addiction. Instead, we asked Burroughs to elaborate and clarify several points he had made in this and other works, and to talk about the relationship between drugs and writing.*

What year did you first begin using morphine? Was it 1942? This is one of the things that's not specifically mentioned in Junkie.

No, I think it's a good deal later than that, near 1944 or '45, around in there. Actually, I used drugs off and on for a while, but I think it was in 1944 or '45: the war was still going on, so it must have been around in there.

In Junkie *you report that the first time you took a shot of morphine your reaction was fear and nausea. That being the case, why did you take the second shot?*

Well, if you read that again, you'll see that it was certainly not unmixed fear and nausea. There's usually a degree of nausea, of course, when anyone takes a shot for the first time. The fear also had an interesting aspect to it: there were these sort of visions, and sensations of moving at great speed. So I would say that it was certainly not a completely unpleasant experience; certainly not enough to deter me, because I remember the second shot was very much more pleasant. The nausea was gone, and there was very little fear.

When I went from morphine to Mexican heroin, I didn't notice very much difference. Of course, morphine is characterized, like Pantopon, by a sort of pins-and-needles reaction, which you don't get with heroin,

---

7. Published by Ace Books as *Junkie* (by "William Lee") in 1953; republished in a complete and unexpurgated edition as *Junky* [*sic*] by Penguin Books in 1977, using Burroughs's actual surname.

or with Dilaudid either. Or with injected methadone. So there is a difference, yes. It's sort of like the difference between gin and whiskey, or
something like that. You would know right away which is what, whether
it's morphine or not, though it would be hard to distinguish between
heroin and Dilaudid. I have used morphine for long periods, but I'd say I
preferred heroin somewhat. I don't particularly like the pins-and-needles
reaction to morphine.

In Junkie, *two of your hustles were lush-worker and dealer. Were there any other
hustles that you practiced at that period of time?*

No. I was never very good at any of them—I was never very efficient.
I was able to avoid being busted while I was in New York City, but that
wasn't too much of a trick.

*Why did you have to hustle at all, given that you had a fairly substantial private
income of one hundred and fifty dollars a month? That would have been a fairly
substantial amount, at that time.*

It wasn't really enough, when you consider. You couldn't get by for
less, really, than ten dollars a day; ten dollars a day is, after all, three
hundred dollars a month, and then living expenses. No, it wasn't enough.

*Some of the people we've spoken to were able to scrape enough money together to
pay for their habits—in the thirties and forties anyway—by absolutely slaving
at some job or another. But you found it necessary to supplement your private
income?*

Yes. But that was only a brief period, you see, when I was in New York.
The period of supplementing my private income with any kind of hustles
was only a matter of months, really. Then, when I was in Mexico, there
was no necessity. I never registered as an addict, but I knew someone
who had a government script, so I'd pay for it and we'd split it. It was
cheap. Besides which, of course, an American cannot hustle in Mexico
very satisfactorily. You just don't get mixed up in that situation.

You make the remark in Junkie *that, if the wholesaler is an Italian, he is almost
sure to give you a short count. Why was that?*

They just had that reputation. The Jews were in it for a while, and they
had the reputation of giving a good count. But the Italians *always* had the
reputation for squeezing the last nickel out. Of course, they're the ones
who were responsible for putting it up, and putting it up, until they finally
priced themselves out of the market by creating these heroin panics. I've

seen exactly the same thing as that done with basic commodities, like cooking oil in Morocco. Somebody moves in there, they buy up all the cooking oil, and they put it in a warehouse. They hold it off the market: there isn't any cooking oil. Then it will come back at a slightly increased price. They're squeezing their money out of the poorest people. Well, exactly the same thing is done with heroin, or was done with heroin. There'd suddenly be a heroin panic, when there wasn't any heroin to be had. A week later—not quite long enough for people to get off—but a week later it would be back, at double the price usually. That happened, as we know, a number of times, until finally they priced themselves out of the market. It's just recently that other people have moved in and the price has gone down. It's now down to about thirty dollars a day, whereas about eight or ten years ago, in the 1970s, it was getting up to a hundred dollars a day, and people just couldn't do it.

Cartel

There weren't any Jews still dealing when I became addicted. This is sort of folklore. See, the Jews had been forced out of most of the rackets at that time; they were really forced out in the thirties—like "Dutch Schultz," Arthur Flegenheimer. The same sort of *putsch* that ousted him and his gang was the point at which the Mafia forced out the Jews.

In the late forties, when you were out of New York City, it was very difficult to get stuff. Doctors absolutely would not write prescriptions; there just wasn't anything to be had.

We spoke to several people who specialized in making small-town, southern doctors. But that was a little bit earlier. They said that the doctors would write fairly easily.

They would at one time. But they really began bearing down on the doctors after the war. By the late forties and early fifties it was very difficult, even in the small towns. On the occasions that I did make a doctor, I noticed that the older doctors were more likely to prescribe than the younger doctors. The old doctors had been used to prescribing and, of course, the young doctors had been indoctrinated.

common thread

I stayed off opiates for quite long periods of time after 1957, although I relapsed in 1967. I didn't use for very long: six months, or nine months, then I got off again. I decided to kick for various reasons. I've often found that you get to a point of diminishing returns, and I find that when I kick I get a sort of new perspective, which was useful in writing.

Could you elaborate upon that a little bit? Do you find it, for example, easier to write when you're off?

No, I wouldn't say that. I have found that, while I was off, I was more, should we say, creative? I got more, better ideas and concepts, more vivid

Increased creativity

descriptive passages. In other words, I found that being off was better for creative work. Most of *Naked Lunch* was written when I was off, not when I was on.

The opium dream as a stimulus to creativity is definitely a myth—although it's not a simple situation, you see. De Quincey knew that if, say, he built up a very heavy habit, when he got down to a much lighter habit, he'd have this renewal, and then he felt like writing. It was a real, creative renewal, although he didn't get completely off. He hardly ever did, except for just a few months.

If you had your life to live over again, would you stay away from drugs?

Well, I always feel that you don't have your life to live over. It's like people coming back from the racetrack: "If I'd bet on so-and-so instead of so-and-so, I'd have my pockets full of money." And then it would depend on what kind of a life. Where? There are some cases where I feel that narcotics can be an absolute blessing, like old, infirm people. Some people just from sheer, grinding horrible poverty: a lot of the Indian farmers are addicts. They take a little opium in the morning, and a little in the evening, just to keep them going. So I think it's a very difficult question to answer. I'd have to say what life, where, and what would I be doing?

Let me ask it in a slightly different way. Even without drugs, would you have become a writer? Did you conceive the desire to become a writer before you began using drugs?

Yes. Yes, I did. As a child I always wanted to be a writer, but I couldn't seem to get started. You see, *Junkie* wasn't published until 1953, and I was born in 1914. I think that sort of got me started—there's no question about it. I don't know whether I would have gotten started without that, or what experience would have had any comparable impact to get me started writing. So it certainly was very important. But drugs won't make anyone a writer. Nor will drugs like LSD make anyone a writer or a poet.

How much of Junkie *is true, and how much is dramatic invention?*

Most of it is true. I stayed sort of close to the truth, but then, in the next book, I went on to take a real episode and just stretch it as far as I wanted, fictionally. *Junkie* was mostly autobiographical: I sat down to write an accurate account of my experiences with addiction and with drugs.

Were you consciously mimicking De Quincey?

Oh, no. No, no, no. But I was familiar with his work; I'd read it many years before. I've reread it—I still have it. I find that it is still one of the most accurate books written, because it covers so much. It covers the phenomenon of overdosage, of running up these big, unnecessarily large doses, and how very unpleasant and nightmarish and depressing that can be.

What were the influences on your work?

Lots of them. Well, Conrad, Graham Greene, Kafka; someone named Denton Welch, who very few people have heard of, who's sort of out of print now.[8] He was a very strong influence. And people like Chandler: I have a whole strain of tough-guy detective throughout my books. There were lots of influences. I did a great deal of reading. Of course, I've read Joyce. I read *Ulysses*, but I couldn't quite make *Finnegan's Wake*. Twenty years, and a great book that nobody could read. There's a lesson there, I thought.

One of the things that impressed me about Junkie *is the fact that it's incredibly condensed. We're really talking about, what, a nearly eight-year period of time, and yet it almost seems like a short story. I gather that you left out and compressed a great deal.*

Yes! Yes, I was just trying to hit the high spots, a series of episodes that would hold together, and be interesting and readable.

You mentioned to me earlier that there was a great deal of fiction in Kerouac's books, and that his "portraits" of you were really fictitious.

Yes. He was always saying that I had a "trust fund"—everybody assumed that I have a trust fund, which I never did have. The money that I got was a pure allowance from my parents, who ran a gift and art shop, first in St. Louis, then in Palm Beach, Florida. It was not a trust fund. And so on: he had me married to a Russian countess, and all sorts of things. Well, people assumed that this was accurate, when it isn't. It is fictional.

8. Maurice Denton Welch (1915–48), an English writer known for his sensitive and impressionistic autobiographical novels and stories, characterized by sexual candor and striking descriptive passages.

With *Junkie* I was just trying to relate facts. Subsequently, I just took all these actual episodes and expanded them into any sort of fanciful variations. But I can't think of anything in *Junkie* that's really fictitious. The chronology may be a little bit off; I may have had something here that happened there, or put two incidents together, but essentially it was factual, or as related to me. You could put a real name next to every character in the work.

You've written that "addiction is an illness of exposure."[9] You were exposed, basically, because you were on the fringes of the underworld in New York City. How did you go from Harvard to the fringes of the underworld?

Well, that is sort of a long story. I came out of Harvard at a time when it was very difficult to get any sort of job, and I sort of drifted into that particular group of people, and became addicted. It was chance, I guess. In my experience in high school and at the university, it was just absolutely unheard of for middle-class people to use anything but alcohol. Marijuana was unknown. I managed to get a hold of just a little bit in the 1930s; it was fantastically good. I sort of enjoyed it, but not enough to want to use it regularly. It was something I did just once and again. I was unique in this: most college boys would have been absolutely horrified at the thought of anything that they called a "drug"—as if alcohol wasn't a drug.

9. "Kicking Drugs: A Very Personal Story," *Harper's* 235 (July 1967), 40.

11.

Busted

Even for addicts holding down steady jobs, arrest was an ever-present danger. They could always be prosecuted for possession of drugs, regardless of the legal nature of their occupations. For those who supplemented their incomes by hustling, or who did not work at all, the odds were so much the worse: they could be arrested for possession of narcotics, for various property crimes, or, if prostitutes, on morals charges. No matter how smooth their operations, they eventually got caught for something. Most got caught repeatedly.

Some of these arrests were of the revolving door variety, but others resulted in jail terms, and that meant withdrawal, either gradual or rapid. A few addicts were lucky enough to end up in prisons with medically supervised detoxification, but these were the exceptions. The rule during the classic era was cold turkey: kicking it out on a stone floor. Addicts could sometimes forestall this by scoring drugs from other inmates, but in-prison supplies were irregular and expensive. Their only other hope was to make bail, either on their own, or with the help of family and friends.

That is, if they had any. Addicts on the bust-prison-freedom-bust treadmill found it difficult to maintain personal ties. Relationships were necessarily precarious: the unexpected frisk, the knock on the door, could cause someone to disappear suddenly, indefinitely. It was a world of impermanence, of changing faces, of plans and expectations that seldom extended beyond the next shot.

TEDDY

"I couldn't tell you how many arrests I had," Teddy admitted. "My yellow sheets are a few inches thick. I had four felonies alone." The first three felonies netted him five years in the penitentiary; the last one, in 1965, thirteen. "Then, if you throw in the little three-month and thirty-day bits, I guess altogether I got about

twenty years." At various times Teddy wrote numbers, dealt heroin, shoplifted coats and radios, and even robbed payrolls. "My sentences were all narcotic-related," he said. "If it wasn't for dealing, it was for getting the money, one way or another, to buy narcotics."

My first arrest for narcotics was in 1945 or 1946, before I went into the army. The police busted us for dealing, but they didn't have a clear-cut case, so they threw it out. But in the meantime I cold turkeyed in the Tombs. In those days there was no methadone. You were lucky if you got a tranquilizer. Asking for an aspirin, you might have got your head busted. When they took you down to the Tombs they sent you up to the ninth floor and you grabbed a corner, and you squatted in that corner for three days. After three, four days you started feeling a little better, but, boy, during them first two days the best you could do was stand it, naked in that corner. It stinks, you vomit, you go through days and nights squatting in that corner. You don't move. There was no help, unless maybe you were fortunate enough to have a lawyer, and he could come down and get you to a hospital where you could get a shot of morphine. But it still didn't make no difference: you were eventually going to cold turkey anyway. So you go ahead and take it, and get it over with.

They turned us loose. I was on 134th Street. I was with this fellow, Pete, who was dealing. I was in his house when the feds raided it, and they caught us. The FBI rounded us all up, and they came up with a book. One of them said, "Oh, you're listed here as a draft dodger. They're looking for you." I said, "No, I never received no papers." I *had* received them actually, but I had sent them back "address unknown." The only thing I had was my draft card. I wasn't even eighteen when I got my draft card, but I kept it because, everywhere you went, if you were asked for I.D., you said, "Here, I've got my draft card." That was its only purpose. I had no intention of going into the army. But, anyway, the FBI was going to say that we were selling narcotics. We said, "Oh no, no, no." They said, "Well, look, we'll settle this if you go in the army. You go to the army, or you go to jail." I said, "Oh, I'm not even eighteen years old." They said, "But you got a draft card." I said, "Go talk to my mother." So they got my mother, and she said, "Yes, send him in the army. Better for him than jail." I said to her, "Don't sign them papers!" She signed them. That's how I ended up in the army.

I went in January of 1946 and came out January of 1947. I was sent to Fort Dix.[1] I went AWOL. Army life didn't appeal to me, and I was homesick —this was the first time that I ever was away from home. I didn't know anyplace but New York; when they took me out I was completely lost.

---

1. Near Trenton, New Jersey.

So I said to myself, "I'm going back to New York." I came home and I started snorting stuff again. But at that time they had the MPs patrolling the streets, you know, walking Seventh Avenue. I was in Small's and, like a fool, I hadn't taken off my uniform. The MPs asked me for my papers. I said, "What papers?" They said, "You got to have papers." I said, "I ain't got no papers." So they scooped me up, locked me up on 110th Street, and then sent me back to Fort Dix. Then they put me on a train and three days later I wound up in Fort Lewis, Washington.[2] I thought, when they said "Washington," that it was Washington, D.C. I had never knowed that there was another Washington in this country. At first I thought that there'd be narcotics out there, because it looked like everything was run by the Chinese. But there weren't any.

I went AWOL again. They caught me in Texas, but meanwhile my outfit got shipped out to the Pacific—they were like clean-up forces. When I got back to Washington they were gone, so they put me with a shipment going to Europe. The war was already over, but they still had what they called "constabulary forces" over there. It was bombed out. Man, the place was a wreck. We were guarding camps, and I was hauling stuff for different outfits. I was a truck driver. My unit was segregated: black men, white officers. We were separated even back in Jersey. I accepted this. That's the way it was, you know. You figured anytime you got ready to leave New York, you might as well get ready to face it.

I was all over Europe, in England and France and Germany. I stayed drunk most of the time. I never really liked alcohol before I went into the army, because I used to look at people who drank and I'd say to myself, "Oh, look at this guy here, he's all fucked up, actin' stupid and hollerin' loud. That ain't cool at all." A guy who snorts heroin, or coke, or shoots up, he's cool. He can get high, but if you don't nod, nobody will know what you're doing. If I could have got some narcotics, I'd have shot narcotics. But at the time I couldn't get no narcotics. This is why I went into the alcohol thing. I drank because I wanted to get high, to feel good. Like, in the army, when you go to town and there ain't nothing to do, you say to your buddies, "Oh, let's go get us a bottle. Let's go." I was getting high, drinking every day, just killing time. I think that's the reason they discharged me out of the army. They shipped me back to the States because they said I had the D.T.'s, but a lot of it was my acting to get out of the army.

I had about three thousand dollars when I got back to New York. I was stuck into the alcohol thing; I started drinking real heavy. Then a friend of mine said, "Listen, let's start writin' numbers." We started at 133rd Street, 132nd Street. He worked one side and I worked one side.

2. Near Tacoma.

We were making good money, but we weren't saving any. By good money I mean about three hundred dollars a day for myself, three hundred a day for him. See, we had every house in the block playing numbers. Any number that was played for a dollar or more, we figured we couldn't pay, so we turned it in to another controller. We didn't have a banker; we were controlling our own numbers. So if you hit, we'd pay it off ourselves. Say you bet five dollars. We can't pay this kind of money, so we'd go to another banker and take your number and play it with him.[3] You wanted to play 354? We'd go to this other banker and say, "Oh, listen, 354 for five dollars." So if the number comes out, he's got to pay us. [Laughs.] But you'll never know it, because you think you hit with us. And them little numbers, we just banked them and kept all that money ourselves. At the end of the day we split it up.

Together, we had a six- or seven-hundred-dollar book. Then we sold our territory to this other guy. See, we controlled this: nobody was going to play no numbers unless they played with me or my partner. This guy came in the morning and tried to write numbers, but the people said, "No, we don't play with you. We play with Teddy." He wanted to get in over here, so what he had to do was buy us out. But he didn't know that we were working for ourselves. We told him, "No, we can't sell out to you because we owe so-and-so some money." It was a game, you know what I mean? He said, "Well, how much do you owe?" I said, "Well, about eight, nine hundred dollars." He said, "OK." He bought us out.

We were doing so well my partner said, "Listen, let's get into some dope. We got the money, let's buy us a piece of stuff." I said, "No, I don't want to get into no dope." So we split. So he gets into narcotics, and he gets big, becomes one of the big people uptown. Eventually, I started dealing for him on a small scale. He said, "Teddy, come on, why don't ya?" I said, "OK." But I'm not using the dope. I'm still drinking. I was drinking nothing but Canadian Club, at least two pints a day. I always carried a pint in my pocket. But then I started to get the shakes and stuff, you know. I said to myself, "Man, I got to cut this out!" To ease off of it, I started snorting stuff again, and I wound up getting hooked.

At one point I was dealing three-dollar bags. I sold from my apartment. I had a small trade of my own, but it got to the point where I had to get out of it because too many people were coming to my house. Everybody was saying, "He's got a good bag." This is another thing I learned: if you're going to deal narcotics individually, the best way to avoid having your stuff pile up on you is to have a good grade of stuff. If you have good stuff, you have no problem getting rid of it. The word will spread [snaps

3. Winning numbers were generally paid off at six hundred to one. A five-dollar bet might return three thousand, hence the need to find someone with a bigger cash reserve.

fingers] like that. People will come on the corner and say, "Who's got it?" Someone will say, "Teddy's got it. His horse is smoking'. It's boss." And everybody will come to you. But this is a tip to the police. All they've got to do is sit there and say, "Oh-ho, something's going on in there." He can see the traffic that's going in there: it's telling on itself. So I had to quit selling out of my house. I thought, "Rather than being trapped in there, if I've got to sell it, I'll sell it out in the open. That way I may have a running chance. But if I'm in the house, I ain't got a chance in the world." And, I'll tell you, if I'm running and they don't get me in a short time, they ain't going to find *nothing* on me, unless they've got marked money. This is why I went to dealing in the street. Then I said, "Well, what the hell, I might as well sell to everybody else—everybody else is selling too." So it was no more of an undercover thing. The only thing you tried to do was to, like, not sell it on Seventh Avenue. I sold it over on St. Nicholas Avenue, by the park. That was my area over there.

I had a dog, a Doberman. He was a vicious dog: a friend of mine had him, but he got busted, so he gave the dog to me. *I* was scared to death of him. [Laughs.] If he looked at me hard, I punked out. I kept this dog with me when I was dealing, on a leash and collar. When I was in the house, going up in the hallway, or coming out, I'd take him off the leash, because if anything is on them steps, big trouble. I didn't have to worry about nobody waiting up there to mug me, unless they took him off first. And if they took the dog off, then I'm not coming out of my apartment or going no further up the stairs.

But even with the protection of the dog, I wound up going to jail for narcotics. In 1965 I was arrested for robbery and attempted murder. A friend of mine got killed over some narcotics. The people who killed him came looking for me. I wasn't involved in this, but these people thought, "Well, Teddy and him were so tight, he's *got* to know about it." I'm not really implicated in this, in no form or shape, you see, but if they're looking for me, there's no way they were going to believe what I was going to tell them. So what I did was to turn around and I went looking for them. I found them in a bar, and I tried to tell my story. "I don't know anything about this," I said. They wouldn't go for it. It became a scuffle, then it became a shooting. I shot the guy, but I didn't kill him. I got away from the bar. Later I found out that they also had robbery on me. This bar happened to be down with the guy I shot, so they said that I robbed the bar too.

They busted me and took me to court. I already had three felonies; this was my fourth. They offered me a trial, but I couldn't go to trial, because they had positive witnesses saying that I went in there, robbed the bar, and then shot the guy. It was a frame-up. I admit that I shot the guy, but it was no robbery. I didn't take nothing, because I was too busy trying to get out of there. But I couldn't beat the case, so I copped out. If I went to trial on attempted robbery and attempted murder, I could get from forty to eighty years. With that, I wouldn't even get to the parole board until I did twenty years.

As it was I didn't get out until 1977. I went back uptown, and there was a complete change after thirteen years. Harlem wasn't Harlem no more. I looked at it and I couldn't believe it. I got back at night, around eleven o'clock. I saw that the trains were all marked up with grafitti, and that the platforms were dirty. I said to myself, "What the fuck has happened?" I got off the subway at 135th Street. I looked at the neighborhood and there weren't any more houses, just bricks and garbage and shit piled up. I said, "Goddam!" I walked down another block, and I saw that all the stores that weren't closed up were barred up. You couldn't see anything in the windows no more. There weren't any people in the street, and this was summertime. When I left there were people all over the streets. You could hear music, and kids laughing. Now it was almost like a ghost town.

I went home. When I hit the hallway of the house where my mother lived, I saw the plaster falling off the wall and the garbage behind the steps. The lights were hanging down, the walls were marked, the halls smelled like piss. I said, "Wow!" At the time I left, this was a decent house on Seventh Avenue, one of the best avenues uptown to live on. I went into the apartment and said, "Mom, what's going on." That apartment used to be spotless, but now the plaster and shit were falling down.

I went to bed. When I woke up the next morning and looked out the window . . . it was just completely turned around. Across the street the houses were boarded up, nailed up. And the first thing I see is a guy out there selling dope.

STICK

The longest prison term I had was for robbery. I was carrying dope, transporting it. I stopped in Pennsylvania to send a telegram to my girl. Since it was during the Christmas holidays, I stopped to bullshit in a bar with some dudes I knew. We had some coke 'n' dope 'n' some girls up at the hotel. One guy said, "Hey, man, I know where to get some money at, but I need a pistol." I said, "Well, shit, I got a pistol." So I lent him my damned pistol. He got into his father's car. But, instead of me letting him go to get the damned money, I followed my damned pistol—I didn't want him to run off with my pistol, right? So I got into his father's car with him. He went to this joint and stuck the damned place up. He came out with cash money and jewelry and jumped into the car.

It was a dark, rainy night. He turned up a blind, dead-end street. But, instead of his taking his time and backing out of the damned street and going where he was supposed to be going, he was burning rubber backing out of this alley. The police happened to be driving by, and they stopped us. They got this shopping bag, goddamn it, full of this bullshit.

There wasn't any dope in the bag, just jewelry and money. We had shot the dope and the coke back at the hotel, me and him and two more dudes and four girls. *He* was the one who had run out of money. I had money—I had a shoe box full of money. If I'd have given him the pistol and let him go ahead, I'd have been all right. I didn't have to go with that sucker. But I did, and that's how I got busted for robbery.

I got five to ten years. I did eight years and nine months, but in different places: four years in Western State Prison in Pittsburgh; Huntingdon, Pennsylvania, for two years; and Graterford, Pennsylvania, for a couple of years. While I was at Graterford I spent nine months in solitary for inciting a riot. That was when Elijah Muhammad was going strong, and he was recruiting all these guys from the penitentiary and turning them into Muslims. I wasn't a follower, or a member, but I was a sympathizer to his cause. There was a big beef because the guys in prison wanted to get religious material, and they wouldn't let it come through the mail. They wanted to get the Muslim bible, the Holy Koran. They also wanted to get a kosher menu in the mess hall, because there were enough guys there who didn't eat pork to warrant a separate kosher line. Everything they cooked in the joint had pork in it, so these guys were literally starving themselves to death, living off crackers and coffee and stuff. That was the main beef, and then there was a lot of other stuff. Well, I was one of the pro-Muslim speakers—you know how guys get up on the soapbox and harangue the crowd. A "rabble-rouser" I guess you could call me at that time. That's why they busted me and put me in solitary.

Every jail's got its own particular thing, but in Graterford they had a jail-within-the-jail: off in the corner, inside the main wall, they had another wall with another jail in there. In solitary, you had two walls separating you and freedom. The cells were regular sized, maybe seven or eight feet long, and maybe five feet wide. They'd take us out and let us take a shower once a week. The rest of the time we were in the cells. A guard might come in and, if he felt like it, let us out two at a time to walk up and down in front of the cell for fifteen minutes. But we had to keep walking; you couldn't come out and lean up against the wall. And the food—hey, this'll be interesting—the food was served in this way. They'd bring it to the solitary cell on a wagon that was capable of keeping the food hot. But the officer who had the wagon this particular day—or any particular day, because there were quite a few of them taking turns—the officer would come in front of your cell and beat on the door. "All right," he'd say, "You want breakfast?" You'd get up and you'd look: "What d'ya got, man?" He'd say, "What d'ya want, eggs?"—and he's digging in his nose, or scratching his ass, or something. Then he picks up your egg with his hand and slaps it on your tray, just slaps on a fried egg, and some bread and a slab of butter. "You want some bacon or some coffee," he'd say, and he'd give it to you with the same dirty hand. That's the way they served you.

Like you were an animal.

Like a dog! Like a dog! Like a dog! They'd just throw it to you. They may just as well have thrown it on the floor, like they were throwing a bone to a dog. "Here, dog." Yeah. Yeah. Yeah, man, I'm telling you—whew!

These were white guards; the prison population was mostly black, 75 or 80 percent black. They had one black guard in Graterford, and every white officer was fucking his wife, the bum bastard. 'Cause they all lived right around that little creep town, you know. Shit, he was the only black guy working there and every fucking guard in that damn prison was fucking his wife. Shit, man, I'm telling you. . . .

They had a thing in this same jail, they called it "the glass cell." Dig it, if you got busted again, after you're already in solitary—if somebody sneaked you a cigarette or something—they'd put you in this glass cell. Here's what it consisted of: it was a regular cell, but in front of it there was a glass windowpane, a big sheet of glass. That was to prevent you from throwing shit out at the guard—there was a guard that sat right out in front of the cell. It was constant, twenty-four hour surveillance. They put you in this cell, right? He sits there, and you're in your cell. If you *breathe*, he's going to know that you're breathing.

I was in the glass cell three times, for talking and smoking—all that kind of dumb shit. When I went in there all I had on was a pair of white overalls. No drawers, no socks, no shoes—you had on them little cloth shoes that you wear in the hospital. That's all you had on, winter or summer. That's it. Only other things you had were your toothbrush and toothpaste. No soap. Only soap you got was when you took that one bath a week. What I'd do is go into the cell and fix my bed the way I wanted it—I didn't have no blankets or nothing, just a bed and a mattress—I'd fix the bed, sit down, and look at the guard. He'd sit there and look at me and I'd sit there and look at him. That was the only way to do it.

They'd try to bug you. Here were this guy's exact words: "We gonna break you before you get outta here. We done broke better men than you." I said, "Oh, that's what you're here for? To 'break' people? Is that what you're here for, man? That's your job, to break people? Wow, man, you must be proud of yourself—'I done broke better men than you.'" Hmmph! Yeah, rehabilitation.

It's just like this Ramsey Clark said, the only thing we can do to better the penal system in America is to tear down every goddam jail we have and destroy them. You can see me saying that, because I'm bitter and I'm a "malcontent" anyway. But, hey, Ramsey Clark said that. What about *him*?

MICK

This broad I lived with in Harlem was married. She had two daughters, two beautiful daughters. She was educated. She'd graduated from high school, she went through business school. Her family was above average, more like a middle-class family. Her father was a teacher in Warwick, New York, at the training school up there.

But she married an addict. He broke her in. She was only at that time about eighteen, nineteen. He was a house painter. He had a good job, made good money, had plenty of work. And his family had money—his father was a chef at one of the hotels in New York. So they started out pretty good, and she wasn't addicted in any way then. But, as far as I know from what she was telling me, he started her off—"Come on, take a fix," or something like that. Then she got so she liked it so much that she became really addicted.

Then he got locked up. He committed some job, grand larceny. He was in some house and stole all the jewelry and stuff. He worked for a contractor. He'd case the house while he was painting. He took everything out of there. There were several jobs he did like that. But, finally, they caught up with him. So he went to jail, and when he went to jail she went on relief, like what usually happens. She went on relief with the kids. She wasn't really in the life then. Like, she wasn't out selling herself yet.

"The life"? When you're "in the life" up there you're a junkie, you use drugs, you bet numbers, you drink, you're in with all the racketeers, you know, in the life. That's the life. That's what the blacks call "the life." It's not a white term. It's a black term: "Aw, you're in the life," "She's in the life"—the life of a prostitute, or so forth. In other words, you'd do anything for a buck.

For a while this woman managed to stay off the street. Then she went into the street. That's how I met her. I was having a couple of drinks somewhere, in a bar. She came up alone and asked me to buy her a drink. That's how I got to talk to her. I talked pretty sensible to her and she said, "You talk a lot different than these other guys. All they're looking for is this and that and the other thing." And I said, "Aw, don't give me that bullshit. What are you trying to tell me, that I'm an angel or something?" But I found out that she was pretty sincere in her ways of talking and by her actions. And I had a few bucks. I teamed up with her. We went to her room, and so forth—we got to know one another, to hang out like that, to stay with one another. I stayed with her a couple of years. I met her father and all like that. He knew.

While she was with me, she never messed around, you know what I mean? She stayed off the street. We had our own room. I took care of her. Yeah, I'd score, I'd make the pickups. She could make the pickups too. She could enter a place where I couldn't: because of her color, it wouldn't seem as odd. She was dark—she was a Panamanian. She wasn't no Puerto, she was a Panamanian. She could go to, like, shooting galleries.

The shooting galleries were in Harlem, right up there on 112th Street, 113th Street, and up that way, off Lenox Avenue, St. Nicholas Avenue, and all through there, that whole section. And 116th Street, 117th Street —that was junkies' heaven then, all them houses, all them basements and cellars. On the East Side it was 117th Street between Third and Lex— that's when the Puerto Ricans started to move in—and on the West Side it was 117th between Lenox and Seventh. That's where the blacks were, and along Madison and Fifth. The blacks and the Puertos didn't get along too good, you know, because the blacks figured the Puertos were taking their customers, and they didn't like that.

The fact that I was white didn't keep me out of all of these places. I could go into some of them where I knew the blacks, where I knew the guys. Of course, in a shooting gallery, there was always like one guy, he was a majordomo. If you didn't give him a fix, you didn't get in there. You had to give him a fix or you had to give him a buck, see. And if you wanted to use his spike you had to give him another dollar.

I could have shot up in my own place, but I went to these shooting galleries because that's where the stuff was available, and it was handy. Like the time when I had a room in Long Island City: why go from Harlem to Long Island City to shoot up when you could just buy it on the corner and go down in the cellar and shoot up? And then when the broad and I had the room in Harlem it was convenient. Right there.

Of course the cops used to come into these galleries, raid the joint and bust you all up and everything else. Kick you around a little bit. Yeah, and a white guy in there with all them blacks and Puerto Ricans—they'd murder you.

I was caught in several of them. When the cops came in and raided the place, one of the detectives would go, "Get out of here you son of a bitch. Don't ever let me see you here again or I'll break your chops. I'll tear you apart." See, I got out because I was white. The black and the Puerto Rican addicts, they knocked the piss out of them. Took them. Locked them up. Booked them.

This happened twice. One time in 117th Street . . . you might have heard of this here Egan, he was a guy who used to dress up like Santy Claus and go in the bars. Yeah, that was the guy that was in the movie *The French Connection.* He didn't bust me, but he was the guy that chased me. He said, "You white bastard, get out of here before I knock your head off." And he could do it too. He had all them niggers and spics lined up against the wall there. And, boy, they didn't even look cross-eyed, because he was a mean bugger. Mean. I mean, *mean*. He didn't care if you were four foot tall or four foot wide, he'd beat your brains out. Tough bastard. He let me go. "Get out! Get out!" he said.

But he had the broad there. I was with the broad. The broad had to stay.

Racist -

ARTHUR

I lost count of the number of times I've been arrested. Between six and eight times, I would guess. You could get a yellow sheet and see. All possession arrests—no, one was not possession, one was forgery. I used to buy stolen government checks at 50 percent of face value. At 123rd, 124th Street there was a little printing shop there; you'd bring him a check and he'd make you up a beautiful set of I.D.s to go with this check. Whatever name was on the check, he'd make you I.D.s for it. Of course, he's not there no more. This is back in the thirties and forties.

June 18, 1937, was my first arrest for illegal possession. I was working at 128th, 129th and Lenox Avenue, and I was copping at 122nd Street between Seventh and Lenox. There was a guy there who had no legs. He walked around on his knees. When he came out on the street, he put on artificial legs.

At that time the police narco squad had a quota system. I suppose you're aware of that: they had to make a certain number of arrests a month. Now, if they knew, for example, that you or I were selling drugs here, do you think they'd come in here and bust you? No. They'd park across the street or around the corner or someplace and they'd just watch. Everybody that'd come in here and go out, they'd bust 'em. When they get enough, then that's it. They'll let you stay there and sell as long as they keep making arrests.

That's what happened with me in my first bust. I came out, walked down Lenox Avenue to 122nd Street, went up to No-Legs's private dwelling, and knocked on the window. He handed me a little bottle— at that time they used to have dollar bottles with the powder in it. I'm coming back and at 124th Street these two big detectives step in front of me. One says, "Pardon me. Do you have any policy slips or numbers or anything like that?" I said, "No sir, no sir, I don't," and started off. He said, "Wait a minute, wait a minute. What are you rushing for?" I said, "I'm on my lunch hour," which it was. I used to go across the street to the Empire Cafeteria on 125th Street and go in the bathroom and shoot up and go back to work. So he said, "Well, if you don't have any numbers or anything on you, you don't mind us looking you over, do you?"

Well, listen, what could I do? I had it right here in my pocket. It came

out and they said, "What is this?" I said, "Tooth powder." [Laughs.] You
know, my first bust, I don't know nothing about this. Well, he says, "*Tooth
powder?*" They took me—and I had just paid down on my first automobile.
I showed them: I said, "Look man, I'm just buying a car, I'm doing all
right, I'm working every day." They busted me anyway.

They took me down to the old Tombs. At the time they had something
they called "Magendie," and they'd shoot you up. I don't know what it
was. It was some drug. It would straighten you out. It got you high.[4] They
started you off with fifteen milligrams, then they cut you down to ten,
then they cut you down to five. It took two weeks before they finally get
you down to five milligrams, then they send you over to Riker's Island.
You have no habit when you get there because you've kicked it down in
the Tombs with Magendie.

I was one of the first arrivals at Riker's Island. When I got there, the
fixtures—you know, the mirrors and stuff—didn't have the paper taken
off. Brand new fixtures. There were only three blocks occupied at the
time, in 1937. They had just brought everybody from Welfare Island, I
believe it was, when they closed down that prison. They were moving
people up there. It was a beautiful place.

Everybody in my family knew I was addicted, yes. They weren't upset
about it. They were very cooperative. If I got busted at twelve o'clock, at
four o'clock I'd be in the street. My mother would be down there with a
lawyer and a bondsman. I'd say, "Mom, you don't have to bring a lawyer.
Just bring a bondsman."

They'd found out about it before I was arrested. They objected about
it; they didn't approve of it, no. But they went along with me. Whenever
my mother got me out of jail, I didn't have no money, she'd reach in her
pocket and give me money to go and cop. I had to have it, see.

My wife died July 14, 1945. We were not married legally. She was
sixteen and I was twenty-one when we started living together. She was
also an addict. Definitely. That's what she died from, tetanus. When she
died in Bellevue Hospital the doctor told me, "Make sure you do not use
the needle that she was using. That's what killed her, tetanus." I went
home and took the same needle and kept using it, using it, using it, trying
to get hepatitis or tetanus, but, unfortunately, I didn't get it.

There were two suicide attempts to my credit. Once they saved me in
Sydenham; once they saved me in Bellevue. My first suicide was September
2nd, 1945. That was her birthday. Every one of her birthdays we
always did something big, we went out to dinner and a show. Always on

---

4. Magendie's Solution, named for the French physiologist François Magendie (1783–
1855), contains morphine sulfate.

her birthday for the eleven years that we had been together. So this was the first birthday that I'm by myself, you see. I came home that day by myself. I fixed my shot. I'm sitting there thinking, "Gee, this is Baby's birthday"—I used to call her Baby, she used to call me Daddy—"I have to do something big to celebrate Baby's birthday." So I hollered out the window, I saw a guy going by. I said, "Go up to 128th Street and buy me some coke." He went and got the cocaine and I got the heroin—you know, they call that a speedball. I shot that and then I went upstairs— the kitchen was upstairs, it was in a brownstone—and I locked the door, took the ladies' curtains and the washcloths and things and stuffed them all along the bottom, the keyhole, the window, turned on all the gas jets, turned on the oven, took paper and started to write four suicide notes: one to my mother in Spanish, one to her mother, one to my favorite sister, and one "to whom it may concern." I wrote a little bit here, a little bit there, a little bit in Spanish, a little bit in English. They showed me the papers later, after the cops got me and took me out of there. When the gas began to take effect, you could see where my handwriting began to go off: "I have to hurry up now, I don't have too much time left . . ." When I finished finally I took off my t-shirt and made it like a pillow and stuck it in the oven. I laid down on the floor—it was one of those ovens that opened down—and I stuck my head in the oven. I'm ready, I'm going. Then the last thing I heard was something that sounded like knock . . . knock . . . knock—like somebody lightly tapping on the door. That was the emergency police with sledgehammers breaking down the door. Somebody had smelled the gas and then called the police. They smashed in the door and then took me to Sydenham Hospital. That was my first suicide attempt.

The second suicide was a foolish thing. I went into the drugstore and bought everything that I saw marked "poison." Poison for rats, poison for bugs, poison for this, poison for that. I bought eight or ten different things just because it said poison. I went home and dumped it in a glass and put water in it, but it was so thick you couldn't drink it, but you could eat it with a spoon. It was blue, the color was blue. I gulped as much as I could and I passed out. My neighbor or somebody came in there and they found me in that condition. They called the ambulance and took me to Bellevue. When I go to Bellevue I hollered, "I want to die! I want to die! I don't want to live, I want to die! Next time I'm going off of the building. Next time I'm going to jump under the train." They wrapped me up in one of those strait jackets. This was the same year, 1945.

It was my wife's mother who is the cause of my being here today. She used to come and visit us every Monday. She knew we were both on drugs. When I used to come in at lunchtime she would just turn her back and keep talking to her daughter. And her daughter would fix the stuff,

I'd drop my pants, and she'd hit me in my leg. Then I used to fix the stuff and hit her. Then her mother would turn back and keep talking to her daughter and I'd go back to work. That was my lunch, a shot.

After her daughter died, she still continued to come and visit me every Monday. She said, "Arthur, you going to keep up with this suicide business? One of these days you're going to succeed, if you keep on. You think when you die you're going to meet Baby again?"

After my second suicide attempt, I went to Puerto Rico. My family wanted to get me away from the environment, and my brother was in Puerto Rico. But the late forties were very bad years for me personally. I lost my entire family then. My wife, my mother, my sister, and my father: '45, '47, '48, '49. Then, in 1950 I went into the navy. They bounced me in 1951. When they bounced me I was in jail in Germany. I got busted in Germany coming through customs.

I was in the steward department. I volunteered for the navy because I heard that overseas drugs were plentiful and easily available. It was so rough here, you see, I figured I'd go over there. That's how I went down to Fifty-eighth Street, the army base in Brooklyn, and signed on as a waiter. I just wanted to get on; I wanted to go to Europe. When they reviewed my application and they saw I had an extensive background in the food line, they said, "Mister, you have experience here. We need a butcher. Would you want to take a job as a butcher instead of a waiter? You get twice as much pay, practically." Well, I would take a job doing anything to get on that ship. And it happened so fast . . . the next day I had to go back and get an examination and get shots, you know, the shots they give you to go overseas. About two or three days later—bam!—I was on the USS *General S.D. Sturgis,* troop transport.

Drugs were plentiful on the ship. What kind? Morphine. That's why I say I'm glad, thank God, we never got hit with a torpedo. Because if they put people in those lifeboats . . . you know what "tartrates" are? A little tube, looks like toothpaste, with a needle on the end. You stick somebody and squeeze the morphine out of it. Well, they had tarpaulins covering all of the life rafts or lifeboats. I don't know who, but somebody used to go through all of those lifeboats and tear up the tarpaulins and steal all the morphine. Practically all the crew members used to use morphine on the ship.

When I got to Batavia, in Java, I bought some pot that was out of this world. We used to come into customs and I'd see a kid walking down the street with a stack of green tissue paper packages under his arm, from here all the way up to there. He was crying out, "Mar-eee-wana, mar-eee-wana, mar-eee-wana." I said to the tailor, the guy behind me, "I could have swore that guy said 'marijuana.'" The tailor said, "That's just what he did say." I said, "There's the cop on the corner, man, how could it be?" He said, "If the kid wasn't there and you wanted some marijuana, you ask the cop. He'll tell you where to go. It's legal here. And that's what I got busted with later, in Germany.

I also figured out a little racket for myself on the ship. I was a loan shark. With the navy, you get paid on the seventh and the twenty-second of every month on the ship. I don't care where you are: in the middle of the Pacific, up in the Arctic, any place in the world, you line up at the purser's window and they pay you in cash. No checks—cash money. The result is that there's a poker game and a crap game going twenty-four hours a day on the ships. Those who work nights gamble all day; those who work days gamble all night. After they'd get broke, I'd loan them. The seventh and the twenty-second at the purser's, everybody's getting paid, and I'm standing there with my little pad. "How much do you owe me? Thirty dollars?" Then I used to deduct five or six dollars —20 percent. I wouldn't loan no less than ten dollars.

On the ship they have currency for every country you go to. You go to Germany, they've got marks. You go to England, they have pounds. You go to Japan, they have yen. You change how much money, approximately, you're going to spend on the ship before you go ashore. You're not supposed to take American currency ashore. However, everybody's got a money belt, and it's full of money.

When I went ashore I also used to have about eight, ten packs of cigarettes stashed all over me. Any kind of cigarette on ship costs a dollar a carton. One dollar from the government. So everybody had fifteen, twenty cartons of cigarettes in the bottom of their locker, and we'd take them ashore. A waiter, a cab driver, anybody would rather have a pack of American cigarettes than a dollar. And it cost us a dime, so we used to use them for tips. When you got to customs, he'd take your pass, stamp it, and say, "You got any American currency on you?" "No." "How many packs of cigarettes you got on you?" "Two, three"—whatever the limit is. Then usually they'd let you go.

But I'm a money shark. A guy by the name of Daniel, he owed me twenty dollars. So, just as I'm getting ready to go down the gangplank in Bremerhaven, he says, "Arthur, in case I get broke tonight, here's the money I owe you." Now, I have my money belt with American currency, but I don't want to go back downstairs to open up, undress to put the twenty-dollar bill in there. So I took it and put it in my sock. I also had seven joints rolled up in a package of Chesterfields, with a few cigarettes in the front.

Do you know that damn German customs guy, after he stamped my pass and I showed him my cigarettes, he started frisking me and went down to my ankle and felt that little hard thing. He said, "What's that?" He pulled a twenty-dollar American bill out—I was taking American currency ashore. "Hey, Hans, or Fritz"—he called another German, he put him on the line. He said, "You come with me." He took me into a

little room and he said, "Give me your hat." I gave him the hat and he
went all around the hat. He was going all through each piece of clothes,
stitch by stitch. When I got down to my shorts, right under my shorts was
the money belt. So I said, "Do you want these too?" He said, "No, that's
all right." So he came over and takes my shorts and starts to go around.
Naturally, he felt the money belt. So—zip!—out comes the money belt. I
had about four or five hundred dollars in there.

Now, after all that searching he'd got the five packs of cigarettes I had
and a stack of American currency. He made a phone call and then he
started to type, type, type. I said, "But, wait a minute. This is our last
stop. We were out for three months. That's my money that I earned on
the ship. I have a wife and three kids in New York. This is to buy them
Christmas presents." I'm bullshitting, you know. I said, "I don't want
to get in trouble with this. Look, you came in here and you searched
me—I didn't have no money, I didn't have no cigarettes. Say 'I didn't
find nothing.' Just let me put on my clothes and go." I'm giving up all
the money, see, I'm giving up the cigarettes. He crossed his legs while
I was standing there saying it. After I finished talking he turned around
and spoke in very rapid German. I said, "Wait a minute man, did you
understand what I'm saying?"

Eventually, he found the marijuana. He also found two hypodermic
needles. I was going to Hamburg to buy some drugs. But he didn't arrest
me for marijuana. He arrested me for "importing American currency into
Germany for black market operations." That was what the charge read in
court the next morning.

I was convicted. The sentence was four months' confinement, but
I actually stayed about two months. I was sentenced on the twenty-
something of October, and I was released on the twenty-fourth of December, Christmas Eve.

I was sent to Mannheim, where there is their version of our Sing Sing.
They didn't detoxify me. I had to go cold turkey. But my habit wasn't too
strong. Using morphine on the ship—it wasn't always available. It wasn't
a daily thing. Whenever we got it, we used it.

The jail was half of what was formerly a big prison. It was an American
jail, all American GIs. There were enlisted men in there who had committed major and minor crimes. There were guys in there for murder, and
there were guys in there for stealing coffee out of the PX. However, the
warden of the prison in Mannheim said, "I don't see why they keep sending you fellows here. We have no authority: all the laws of this institution
cover only enlisted men. You are not an enlisted man. You are a civilian
employee." So I could more or less do what I wanted to. I used to go to
the movies every day, sit in the library and read. But the GIs had to get
up every morning and drill in the yard whether it be raining or snowing.

When I was in Mannheim I got a letter. I will quote it for you: "Dear

Mr. Arthur Smith: Please be advised that it has been proposed to terminate your employment with the U.S. Navy Department for falsification of your application. You answered in the negative item number sixteen, which reads, 'Have you ever been arrested since your sixteenth birthday? Do not include traffic violations for which you were fined twenty-five dollars or less.' We now have in our possession information indicating that you have been previously arrested for the commission of a crime. . . ."

After I was released from jail, I came back to the States. I went right back to work, and selling drugs. The last time I was arrested was ten or fifteen years ago, before I came into methadone. My shortest sentence was four months, my longest, twenty months. Twenty months in and sixteen on parole—three years. Bunch 'em all together, I did about five or six years.

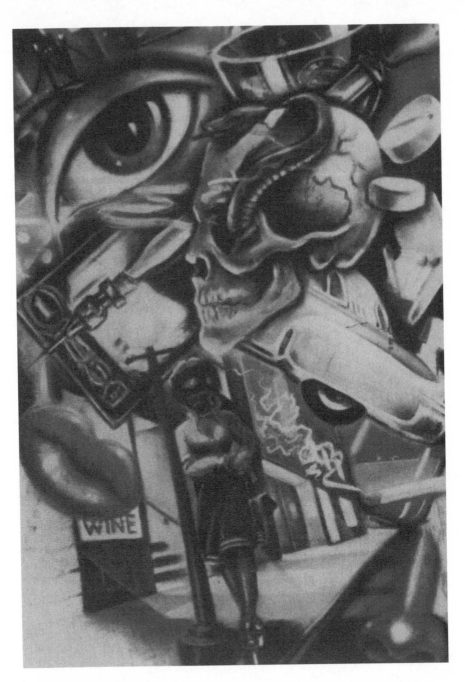

IN THE LIFE

A surreal painting by an addict, which the Bureau of Narcotics used and interpreted as a hellish portrayal of the evils of drugs. By the early twentieth century narcotic use was entrenched in and increasingly confined to the urban underworld, a fact that strengthened the consensus for strict drug laws. *DEA*

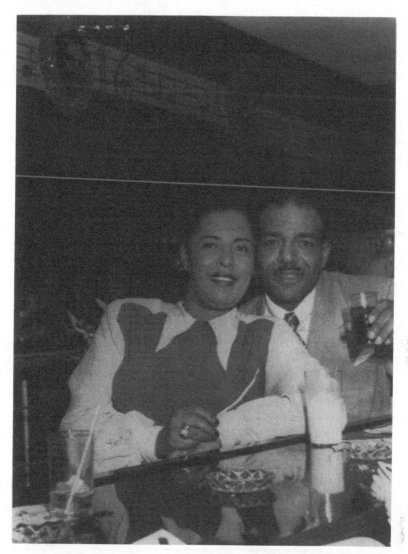

BILLIE HOLIDAY AND FREDDIE GREEN, CLUB ASTORIA,
BALTIMORE, SEPTEMBER 1948
　　Holiday had been arrested and imprisoned for a narcotic offense the
previous year. Green, a peerless rhythm guitarist and Billie's sometime lover,
was arrested on a marijuana charge the same month this photograph was taken.
"Billie Holiday used to smoke [opium] before she used junk," Al recalled.
"She used to come to my house . . . and sing to my kids." *DEA*

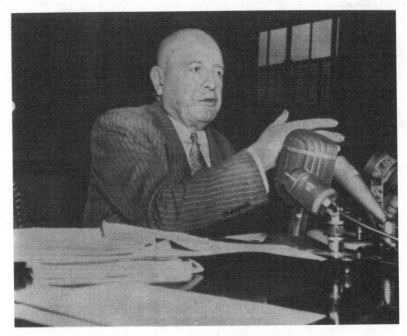

THE MAN

Harry Anslinger dressed like a diplomat, thought like a politician, and acted like a tough cop. "When the Russians land on the moon," Lucky Luciano once complained, "the first man they meet will be Anslinger, searching for narcotics." *Historical Collections and Labor Archives, Pattee Library, Pennsylvania State University*

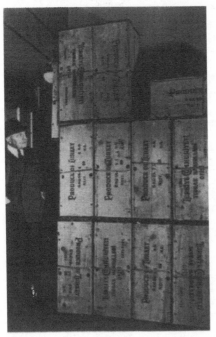

ANSLINGER INSPECTS THE NATIONAL STOCKPILE OF OPIUM

Although not usually thought of as a narcotic purchaser, Anslinger was in the late 1930s the world's biggest. He bought up three hundred tons of opium in anticipation of military medical needs, causing the world price to triple and worsening the "panic" among street users in the early 1940s. Anslinger himself used narcotics late in his life, when he took morphine to control the pain of angina. *DEA*

Beware! **Young and Old — People in All Walks of Life!**

This **[image]** may be handed you

by the friendly stranger. It contains the Killer Drug "Marihuana"-- a powerful narcotic in which lurks **Murder! Insanity! Death!**

WARNING!

Dope peddlers are shrewd! They may put some of this drug in the 🫖 or in the ☷ or in the tobacco cigarette.

WRITE FOR DETAILED INFORMATION, ENCLOSING 12 CENTS IN POSTAGE — MAILING COST

Address: THE INTER-STATE NARCOTIC ASSOCIATION

(Incorporated not for profit)

52 W. Jackson Blvd.   Chicago, Illinois, U. S. A.

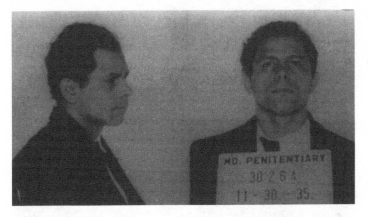

THE KILLER DRUG

Above: A billboard outside of Chicago in the mid-1930s. *Dorothy Dusek Girdano and Daniel A. Girdano,* Drugs—A Factual Account, *2nd ed. (Reading, Massachusetts: Addison-Wesley, 1976), with permission from Random House. Below:* A cautionary tale by the Bureau of Narcotics. In 1935 this man, a Puerto Rican seaman and "marijuana addict," was convicted of rape and carnal knowledge of a minor. He was hanged the following year. The original crusade against marijuana was based on claims that the drug fostered criminal, or even maniacal, behavior; later, in the 1950s, marijuana was deplored as a precursor to heroin use. *DEA*

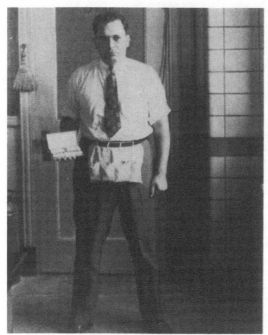

RETAIL MARIJUANA

An agent of the Alcohol Tax Unit in Philadelphia displays an apron containing a gross of marijuana cigarettes and a cigarette case with forty-five reefers. Both were taken from a twenty-five-year-old black dealer, who kept the apron under his trousers, attached to a belt that he also wore under his trousers. *DEA*

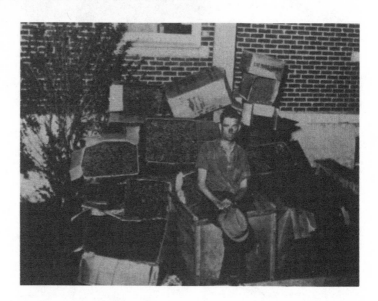

WHOLESALE MARIJUANA

Defendant arrested with a ton of marijuana, Blue Mountain, Mississippi, sometime during the Depression. *DEA*

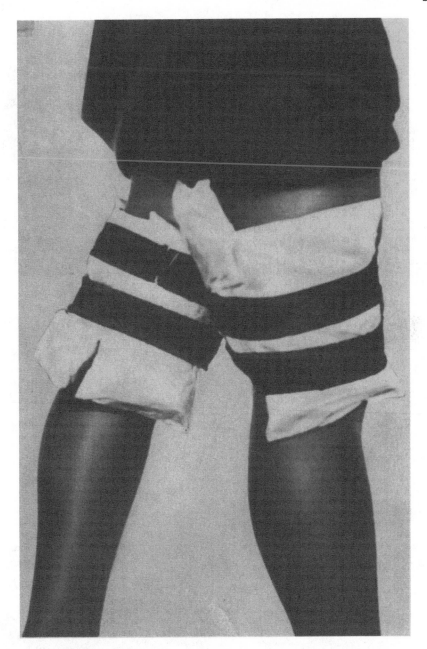

CONCEALED HEROIN

Written on the back of the photograph: "A 'clothes up' or 'close up' of heroin smuggled by Japanese woman on Pacific Coast." The compactness and value of heroin made it the ideal black market commodity. *DEA*

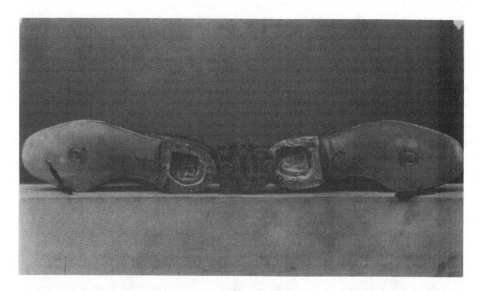

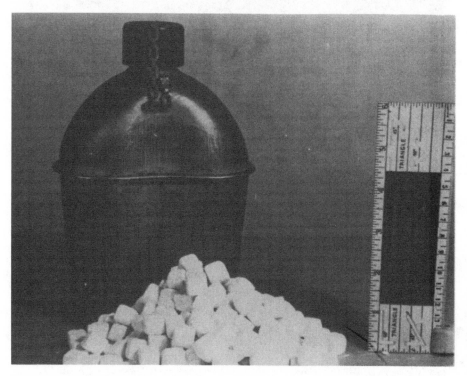

SMUGGLING TECHNIQUES

Above: Hollowed-out heels used to conceal three hundred grains of heroin intended for the inmates of a New York prison. *Below:* Morphine cubes stolen from a hospital supply dump in Nuremburg, Germany, and brought to Portland, Oregon, in an army canteen. *DEA*

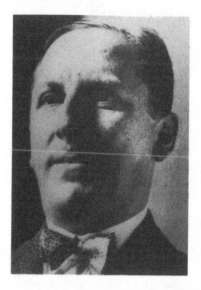

ARNOLD ROTHSTEIN

Widely known as a gambler and fixer, Rothstein was also a leading narcotic importer in the 1920s; according to some interviewees, his death brought to power a new and more ruthless generation of traffickers, who hiked prices and adulterated drugs to unheard-of levels. The New York Times

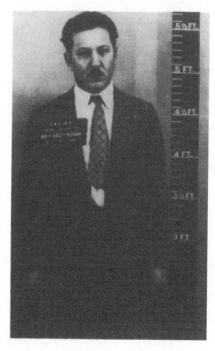

LOUIS "LEPKE" BUCHALTER

A small man with a long reach, Buchalter arranged contract murders, engaged in labor racketeering, and sold narcotics on a large scale. In 1944 he became the first—and last —top-level organized crime figure to be executed in the United States. DEA

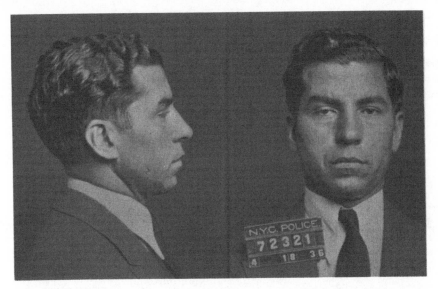

LUCKY LUCIANO

A natty dresser with a taste for silk underwear, Luciano was an international narcotic trafficker and archenemy of Harry Anslinger, whose name he contemptuously mispronounced as "Essingler." *Collections of the Municipal Archives, Department of Records and Information Services, City of New York*

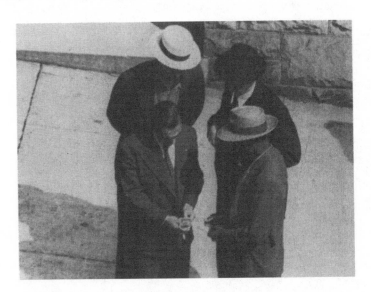

MAKING A BUY, BALTIMORE, 1941

Jaushawau [*sic*] L. Taylor, lower right, was a legendary black narcotic agent who went by the street name of "Cyclone Thompson." He has just purchased heroin from a dealer named George Presto, who is counting the cash from the transaction. An informer, smoking a cigarette, looks on. Despite its reputation for conservatism, the Bureau of Narcotics was one of the very few federal agencies to employ blacks in other than menial or clerical jobs before World War II. *DEA*

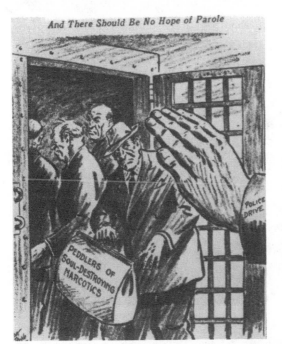

And There Should Be No Hope of Parole

THE HARD LINE
Classic-era editorial cartoonists were fond of caging, skewering, bashing, and otherwise destroying narcotic dealers, whom they portrayed as Mephistophelian thugs or loathsome animals like snakes. Such cartoons reinforced Anslinger's stand against maintenance by showing narcotics to be inherently destructive. New Orleans Times-Picayune, *September 23, 1937*

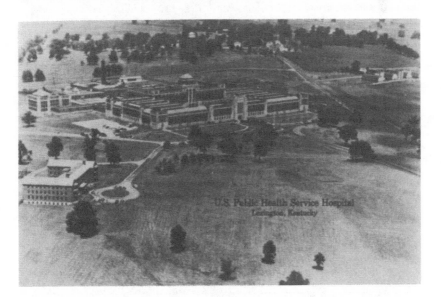

LEXINGTON
The institution's dual nature as a prison and a hospital is well displayed in this aerial photograph, which appears to have been taken during the 1940s. *DEA*

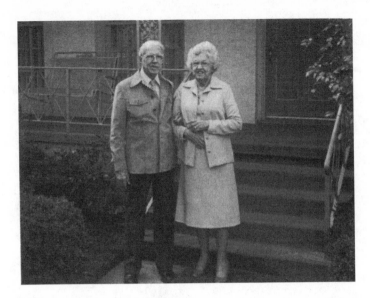

DR. AND MRS. WILLIS P. BUTLER,
SHREVEPORT, LOUISIANA, 1978
The closure of Butler's morphine maintenance and treatment
program in 1923 marked the beginning of four decades of nearly
absolute narcotic prohibition for addicts. *David Courtwright*

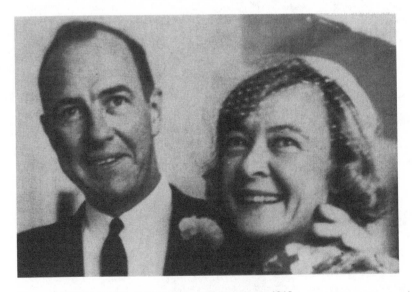

DRS. VINCENT DOLE AND MARIE NYSWANDER, 1965
Their work applied the coup de grace to the antimaintenance policy and
brought the classic era of narcotic control to a close. Dole and Nyswander
were married in September 1965. *Courtesy, Vincent Dole*

PART THREE: TREATMENT

12.

The Clinics

The treatment of narcotic addiction in the United States has passed through several distinct stages. Prior to the 1830s little was known about addiction and there were few reported cases; it was more a medical curiosity than an object of systematic inquiry and treatment. The toxic properties of opiates were of greater interest, since the average practitioner was far more likely to encounter an overdose case than one of chronic use.

During the last two-thirds of the nineteenth century, medical attitudes changed. Opium toxicology was still important, but there was a new and growing emphasis on the problem of addiction. The introduction and popularization of hypodermic injections, the physical and emotional trauma of the Civil War, the mass marketing of patent medicines, and other factors helped to bring about an epidemic of morphine addiction in the United States. Physicians began to specialize in treating addiction, and to develop theories about it. They debated its etiology: whether it, along with alcoholism, was symptomatic of a more general nervous disorder; whether gradual or rapid withdrawal was to be preferred; whether withdrawal could or should be palliated with nonnarcotic drugs and, if so, which ones. A hundred years later most of these issues are still unresolved.

Nineteenth-century physicians interested in addiction were handicapped by the embryonic state of medical science—they knew nothing of drug receptors, or endorphins, or narcotic antagonists—but they did have at least one advantage over modern researchers: almost total freedom. There were no federal regulations, no bureaucracy to deal with, and medical institutions, such as they were, largely steered clear of the problem. So doctors were at liberty to experiment, to prescribe purges, baths, electric therapy, dietary regimens, and various exotic concoctions for their addicted patients. Many of the leading authorities in the field operated private asylums, where the treatment was tailored to their particular theories of addiction.

Addicts, too, had a fair amount of choice. They could stay at one of the private asylums or attempt withdrawal as an outpatient under the supervision of a physician. Some bought "opium habit cures," patent medicines which were often laced with narcotics, and hence no cure at all. Or they could do nothing and simply continue to use undisguised narcotics. Few addicts were legally committed to institutional treatment. When they made an effort to quit, it was generally motivated by a sense of disgust, combined with health and financial worries and pressure from family and friends.

With the legal changes of 1909 to 1919, the freedom of both physicians and addicts began to disappear. Government officials assumed that, if addicts were denied access to drugs, the problem would resolve itself. They therefore discouraged both ambulatory treatment and maintenance by physicians; what they envisioned was institutional detoxification followed by enforced abstinence. When the Webb case was decided in 1919, they had a legal precedent upon which to base this policy.

The Webb case, however, involved individuals who had allegedly conspired to violate the Harrison Act. What would happen if maintenance programs were instead organized by municipal governments? This was the issue that was disputed during the famous clinic era of 1919–23. Following the Webb decision, some thirty-five municipalities in twelve different states opened up "narcotic clinics," so named because they sold morphine cheaply to their registered patients. A few also sold cocaine or heroin. What is sometimes misunderstood about these clinics is that they were not homogeneous, that their methods of operation varied. Some were geared toward indefinite maintenance, others toward detoxification through gradual withdrawal. Some were run for profit, others merely to break even. Some were models of efficient administration, others were fly-by-night operations.

One thing, however, they did have in common: all were eventually closed by the federal government, most within a year of opening their doors. Treasury Department officials, determined to eliminate both licit and illicit sources of narcotics for addicts, viewed the clinics as dangerous precedents and potential obstacles to the rigorous enforcement of the Harrison Act, as recently interpreted by the Supreme Court. So they moved to abort them through a combination of critical inspections, threats, and legal pressure. The clinics obviously touched a deep nerve, for, more than thirty years after they closed, the Bureau of Narcotics was still declaiming against them.

WILLIS BUTLER

Willis Pollard Butler was the most celebrated and controversial of all the early clinic doctors. Born in modest circumstances in Gibsland, Louisiana, in 1888, Butler moved with his family to Shreveport in 1899, where he took a summer job as a drugstore delivery boy. (Ironically, his chores included the delivery of dram bottles of morphine to the local addicts.) He eventually worked his way through Vanderbilt Medical School, graduating in 1911. Returning home, he applied his talents as chemist and bacteriologist for the Shreveport Board of Health, until he *was elected parish physician and coroner in 1916. He served in that capacity for no fewer than forty-eight years. When interviewed in 1978, he was over ninety years old.*[1]

Butler was above all else a superb politician. He was handsome, charming, articulate, and on a first-name basis with everyone who counted in Shreveport. That, together with the efficient and discriminating manner in which his clinic was run, assured local support and temporarily frustrated the designs of interloping federal agents.

Although Butler's memory was phenomenal for a man of his years, it should be borne in mind that his is only one side of the story, that the agents who hounded him and the doctors who turned on him can make no rebuttal. As Butler himself observed, "I don't know anybody connected with it—top, bottom, or middle—still living except me." For the sake of confidentiality, the names of addicts mentioned by Butler have been changed, as have the names of those who may have violated the law.

I was health officer, medical examiner for this district, and parish physician. One day—it was the third of May, 1919—Dr. Oscar Dowling, president of the state board of health, came to Shreveport. As usual, he called me, because I was representing the state board of health up in northern Louisiana. He asked me down to the hotel to make a culture of his throat —he had a sore throat. I went down there to see him and, as we walked out of the hotel, he said, "Butler, you having any problem up here with addicts?" I said, "Yes. I don't know about particular problems, but we got a lot of them. I'm having trouble with them in jail, and there's an awful lot of thievery and that sort of thing going on, and the police say that a lot of them are responsible." He said, "Well, we have opened up a clinic down in New Orleans, under Dr. Marion Swords. I suggest that you come down there and see how it's being done, because we have the approval of the government and the Treasury Department Narcotic Division. Maybe you could start the same thing up here."

Well, I went to New Orleans. I knew Dr. Swords quite well; he was secretary-treasurer of the state board of health. He had this clinic right across from the courthouse on the corner of Conti Street; it looked like a little alley down in the French Quarter. What I saw was a bunch of derelicts coming in, and they were giving them a little vial—it looked

---

1. This was not the first time Butler had been interviewed. Portions of a previous interview appear in Dan Waldorf, Martin Orlick, and Craig Reinarman, *Morphine Maintenance: The Shreveport Clinic, 1919–1923* (Washington, D.C.: Drug Abuse Council, 1974). The anecdotes related in the two interviews are generally similar, although details and sequences occasionally vary. Anyone wishing to explore the Shreveport episode further should compare both versions, as well as the account in Musto, *The American Disease*, 167–75.

like it might hold 15 or 20 cc. He said that they were putting morphine in there, a certain amount according to what they wanted them to start with. The next day, they would put in a little less, but the same amount of water. They were going to get them off of it by reduction. I said, "You don't know much about addicts if you think that you can fool them as to whether they're suffering or not." I said I'd have nothing to do with that sort of thing at all, and I told Dr. Dowling that I did not want to assume any such responsibility.

So they called a meeting of the board of health in New Orleans. Governor John M. Parker was there—he was a running mate of Theodore Roosevelt for vice president. At the meeting I could see that the governor knew nothing about addiction at all. When I told him of the seriousness of the situation he said, "Well, why not just send them all up there to you?" That was ridiculous, of course. I said, "Governor, have you had any experience with addicts?" He said, "Well, I'll tell you what happened to me as I was getting on the train this morning in Baton Rouge. A lady, a rather nice-looking lady, came up to me and said, 'You're Governor Parker?' I said, 'Yes, ma'am.' She said, 'I demand that you give me permission to get some morphine. I've *got* to have it; I'll die without it.' I didn't believe it and said, 'What would you do to get it?' She said, 'If necessary, I'd cut your throat.'" Then he said to me, "It must be sort of serious." I said, "You're just beginning to learn."

I came to Shreveport, and in the meantime I thought, "Well, this is not such a big proposition. I'll write prescriptions." For a short time, for each one that we examined once we had our organization set up, I wrote prescriptions and had them filled at one drugstore, the Shreveport Drug Store, by a Mr. John Scott, so we could keep the records straight. Well, I saw in no time that that was impractical. Then, just by trial and error, I worked at it and devised what finally developed into the outpatient and institutional treatment. Dr. Dowling gave his strong affirmation of the work—although he lied later and stated that he did not do it.

Some interesting complications came up because many very prominent people here didn't know anything about narcotic addiction; all they knew was "dope fiends" and street characters and "hopheads" and that sort of thing. They didn't know that, out of the sixteen hundred patients that I had, that many of them were the very most prominent people—financially and socially and politically—in this whole community, including two previous United States district attorneys, preachers, lawyers, doctors, nurses, real estate people . . . All of these were kept secret. I didn't want to hurt anybody that would be on the clinic by exposing them to people who didn't understand what it was all about. So I allowed them to sign their right name in a locked book that I kept secret, and to use an alias on the public register every time any dispensation of drugs was made. And, by the way, this dispensing was in order to prepare them to be placed in an institution that I established here, in which we detoxified over four hundred. Now, that was unless they were aged, infirm, or incurable. They all had a doctor's certificate—and I had seven doctors sign, as a rule.

Our federal judge for the western district of Louisiana, George Whitfield Jack, came out and looked into it personally, because he was a very close friend of mine. Judge Jack said, "Well, I've never had anything quite like this, but it's humane and it's right. Looking over the names of these people, some of them that you have here, I'm thoroughly amazed."

One day I was in the police station on some sort of business. Captain Bob was commissioner of public safety. He was a very wealthy oil man, elected to office as a plaything, more than anything else for him. He said to me, in the presence of two rather prominent local men, "Doc, you know I think it's a shame the way you're taking care of these hopheads, drug addicts, and scum around here in Shreveport. Tell you the truth, I think every one of them ought to be run in the river." Well, I made no comment, except, about that time, these gentlemen excused themselves and went ahead. I said, "Cap'n Bob, let me speak to you personally in your office." We walked into his little private office, closed the door, and he sat in his desk chair and I sat in another. I said, "Now, Cap'n Bob, you and I have been friends for many, many years. When I make a promise of secrecy, I do my best to keep it. Sometimes an occasion arises when you've got to apparently violate that promise. You said that all these people on my clinic ought to be run into the river." He said, "Yes." I said, "Well then, would it surprise you to know that your mother has been on that clinic for two years?"

He dropped his hands and looked at me. He said, "Doc, do you mean that?" I said, "I don't say it if I don't mean it, Cap'n Bob. You want to see the record—you're entitled to it. It's private, but if that's what it takes . . ." He said, "No, your word is good."

After a few minutes of silence he said, "This startles me. Did anybody know this?" I said, "Yes, four people: me, your father, your mother's family doctor, and John Scott, who's a pharmacist that dispenses it. The other names I can't give you, because she buyed it from bootleggers, in the alleys and so forth." He said, "Well, that clarifies something in my mind. My mother is a wonderful, wonderful fine Christian woman. I've never given her any trouble. I've taken care of her, and I'm proud of her, and I love her. Just to think that she's been going through this and I didn't know it. And I have wondered—although it didn't bother me—I have wondered why she had needed so much money in the last few years. She had no expenses." I said, "Well, she's been getting this money to pay bootleggers from one to three dollars a grain for codeine, mostly."

He said, "I want to say something to you. From now on, if there's anything in the world I can do for you, if you ever need help, you can call on me." I said, "You mean that?" He said, "Yes, I do." I said, "I'll tell you what I want right now. Captain John Hudson is your chief of detectives. I want him assigned to my clinic as an inspector. I'm going to select Ted Voight of the health department as the other. I want these two men to work together and investigate, with any help they want, every person on that clinic." He said, "No more said than done," and up the hall we went. He got John Hudson—Cap'n Hudson, he was—and said, "You're working for Dr. Butler from now on." He got Ted Voight and told him the same thing. And I'll say that every morning when that clinic was open those two men were there. They checked on *everybody*—no matter who, good or bad—in the first place, to see if they were sick, if they were legitimate, needed medicine, and so forth.

One way I checked on them, I fingerprinted every single one of them. We took their histories, we fingerprinted them. At that time, the FBI wasn't organized like it is today; it was in Leavenworth, Kansas. I sent as many as six hundred sets of fingerprints up there at one time and got a report on every one of them—to see if they were wanted anywhere, you know. The first time I sent a batch off to Leavenworth, by the time I got the report back, fourteen of my patients had left town. Every one of them was wanted somewhere. That's the way we cleaned up transients from coming through here. Then we limited it to our own citizens, unless there was some reason.

We learned pretty early in the game that Shreveport was sort of being made a mecca to bring them in from other states here. That's why I instituted the fingerprints and got the investigators on the job. Not only did they investigate them, but they went to verify if they worked where they said they'd worked, lived where they said they'd lived. They gave me reports—not always written—but if there was anything wrong they'd always let me know and we'd take action. If they weren't wanted somewhere, we'd take them on at the clinic. Until, until—I don't know what date—but later on we did limit it to Louisiana. But I wouldn't be too sure we weren't imposed upon. You know, it's pretty hard: somebody comes here to Shreveport and lives here and they've got a residence and somebody's going to tell you that they're there . . . In all of this time, remember, I didn't have one solitary single dime from the government to run this thing with. I was buying the medicine from a St. Louis wholesale house; I was paying about two to three cents a grain for it, and I was letting them have it at five or six cents—it varied. Well, that little difference in there is what paid running the clinic.

Now, in combination with this clinic, and as a very essential part of it, was a venereal disease clinic. A tremendous number of people had venereal disease. Syphilitic aortitis was just as common . . . we don't see it now like we used to. I was one of the three in the whole United States that had charge of Salvarsan and Neosalvarsan when Ehrlich discovered it. I started using it here in Shreveport—nobody'd ever done a Wassermann before I came here. It could have been that some of these people came to be treated, not only for their drug addiction, but for their venereal disease. But, anyway, whether they did or not, we found out whether they had it. Every single one of them had a VDRL or a Wassermann test made on them. If we found that they had a disease of one kind or another, we didn't try to take them off the drug. We let them have it until the remedy was there. Then, when they had no other reason, you could take them off with the expectation they'd stay off.

The clinic started on May the third, 1919, and ended on March the thirteenth, 1925.[2] They ordered me to close it two or three times and I said, "I'm not going to do it." The crooked narcotic inspectors came here with the deliberate purpose of doing what their superiors had told them to do, "Go there and get Butler. He's got the only clinic left. We've ordered him closed. We're going to stand behind that order, right or wrong, and he's got to be closed." I just didn't knuckle down and close. I fought it for two years, until I got down to twenty-one incurable, old, infirm patients. I turned all of them over to their own family doctors to take care of and then I deliberately closed the clinic myself.

The situation got so bad here after I closed the clinic—it was worse than before it opened. I didn't try to follow it up too closely, but the police told me and the papers had reports about thievery and robbery. And I recognized plenty of the names.

The majority of the inspectors sent in here were just such crooks and scum and scalawags and downright . . . well, there was nothing they wouldn't do. And I caught one or two of them. As an illustration, there happened to be a Dr. Wilcox in New York, who was a friend of Dr. Terry's.[3] Wilcox was a man evidently of some means and standing. He had by carelessness and self-medication gotten himself to where he needed help. He didn't want to go to somewhere in New York City to do that, so Sidney Howard[4] and Dr. Terry got me to let him come down here. When I met him he had the credentials to show who he was. He proved to be a legitimate doctor and a very nice man, younger than I was.

When he got here he had a glass jar with a ground glass top full of white powder—I would say there were about six ounces in there—which proved to be morphine sulfate. So I took that. Everything we confiscated we labeled, saying where we got it and what it all was. Then, after I had

2. The dispensing of drugs actually ceased on February 10, 1923. Only the detoxification facility remained open until 1925.

3. Charles Edward Terry, an authority on addiction who admired and supported Butler's work.

4. A journalist and dramatist who published a favorable account of Butler's clinic, "The Inside Story of Dope in this Country," *Hearst's International* 43 (June 1923), 24–28, 116, 118–20.

weighed it and measured it and knew exactly what it was, I turned it over to the federal district attorney, so he'd give it to some inspector.

In a few days, an inspector came by to pick all of this up from the district attorney. Well, this inspector happened to come into my office one morning—his name was Cutler. He had with him a state narcotic inspector and another federal narcotic inspector. He introduced himself, showed his credentials, and told me who these other gentlemen were —they sat silently there. He said, "I want to look through all of your records." I said, "All right, it's about ten o'clock in the morning now." This was at the Schumpert Sanitarium, where I had my clinic. I watched him and he looked through things carefully. The other men said nothing. Finally, as the morning wore on, I noticed him getting a little bit shaky— he was using a pencil and a tablet to write things down on. After a little while he said, "Well, Dr. Butler, it's time to go to lunch. We'll go to lunch and come back." I said, "No sir, it won't be convenient to me at all. You stay here till you finish, whatever time it takes. It's open to you now, but it won't be open all day long. I can't do that. We've got work to do here, patients sick, and so forth." He said, "Well, all right." He got a little bit more shaky, and I saw then that he was in the withdrawal symptoms.

I said, "Mr. Cutler, you have asked me an awful lot of questions. You went over to Miss Skelton's home—she's a hunchback, cripple, incurable; and you went to Mr. Meyer's home—Mr. Meyer owns the Meyer Building, he's one of our most prominent and wealthy citizens; and you went to others and you demanded that you would be able to inspect their homes and see what they had in there with no warrants or anything. I want to tell you that I resent it. Now I'm going to ask you something: how much morphine do *you* use a day?"

Well, he shook and dropped his pencil and pad on the floor. He picked them up and he said, "I won't stay here and be insulted." I said, "Insulted, nothing. I just asked you a plain question. I know you're an addict. I know that you're taking it; you're in withdrawal symptoms now—that's why you want to leave. And you're not leaving here till I'm satisfied about it."

Now, I spoke awhile ago about this Dr. Wilcox coming from New York and bringing his morphine with him, and how I measured it and it was later picked up. The district attorney had gotten it back, and when I measured it again, it was about a dram and a half short. I knew this when Cutler was sitting there in my office. I accused him of being an addict, then I asked him, "What happened to the medicine? I'd like for you to know that I measured it before I turned it in, and we've got it back and there's a dram and a half gone out of it. Nobody had it but you." Cutler said to the other two, "Come on, fellas," and out they went. Just as they were leaving, my secretary and bookkeeper and some of the technicians who were training there said, "Dr. Butler, we're afraid you've made a big mistake." I said, "No sir, I know better. We've got a jail full of that sort."

About that time the phone rang. I answered it and said, "Dr. Butler."
The speaker said, "This is Mr. Ernest. I'm one of the men with Mr.
Cutler. You don't know how glad we are of what you told that man.
You're right. If it becomes necessary, we'll back you up in it. But you're
completely right." I said, "I feel sure, and I appreciate it and I thank you
about it, and I'm going to get a warrant out for him if I can catch him."
And I notified Attorney General Palmer in Washington about it. But the
attorney general didn't do a thing in the world except transfer him to
Indianapolis, Indiana.

I got no support from the federal government at all. Now, they did
send one man here named Fraser. This man Fraser was, I think, next to
Colonel Nutt.[5] He came down here—he proved to be a perfect gentleman
in every way. I drove him around and he told me about little things that
might happen that would be all right but could cause me trouble. He was
really very helpful. He showed that they did at least have one man who
was honorable and honest and all. But, unfortunately, he left here and
they moved him to Pensacola or Jacksonville, Florida, and his wife shot
him in a post office. [Laughs.] I don't know what that was all about.

Huey Long and I were pretty close together for a long time, till I
learned him. If he couldn't use you, he didn't need you anymore. But,
anyway, we were strong friends and supporters for a long time. Huey
Long walked into the federal courtroom one day and told me, "Doc, why
don't you tell your friends when you're in trouble?" I said, "What do you
mean, 'in trouble'?" He said, "I'll tell you: the federal grand jury." Well,
I thought about that. I went on downstairs to the elevator and there was a
man standing there. He said, "Dr. Butler, my name is Knight"—a well-
known family up here from Benton—"I'm not supposed to say anything
about this, but somebody's trying to pull off something pretty dirty against
you. I just wanted you to know about it." Well, I didn't know what it could
be, and I went on home still wondering.

About seven o'clock the phone rang: "That you, Doc?" I said, "Yeah."
"This is Huey. Can you come down here?" I said, "Who's there with you,
Huey?" He said, "Alice Lee." Alice Lee Grosjean was his secretary and
lady friday—at least.

When I walked in there, Alice Lee went into her own office, but I saw
an old gentleman sitting there. I don't mean this in a derogatory sense at
all, but you could see he was "rural"—he was roughed up a little. Huey
said, "Mr. Ewell, this is my friend Dr. Butler. I want you to tell him
just what you've told me. You can trust Dr. Butler. You tell him." Mr.
Ewell said, "I'm a member of the federal grand jury, and I know I'm not

---

5. It is possible that Butler misrecollected this name. We have been unable to verify
Fraser's position in the Prohibition Unit. Butler is correct, however, in identifying Nutt as
the head of the operation.

supposed to talk, but Dr. Dowling has come up before the grand jury and brought a whole lot of stuff, all against you. I just told my friend Huey here, and Huey said you were his friend." I said, "Well, I don't know what's going on."

Huey said, "I'll tell you what you do. You've got all your records, haven't you?" I said, "Sure, I've got them exactly as best I can up to date." He said, "Well, you get your records all together and turn them over to Tom Hughes"—Tom was sheriff, and I guess my closest friend—"and ask Tom Hughes to give them to Philip Mecom"—the district attorney —"in the morning. I'll take it from there." Well, I called Tom Hughes and told him what Huey had said and gave the records to him. Tom Hughes took them over to give them to Philip Mecom. Then, next thing I knew, the case was thrown out.

Dr. Dowling got on the corner post office steps there and publicly stated, where a dozen people heard it, that he was mad that Shreveport was full of addicts and there were not more than twelve doctors here who were not involved in it [overprescribing]. I didn't hear it, but a lot of people heard it. Rupert Peyton, who was a Louisiana representative, but also a reporter, came and told me. I went to the president of the medical society and told him. He called a meeting for that night of the medical society to expel Dr. Dowling, or give him a chance to make an explanation why he'd make that statement. He did his darndest to crawfish out of it. He also purposely and deliberately got up before the meeting and stated that he had never endorsed this clinic's work. I produced twenty-two letters right there, signed by him, where he had endorsed it. I had very little to say except, "Gentlemen, this is the record: one or the other of us is a liar, and you can determine which one it is."

One hundred and six members were there. It had to be unanimous to expel him, but he got one vote, so he wasn't expelled. Dr. Dowling's partner, Dr. John Scales—one of the finest Christian men and friends that I had—wouldn't vote against him. Dr. Dowling said to me, "I'm going to see that you're sent to Atlanta if it's the last thing I ever do"— there happened to be a penitentiary there. From then on, the poor man, he had a stroke and fell off of a train on a ferry crossing the Mississippi and was crushed to death.

Dr. Dowling was my friend—I thought. He had been in my home, and we had talked about things, being alumni of the same school. I just can't understand it. But, in my own mind, I feel real sure that, when Dr. Dowling got the word that the headquarters up in Washington had made up *their* mind that they were going to close the clinics, he switched just like that and later denied that he had supported it. Dowling was scared of Washington—that's the whole thing.

I don't think I was treated fair, but I'm glad I went through it. I remember coming home one day to my wife, bless her heart. I'd been to

Doctor being turned out of fear of Washington

this medical meeting where Dr. Dowling stated he was going to send me to Atlanta if it was the last thing he did. I didn't know what a character like that might do—if they indict you, they don't expect to convict you; if they can just stir up something, they've done the damage. My wife was on the bed, and I said, "Well, I'll tell you, this thing's just about gotten out of hand. I don't know how much longer I can take it." I said something about "sending me to Atlanta." And her remark was, "Well, if you go, I'm going with you." To me, that gave me one of the biggest boosts. I decided then that neither one of us was going. I hadn't left anything over there in Atlanta, and I wasn't going back for it.

LEROY STREET

"Leroy Street" is the pseudonymous author of I Was a Drug Addict *(1953), one of the minor classics of confessional drug literature. The book (which was dictated to a collaborator, David Loth) is an account of Street's addiction from age fifteen to twenty-three, his frequent relapses, and his final, romantically inspired cure. When interviewed in 1981, he had been off all drugs, save nicotine, for fifty-eight years.*

Street may be the only person still living who attended a narcotic clinic as a patient. What he saw, however, must have differed greatly from the situation in Shreveport. The New York City clinic was large, hastily organized, and overcrowded; its clients were mainly young, male street addicts; it offered a choice of heroin or morphine; and, most importantly, it attempted to detoxify all patients by gradually reducing their daily allotment.

The first people to sniff heroin were the Chinamen. Hopheads: they had opium habits. In 1909 they banned opium coming in for smoking purposes. Some of these Chinamen got arrested trying to get the stuff. A lot of them had a bad cough; when they were in jail they gave them heroin, which is a *marvelous* cure for a cough. But outside of that, it's a hell of an addictive drug.

I started sniffing heroin with my companions in 1910. It only took about a month to get addicted to it. At that time I had pure heroin, but I was mixing it with sugar of milk. What we got came from Germany— Bayer and Bayer—in little bottles. It was 100 percent heroin; we actually had to adulterate it, it was so strong. So we bought sugar of milk—for a couple of cents you get a whole lot of that—and we mixed it up.

After the Harrison Act, heroin became increasingly expensive and hard to get. It created a black market. The big black market dealers? Well, I'd hate to tell the nationality even. They lived in an Italian area of Greenwich Village, to the south of Washington Square Park. Yes, they were Italian, but I'd better not get into it, or they'll have the Mafia after me. The Italians were involved in the beginning, and the drugstores were involved in the beginning. There was one drugstore that gave us Christmas presents. It was really something: a brand-new, shining hypodermic needle with a little ribbon around it and a little card, "Merry Christmas."

The Italian street dealers I was buying from got it from big drug dealers, maybe drug companies where they had somebody working. There was a drug company up on Thirteenth Street, a big drug company, and people worked there and they were in a position to steal. In the early days the street dealers didn't necessarily smuggle it into the country, but they got it from the drug houses, then diverted it onto the street.

I bought from the street dealers and then we found a connection, Barney's Pharmacy, which was on East Fourth Street and Avenue B. He was doing a business already with others, but he was scared. He sold it to us, but he wouldn't give it over the counter. He'd take the money, he'd measure it up, and then he'd say, "You come back in about half an hour and go in the hall." The store was on the corner of a big apartment house: you'd go in the hall and down behind the radiator you'd find the stuff. That way they couldn't get him, though they might catch you coming out. This was the idea of the thing.

He got away with it for quite a while. Then, later on, when I got arrested once for junk, I was walking the flats in Jefferson Market, and who do I run into but Barney. He said, "You people made me do it. You wouldn't let me quit. It's all on account of you guys." Well, that's a poor excuse, because he was taking the money, you know.

The narcotic clinic was on Worth Street. There was a big old building there. It hadn't been used for years—it's where the license bureau is now. When it opened up, there were pictures in the paper of the junkies lining up outside the place. I was among some of them junkies.

When it opened up we all barged in. There were several desks where doctors sat, different doctors. You'd be sent to one doctor; the next one would be sent to another doctor. He'd ask you what you used and how you were using it. You'd show him your arm if you were shooting it. Then he would write out a prescription, and then you would go to the rear. There was a big drug counter. You'd put the prescription down and you'd get the drug. I always got heroin. There was a cop standing there to keep order. It was a new deal for the addicts to be able to go in and buy their junk at a clinic with a cop at their elbow.

They gave you a card where it showed how much they cut you down as you went along—a third of a grain, a quarter of a grain, or something. They kept cutting it lower and lower until I got so, after awhile, I think I was going back there for about three-tenths of a grain, or something like that. Well, then it got so low it was useless to do it.

Before they had reduced very much, when they were still giving us fifteen grains or ten grains, the dealers were hurt. They lost a lot of business. It was only when they started reducing down to a certain low level that we came back to them. The dealers told us that: they said, "Well, you'll come back." And it was true. We went back to them.

[margin note: Reducing was not effective]

S. DANA HUBBARD

Here, for the sake of contrast, is an excerpt from a 1920 article[6] by S. Dana Hubbard, one of the New York City clinic's chief physicians.

They know one another by association; but by name, not at all, perhaps a "nickname," or abbreviated first name, being the only appreciable recognizable fact of a connection between them. "May" knows "Ike," and "Shorty" knows "Whitey"; while "Smoke" pals with "The Duke"; and, as for homes, they have none. They meet in places convenient for secret conference, toilets being the most often selected, and in such dens of iniquity as will tolerate such lounging and loafing. Their hours are as irregular as those of a stray cat, and neither day nor night is of any particular consequence, save that the cover of darkness suits their convenience for obtaining a renewed supply of their drug. As for meals, they depend on the effect of the drug most often to assuage any hunger, but they will eat candy, particularly nut chocolate bars. For these, addicts all display a fondness, and when offered to them, will never be refused.

[margin note: Addictive behavior]

All that this class of drug addicts—the confirmed habitué—appears to care for is to have a supply of "dope," and a place where it can be obtained. Having this, he is as happy and contented, and as apparently comfortable as any blessed mortal on earth desires. Thirst he knows not. When a sensation develops, he regards that as a need for another "shot," and so every thing that would be natural in the usual daily life of the ordinary man, to him, is unnecessary.

Addicts confide in one another—they are loyal, in their own way, stealing from the weak or those that have it, to be in turn imposed upon by others in similar fashion. From their pals, in their set—for there is caste —and the hangers-on of such a group or tribe, they borrow even to the last cent, and it appears to be loaned willingly, even though knowing it may never be returned. If one loans to another, he, in turn, borrows from others more fortunate than himself. They are typical human parasites. The following is interesting as relating to this fellowship: A young fellow, unclean, ragged, and apparently in abject pain and misery, applied, got his "script" (slang for prescription) but on going to the pharmacy of the

[margin note: Loyal.]

[margin note: Hash.]

6. "The New York City Narcotic Clinic and Differing Points of View on Narcotic Addiction," *Monthly Bulletin of the Department of Health, City of New York* 10 (1920), 33–47.

clinic found that the amount of money required to fill it was beyond his financial abilities; he dropped out of the waiting line, mingled with his more fortunate companions, borrowing a penny here and another there, until he made up the required amount. He then returned to the line and secured his supply. Then, as he went toward his retreat to take a "shot," he was accosted by one in lower depths, bent on borrowing; he gave his precious all and returned to borrow enough of the drug from his pals to meet his needs until he could secure another prescription, on the day following.

After one of these borrowing excursions, one of these less fortunate individuals approached one more fortunate and asked "for a part of a shot." The poor addict had his little outfit ready to take a dose; he was pale, anxious, and apparently suffering keenly. He pinched up his skin, turning and twisting the needle point, sent it home, slowly injecting the solution, and when about half accomplished, noticing the despair on his companion's face, he withdrew the needle, and turned his syringe over, half filled, to his pal in misery. The poor chap had felt that he needed a little, but also that he could divide with one who appeared to need it more than he, so he took sufficient to "set" him, and willingly passed over the outfit to his beseeching companion in misery. This beggar seized the outfit, jabbed the needle through clothing and all into his belly skin and slowly shot the contents, to the last drop, home.

Having witnessed this charitable and brotherly act, I waited and, when the outfit was returned, I had it refilled and returned to its owner. This chap dropped to his knees and kissed my shoes. I tried to restrain him, and told him the clinic was intended to aid and comfort those in need. Imagine my chagrin to observe, on the following day, the same game practiced by others, clearly stamping this as a ruse, a frame-up, to obtain the drug without paying, by playing upon the emotions of those in charge. Persons that practice such deceptions to serve their selfish purposes are not "on the square," and cannot be trusted because they incite others to practice further impositions.

Another similar instance of imposition played upon the volunteer workers was the following: Early on opening the clinic, there appeared a lad, surely not over 20 years of age, who had the great misfortune to have had both legs cut off at the hip. He propelled himself by having a board strapped to his torso and attached to the bottom of this board was a pair of roller skates. In his hands he had a pair of wooden handles, like dumb-bells, which he would place on the ground and with a shove he would send himself rolling along faster than one could walk. He was alacrity itself, and agile as a cat. He got about gracefully, followed always by a white spitz dog of the toy type. Like master, the pup was very, very dirty. The boy in his crippled condition, accompanied by his faithful dog, naturally attracted attention as well as keen sympathy. This boy was not particularly pallid, nor emaciated; and, on examining him later, no needle marks were discovered. The addicts who snuffle the drug have a sniffing respiration—a constant catching of the breath on inhalation through the nose which, with the presence of excessive nasal secretion, gives a mucous rattle. This symptom was also absent in this case. We were certain that this cripple was not an addict. What was he? His connection was developed later. The clinic was always crowded—jammed was a better and more fitting description—but on this occasion it was unusually congested. Suddenly the crowd surged to a corner and, thinking some accident (an addict overcome through an over dose) had happened, the floor captain (a lady volunteer worker) went over to investigate, and returned stating that the roller skate cripple had had his dog stolen and was crying bitterly. The sympathy of the captain was aroused and, to comfort the boy, she passed the hat about the building and collected a neat sum of money. The money, naturally, consoled the chap, and he left the clinic with his tear ducts dry.

On opening the clinic, the following day, there was our little cripple and, lo! with him was his spitz dog. I approached him and said: "I thought that you had lost your dog?" "I did," he replied. "How did you get him back so quickly?" He said, "I heard a feller had him and I got my pal to go to him and buy him back—it cost me twenty-five dollars." The story seemed honest, but the price to redeem so inconsequential a "mut" was unreasonable. The chap was marked for more careful observation. We permitted the boy to come and go freely, giving him his supply, and, owing to his crippled condition, he was advanced in the several lines, preference being given him at all times. This kindness was his undoing. One day, soon afterwards, our detectives brought in our little cripple, charging him with acting as a "bootlegger"—selling drugs. When brought into the consulting room he was searched, and, strapped to his back, resting on his roller skate board, was a dirty bag containing "coke decks" and sixty dollars in silver coins—in fact it was the tinkling of this pile of coin that exposed him. To arrest a cripple, on such a charge, in our quarters, where sanctuary had been proclaimed, would make others think that we had "framed" the boy and were not playing the game fair. We decided not to arrest him, but to try and get into his good graces, if he had any. The scheme worked. The little chap was not above par when it came to matching wits, so he was quickly and easily caught and confessed to being a "coke" peddler. Not being an addict, he was excluded from the use of the clinic, and later fell into the hands of the police. In his confession, he said that the dog story had always been successful, and that no one had ever before seen through it. He also told how it had always netted him from ten to twenty dollars a day. He said that, at first, his conscience had bothered him about gulling the ladies, but the money came so easily that, later, he never gave it a second thought, and, when he needed money he would go to some crowded place, hang around until known to have a dog and then a chum, on a signal, would secrete the pup and, the stage being set, he'd break out crying—using glycerine in his eyes to make the tears flow freely. With his dirty, wet face and his deformity he was able, as long as the crowd lasted, to get money from the gullible. As he had played the game so long, and so successfully, we had visions of a neat bank account set aside for the proverbial rainy day, but he gleefully informed us that he did not save anything. That when he found the gang hanging about, he would play craps, and that he was always unlucky and soon lost his day's makings. He was asked how he accounted for his ill-luck, and he laughingly replied, "I guess the blokeys use ponies (loaded dice) on me." "Then why do you keep it up?" "If I didn't play, I'd lose me pals. They wouldn't have me hanging around, if I did not do as they do." This seemed to furnish another key to this problem. As clever as was this crippled chap, his pals knew how he made his money, so they considered it "only fair" to get it away from him for their purposes.

The display of wit and natural cunning by these chaps, to meet their selfish purposes, is positively uncanny. We believed that drug addiction sapped the memory and dulled the intelligence—with the experiences of dramatic cleverness exercised to extract the coin of the realm from the unwary, often times to use for gambling or to obtain a supply of "dope," naturally our opinion now is that indiscriminate largesse is exceedingly harmful to general public welfare. Without the drug, these individuals, male and female, appear listless, weary and apathetic, then as the misery becomes more acute they are restless, peevish and distressingly irritable. One very peculiar and universal characteristic is that they, one and all, are insistently selfish and self-concerned. For others they care not at all. . . . In our opinion, drug addiction is simply a degrading, debasing habit, and it is not necessary to consider this indulgence in any other light than an anti-social one, and that those who are charged with correcting and preventing such tendencies should be stimulated to do so to their utmost, and all efforts exerted in this direction should be free from restraint, absolutely unhampered, and that all physicians interested in the general welfare of the people should earnestly encourage such action. . . .

Ambulatory treatment is farcical and useless, and is only putting off what should be immediately done. Physicians should not be permitted, under guise of treatment, to prescribe narcotics for such indulgence. Laws should be so amended that the narcotic addict, when determined, should be sent by due process of commitment to a suitable institution and held there, until a medical officer considers it safe for him to return to society. That after-care should be in an open-air environment—a farm, or outdoor gymnasium, or recreational institute being preferable—and continued until the psychic phase is entirely passed, and the addict can again resume his place and maintain himself in society. . . .

From an experience with many hundreds, passing through our clinic and hospital, it is our firm opinion that entire withdrawal may, in many instances, be successfully performed. That all that is needed is to have the withdrawal process supervised by a physician, so that those who need medical care may get it when it is required.

Strict, adequate, and proper, as well as uniform enforcement of the law —the Harrison Act—throughout this city and country is now demanded, and is essential towards preventing recruits to these miserable ranks.

13.

Lexington and Its Discontents

The eclipse of the clinics at the beginning of the classic era meant that there were virtually no government facilities for the treatment of narcotic addicts. They either had to remain at large or silt up the nation's prisons, which were ill designed to deal with their problems. The solution, proposed by Pennsylvania Representative Stephen G. Porter and enthusiastically backed by the Hearst newspaper chain, was to construct special facilities to quarantine and rehabilitate addicts. These "narcotic farms" were to be set in rural areas, so that addicts could be removed from the tempting cities and set to healthful work.

Money was authorized in 1929. The first narcotic farm, officially known as the U.S. Public Health Service Narcotic Hospital, was completed at Lexington, Kentucky, in 1935. (Among addicts it was referred to variously as "Narco," "Lex," "Lexington," or simply "K.Y.") A second narcotic farm was opened in Fort Worth in 1938. Of the two, Lexington was the larger and more prominent. It was to remain the single most important treatment and research facility in the country throughout the classic era.

From the beginning Lexington had a mixed institutional character. Federal prison and narcotic officials saw it mainly as a penitentiary where troublesome addicts could be isolated and confined, Public Health Service physicians as a hospital where mentally disturbed addicts could be treated and rehabilitated. Architecturally, Lexington reflected the official ambivalence: its beds and wards were secured with massive gates and intricate locks. As one doctor put it, Lexington was "more like a prison than a hospital and more like a hospital than a prison."

As a dual-purpose institution, Lexington had a dual system of admissions. Prisoner addicts could be sent there involuntarily for confinement and treatment, but voluntary patients were also permitted to check in on a space-available basis. The problem was that the volunteers could leave at any time, while the prisoners would have to stay until they were paroled or completed their terms, which might

Mixed insti- character [handwritten marginal note]

be months or years after withdrawal was completed. The staff, in other words, had little or no control over the time of release.[1]

Classic-era addicts were of two minds about Lexington. To some it represented a haven, a clean and well-run institution where a user could detoxify, receive *medical and dental care, obtain counseling, decent food, work, and exercise. "When I would feel bad, or get mentally disgusted," Mike recalled, "I thought to myself, 'What am I doing? I'm a drug addict. I want to quit.' So I'd go to Lexington, and I'd come out feeling like a million dollars." Altogether he went six times. Others viewed this sort of behavior with disdain. "I never went to Lexington," boasted Jack.*

You want my honest opinion of the people who went down there on their own? They never should have been on heroin. They didn't have the ability to support a habit: either they couldn't make enough money working, or they weren't thieves, or they were afraid to deal. [Laughs.] We used to tell them, "What are you doing, going down to get rescued?"

I doubt if I'm mistaken, but if you'll look it up, you'll find that on average better than 75 percent of the people who went to Lexington on their own repeated. Everytime things got bad—boom!—they were back. See, if you go down there once, I can understand it. Even twice, even three times I can understand, if a guy makes some kind of an effort to stay away from heroin when he comes out. But a lot of users go back to heroin immediately, and then use Lexington as a fallback, a port in the storm.

Jack's estimate of 75 percent is actually conservative; several studies showed that 90 percent or more of those released from Lexington soon relapsed. These depressing figures gave rise to a controversy, muted at first but increasingly contentious by the early 1960s. Different theories of relapse were advanced, attributing it to everything from underlying personality disorders to conditioned responses to permanent metabolic changes. Some even argued that addicts returned to drug use because they missed the intense excitement of hustling and scoring; once they were in the life, everything else seemed boring by comparison.

Whatever the reason, the fact remained that large numbers of patient-inmates speedily relapsed after their release. This ultimately worked to undermine the Bureau of Narcotics' policy against maintenance. The 1958 joint report of the American Bar Association and American Medical Association, which revived discussion of the clinic approach, was explicit on this point. "[T]he exposure of a

---

1. Robert W. Rasor, "The United States Public Health Service and Institutional Treatment Program for Narcotic Addicts at Lexington, Kentucky," in Leon Brill and Louis Lieberman, eds., *Major Modalities in the Treatment of Drug Abuse* (New York: Behavioral Publications, 1972), 2–6.

few months to a minimum amount of psychiatry, social case work, educational and vocational activity, cannot eradicate the deep seated necessity and compulsion for drugs which most addicts seem to have," the report noted. "There are no magic cures at narcotics hospitals."[2]

The relapse rate also raised obvious problems of cost-effectiveness. By the early 1970s it was clear that Lexington had not lived up to its original expectations and that it was a "rather expensive anachronism" in an age when local treatment centers could provide the same services more economically. So in 1974 the Lexington facilities, except for the Addiction Research Center, were turned over to the Bureau of Prisons.[3]

CHARLIE

I was on bail when I went into Lexington—this was in the thirties. My case was going to come up in two months, so I went to 19 Pine Street, in New York, and I told them I wanted to go to Lexington for a cure. They gave me a ticket, told me to go to Penn Station, get on a train, and go to Lexington.

I'm not sure how much I was using before I went down there. I can't say I was using an ounce. Maybe I was using a quarter of an ounce. If the H was good, you used less. If it was no good, more. One day I almost used a half ounce. Big tablespoons full. To feel normal—don't say you're going to get high—you had to use three of those spoons. It was all milk and sugar. Later, during the panic, things got even worse. I paid forty-five dollars for a tin of hop in 1940. I threw that much away when I used to buy three tins for five dollars.

Anyway, I was on the train to Lexington and I met this fellow Tommy from Seventh Street. I didn't know him, he was a perfect stranger, but he got to talking to me. He said, "You're going to Lexington, huh? You're from New York?" I said "Yeah." He said, "I'm going there too. I've got a wife that's got cancer. She gets pills, morph, and she's been sharing them with me. But, lately, I get so sick, and she's sick, I can't take it away from her. So I'm going in for a cure." I said, "That's what I'm doing. I got a case for possession. I figure I'll get clean and then come back."

We got a taxi cab. All the taxi cab people know when they see guys

2. *Drug Addiction: Crime or Disease? Interim and Final Reports of the Joint Committee of the American Bar Association and the American Medical Association on Narcotic Drugs*, 88–92; quotation at 88.

3. John Walsh, "Lexington Narcotics Hospital: A Special Sort of Alma Mater" and "Addiction Research Center: Pioneers Still on the Frontier," *Science* 128 (1973), 1004–1008, 1229–31.

coming off the train—they say, "You're going to Lexington, you wanna to go to the . . ." We said, "Yeah."

Now, we're in a room where we take our clothes off and we see a doctor. They give us a bath; they put us in the tub with cold water. Two other guys come in: Mike, from the West Side, and another kid. Mike turned around and said to me, "You come from New York, your face is familiar." I said, "I come from the West Side. That guy, Tommy, is from the East Side." Mike said, "You know, over here, they ain't gonna give us nothing till tonight." I said, "What the hell! We'll call a doctor and tell him." So a doctor came over and said, "What's the matter?" I said, "We're sick, for crying out loud." He said, "Oh, you'll get something when you go downstairs."

So we got in the tub, dried up, and they gave us clothes. We went into what they called "Population." We met people there that we knew. One of them named Teddy said, "What are you doing here? Oh, you knocked on the door." You know, it ain't nice when you knock on the door—you're supposed to get arrested to go in there. Otherwise, they don't have any respect for you. I said, "Listen, Teddy, they could drop dead. I'm sick, I've got a case, and I want to go in clean." We'd heard of people dying up on Hart's Island.[4] You know, you're kicking it cold turkey, you get pneumonia, and you go. [Snaps fingers.]

But you always meet the devil. There's always somebody in front of you, the devil, that pushes you. We got to talking and this guy Mike said, "I got an ounce of stuff, home. The hell with staying here. After they give us our fix, we'll check out." You could check out of there anytime you wanted. You signed that paper, they threw your clothes at you. So, we checked out: me, Tommy, Mike, and another kid. We came home and went to Mike's house, and he had an ounce of stuff there. [Laughs.] We all fixed ourselves up, and he gave us a little extra.

We suffered for it. Later on, when I went in for the case I got sent up to Riker's Island. The judge gave us a six-month bit.

BRENDA

I went into a doctor's office in Arkansas and asked for a prescription. He shook his head. He said, "I would love to give you a prescription, believe me I would. But there's no way I can." This seemed to be an

4. In March, 1939, a Bronx grand jury inspected the buildings on Hart's Island and declared them to be "a disgrace to the city of New York." The city's other East River prison, Riker's Island, was also notoriously overcrowded and unsanitary (*New York Times*, April 1, 1939, p. 8).

odd way of saying, "I'm not going to give you a prescription." I said, "I don't understand what you mean." "Well," he said, "I know that you need it. I know you need it desperately, but there's nothing I can do about it. Because, as you see, I've been there myself." And he rolled up his sleeves: both arms had the long scars. He said, "I forged enough prescriptions, I was sent to Lexington. Now I have my license back, and I wouldn't dream of writing a prescription for anyone."

I sat in his office talking with him. He told me about Lexington. I had my doubts about what it did for you. I suspected that he was still using something, whether it was narcotics or barbiturates. Also, the woman that he was with—whether it was his wife or not—was intoxicated from something. He was too. Not only intoxicated, but while I was waiting for him, one of the patients that was sitting in the office made a remark, "I hope he's able to open his eyes today." [Laughs.]

But after I sat and talked with him for an hour he said, "Brenda, I'm going to give you a prescription. But I want you to promise me that you will not fill this prescription until you are at least fifty or sixty miles out of the area." Now, I appreciated that he wrote the prescription, and I took it fifty or sixty miles out of the area. At the same time, I talked to my husband about Lexington. I told him, "You know and I know that we can't continue on like this." And this was early—this was '53.

We agreed to go down there. The withdrawal at that time was with liquid methadone. They had a long withdrawal; it seemed a long, drawn-out procedure. Very weakening, very tiring. What bothered both of us was that while we were in Withdrawal, it seemed like everyone that came in was off of narcotics; they were eating, having a wonderful time, listening to the radio, dancing around—and we were dying. The food truck came up with cabbage on it. The smell of cabbage—I was already nauseous anyway, but that kept me constantly in the bathroom. Just smelling that, my stomach would turn. And other people were sitting there eating the cabbage. They couldn't have been addicted to very heavy narcotics. They may have been addicted to street narcotics, but I was addicted to pure Dilaudid.

The first time we went in there I was not only using the Dilaudid, I was backing it up with methadone, so it seemed like a long time before I showed signs of withdrawal. Now, if you were sick when the doctor came around, then he would prescribe whatever the dosage was. But it took a long time for my withdrawal to show through. I don't remember exactly, I think it was the second day, the doctor came around and told me, "I don't think you have a habit. We're going to send you over to Population"— that's what they call it. I was terrified, because in the early days I'd been arrested and I'd kicked cold turkey.

We stayed thirty days. The Sunday after we got our first night's sleep we both visited and my husband said, "Gee, I feel great." I said, "I do too." He said, "Let's go!" And we didn't think we would ever have to take narcotics again.

But when you're confined it's very different than when you hit that street. You have no direction when you come out of the hospital. While you're in the hospital, you have something to do. It's planned. You're withdrawing from drugs; that's your main purpose there. When you go out, if you don't have a definite purpose, the time before you start somewhere is a problem time, because you're still thinking about drugs. Thirty days is a short, short stay for people addicted the way we were.

It took us two days to relapse. The first night back in Chicago we sat down and drank, had a few highballs. The next morning both of us thought we were dead. Me worse than him: because I had a high tolerance to liquor, I could consume an enormous amount. My husband would take two or three drinks and take a long time drinking them, where I was a fast, hurry-up drinker—I would have maybe ten or twelve to his three. Yet, I wouldn't become drunk with all this liquor until a certain point and then, after that drink, I wouldn't even remember where I was any more, or how I got home, or anything else. But the next morning I was so deathly sick I couldn't believe it. And that led right back to the narcotics.

I really don't know whether I drank because there was a need for the narcotic. When you're not under the influence of narcotics, you can't relax, for one thing. You can't be what you are. There is something either you don't want to face or you don't want to see in yourself. It's just something there . . . I can't exactly pinpoint it.

A physical feeling goes with it. We weren't out of Lexington, I'll say two hours, than we both had chills. In the hospital you're busy constantly, but when you leave you have a lot of things to think about, on your way home you think. And whether this is a nervous reaction, or what, you start to perspire—these withdrawal symptoms, I found out later, will go on sometimes for a long time.

We tried Lexington again the following year, '54. During the first week in Population, after lights out at ten o'clock, two black girls got in an argument and the razor blades started. It was terrible, just one of them horrible things to see. The security women seemed frightened of them— and these were very young girls. My husband called to see me the next morning. It shows you how things got to the men's side: he had already heard about that problem on my floor. He told me, "Listen, you got to get off that floor." I asked him, "How would you suggest that I do that?"

We decided to stay for a few weeks longer this time, about forty-five days. But when we came out it was no different. The more often you go to Lexington, the more educated you become about how to obtain drugs. This time we left the hospital with other addicts, people who used the kind of pure medical narcotics that we used. One fellow was from Georgia —about our age, early thirties, white. He had been addicted to morphine for a long time. His brother was a pharmacist, so he was able to obtain it. My husband met him in the hospital; he was there maybe two weeks, and he decided to check out the day we were leaving. We went along with this young guy immediately because he knew where to get some morphine within an hour. He had a stash outside: he had the morphine, the hypodermic syringe, everything, stashed at the airport.

The third time I was in Lexington, around '56–'57, was not of my own accord. I was sent there after a conviction for possession in Chicago. I think I had told you earlier that I had been with a lot of confidence men. They all ganged up together at this one night spot in Chicago—they all knew where the other confidence guys hung out. This one fellow, who had just come into town, came up to my husband one night and said, "Listen, my wife is pregnant, I use drugs, and I heard that you have some. Could you help me out?" My husband told him, "Gee, I don't even know you." He said, "Well, so-and-so knows me," and he introduced himself from a bunch of match players that knew one another. My husband told him, "No, I can't do nothing for you."

Now, he approached him three or four times. In the meantime he told my husband he was picking up heroin on the South Side of Chicago, getting beat for his money. He said, "I bring my money out there and these guys rip me off and give me nothing and my wife's pregnant and I don't know what I'm gonna do . . . ," and he told him a whole big story.

One night he finally ran into him again. He looked real sick. He pleaded and pleaded. My husband called me on the phone, and he said, "Brenda, I'm gonna send somebody over to the apartment. Will you give him one of them half-grain Dilaudids? I'll send him over there in a few minutes." I said, "It will take him from downtown thirty minutes to get here, and I was getting ready to leave." He said, "The guy is in terrible shape. You'll see. He's in awful shape—let him have it." I said, "All right."

Well, that was the downfall. He knocked on the door, and when I opened it I had such a gang come in on me that I thought I was getting robbed. I didn't know it was the police. With their guns and all I thought that he had brought them there to rob me. They started tearing the place apart. I told them, "Just a minute. You can have everything you want—put the guns away." One of the policemen recognized me. He said, "Brenda, don't you recognize what's going on here?" I said, "No." He said, "Well, look in your pocket." I had an apron on, and I looked in the pocket, and the kid that walked in for the Dilaudid put ten dollars in my pocket. The ten dollars was marked money.

Then they took the boy—he wasn't a boy, he was a man about twenty-eight years old—they took him in my kitchen and beat him unmercifully. I didn't know what was going on at the time, why he was being beaten like this. I came to find out later that he had been arrested three weeks before. The police had some heroin connection that they wanted; they released him from jail so that he would bring them to this connection. But he was afraid of these people, so all this time he pressured my husband with the story about the wife, and brought them to me. But when they went through the dresser drawers and found all the legal drugs—these all had seals, all had federal stamps on them—they saw, just like this one police officer told them, "This isn't the place." He had once worked on the confidence detail; he knew that I had hung out with confidence men and that this was the wrong spot.

Needless to say they had plenty there, even if it wasn't what they were looking for. What they got out of that house was unbelievable. We had about one hundred and eighty-six 20-cc bottles of liquid Dolophine, eighty or ninety bottles of half-grain Dilaudid, and a bunch of stolen blank prescription pads in a tin box with a combination lock on it. At this point I had begun to forge prescriptions when we didn't have enough medicine; this was one of the ways we got all these drugs.

They brought the tin box out and told me to open it. I told them, "No way." They said, "Open the box," with their nasty threats. But I wouldn't open it, so they broke it open with a screwdriver. The policeman who knew me opened the box before the other cops saw anything. The minute he saw the blank prescriptions he slipped them off the top and put them in his inside coat pocket. He was the head of the state bunch that came in there. There was also one federal agent—five altogether. He turned around to me and said, "You got enough on you here"—you know, with all that was in the box. He let me know that the others weren't going to get the prescriptions.

This guy was known to be one of the worst and rottenest narcotic men there was. They claimed he was a horror. But he helped me all through the proceedings. He later reported to the judge, "I don't think this woman was involved in any sale of narcotics. I believe that the narcotics were there for her and her husband's own purposes." I didn't know why he was helping us at this time. But later on he told me, "I am not looking for your kind of people. I am looking for the pusher that's out there doing harm." He believed, I guess, that anybody that was out there peddling narcotics was out to hurt somebody.

Before I was arrested, they stayed in the apartment for three hours, waiting for phone calls. They said to me, "If that phone rings, anyone that calls, you tell them to come over right away." I asked them, "Why should I do that?" One of the cops pulled out a gun and told me, "You'll do it or else . . ."

The phone rang. It was a girlfriend that I had known; it had nothing to do whatsoever with narcotics. I don't think they were paying too much attention to me at the time, because the minute she spoke to me on the phone, I said "Lonnie, the police are here!" [Laughs.] I got knocked off the chair and the phone got hung up.

About two and a half hours later the phone rang. This one cop grabbed me by the neck and told me, "All right, now we've had enough with your shenanigans. Whoever this is, you're going to tell them to come up. I'm going to listen to every word." He sat with me in the chair.

And who was on the phone? My husband. Of course, we know one another in conversation very well. He said, "Brenda, what's the matter, you having some problems?" I said, "Yes, I am." You see, the cop couldn't hear what my husband was saying—he was listening to me, to what I was saying. My husband said, "Can't you handle it?" I said, "No, I can't." Now, I'm sure he is picking up that something is very wrong here by what I'm *not* saying, you understand. That could only be the police.

But instead of that, he's thinking that the fellow he sent to me is causing me some serious problems and is still there, and that I can't get off the phone. He said, "Well, I'll be through down here in a short while and I'll come home." I said, "No." He said, "What do you mean?" I said, "*No.*" The cop sitting next to me keeps telling me, "Tell him to come over." I said to the cop, "This is my husband." My husband heard me say that, heard me say, "This is my husband," and he knew that I was talking to someone. And no one was ever in the house with me. He said, "All right, I understand." I took it for granted that he understood the police were there. He hung up.

Sure enough, about thirty minutes later, he walked right in on it. He said, "Oh, my God." The policeman who knew me also knew him, and he said, "She's in serious trouble." My husband said, "What do you mean *she's* in serious trouble?" The cop went on to explain about the guy they had in the kitchen. My husband said to them, "What do you have on her exactly?" He showed him the tin. Oh, by the way, there was some marijuana too, which I never used but my husband did. There were two Prince Albert cans of marijuana in the bottom drawer. The cop said, "Look, what you can do is claim the marijuana, and take that away from her. All of these other drugs are not contraband. That's the only thing that is, and it would be a good idea to claim that if you want to help her." My husband didn't know what to do. He didn't want me to take it all, so he said the marijuana was his.

Because of the amount that was there, I guess they considered it a sale. According to them, they had a million-dollar bust of illegal narcotics. This is the way it went in the paper and on television. I think that was the most embarrassing day of my life, to be taken out of that apartment building in handcuffs, like I had killed somebody.

When I went downtown to the lockup, it wasn't so easy to get me out on bond. After I was indicted and bound over for the grand jury I had a thirty-five-thousand-dollar bond. Now, if you are connected in any way with narcotics, nobody wants to touch that kind of a bond. That's the first thing you find out. We did have some money in the bank. My husband told me, "Listen, if it takes every dime, I'll have you out. But it's gonna take a little time."

By the second day I was in very bad shape. They gave me nothing. I threw up all over myself, my hair, my clothes. When night came I didn't know whether to touch that dirty, crawly blanket that they had thrown on the floor or whether to freeze to death. Like, I had the chills so bad I wanted the blanket, and yet, whether it was or wasn't my imagination, I was terrified of the blanket, thinking it was crawling with bugs. Should I touch it or shouldn't I? It got to the point where it didn't make any difference. I *wrapped* myself in it, crawling or not.

About midnight a matron came around and she said to another matron, "I haven't seen one like this since the early thirties." The heroin addicts they arrested in the fifties weren't in that condition. The heroin was very diluted. She came back and asked me if I wanted some hot tea. I didn't want hot, cold, or anything.

My husband finally got a hold of a bondsman. The bondsman owned a nightclub and knew me, but didn't know I was married to my husband. He said to my husband, "Look, you're going to have to put up fifteen thousand dollars of this money. That's the only way I'm going to take thirty-five thousand dollars. And I'll go down and get her."

The bondsmen came down and they carried me out, dragged me out. I came down on the elevator and I couldn't even walk. The matron and one of the turnkeys had to pull me out. He told them, "No, that's not the one. That's not her." I told him, "Yeah, it's me." He knew me, but he didn't recognize me looking like that.

This was the thing that started the downhill for me, having people recognize that I used narcotics. Up to this point, anyone who knew me personally never knew I was involved in narcotics. Even when I was arrested with confidence men, I would swear that I didn't use drugs when I went into the lockup. Even when I was sick, and they would see it, I would still deny it. I'd tell them I drank; I'd never mention the fact that I was a drug addict.

Anyway, I was convicted of possession. The sale charge was dropped, that was knocked out immediately when I told the lawyer what had happened. But it was a horrifying experience. At that time there was a new district attorney, Adamowski.[5] I'll never forget him. They changed the law

---

5. Benjamin Adamowski, a Democrat who switched to the Republican Party, was elected state's attorney for Cook County in 1956. He was constantly in the headlines for his revelations of corruption, especially in the police department. Mayor Richard Daley engi-

to where sale of narcotics, one sale, was twenty to life. But this was for possession, and the judge let me go to Lexington until they saw fit to release me. My husband got thirty days in the county jail for the marijuana, with a stay of sentence until he could take care of business arrangements at home.

I think I was in Lexington a month and a half when I was called downstairs and told, "The police from Chicago are here and would like to question you." I said, "Concerning what?" Well, the fellow that got that beating over the drugs had been killed. He had been given a hot shot and thrown behind a bar. They found him laying in an alley in Chicago. The reason they questioned me was that my husband, when we were in court, said to this fellow, "My wife had better not do one day in jail"—that's like a threat. But my husband was himself in jail by the time this killing took place. We found out later from the policeman who had been in my house —I saw him after I got out of Lexington—that this fellow had turned the big heroin connection that they were looking for on the South Side. I think the people he turned eventually either killed him or had him killed.

This time I was in Lexington for a total of six months. The withdrawal took me a real long time, even though I had kicked cold turkey in jail. When I came out on bond I was right back on again. I had been using for quite some time before I got to Lexington—we delayed the trial two or three times. I was taking two half-grain Dilaudids at a shot, every four or five hours, and using liquid Dolophine to cook it with, instead of diluting it with water.[6] It was a terrible habit.

I think it was sixty days before I felt I was really coming out of things. Even in two months time I was still getting up every morning freezing, with them unbearable chills. My nerves were real bad. The whole time I was there I was on edge constantly. All I could think about was, "Oh, my God, if I only had a shot."

I went to work as an aide in the hospital. I worked seven days a week, twelve hours a day, the whole time I was there. They couldn't give me enough work to do. That was nerves. I couldn't sleep, and I'd rather be doing, doing. I couldn't sit still. Just thinking about it now unnerves me [laughs], just going back, remembering that period.

At mealtime the girls used to get in the hallways and scream and carry

neered his defeat in 1960, allegedly through fradulent means (Mike Royko, *Boss: Richard J. Daley of Chicago* [New York: Dutton, 1971], 108–14, 118–20).

6. Dissolving Dilaudid with liquid Dolophine is like watering Scotch with Drambuie. This combination of drugs explains, not only why Brenda had such wrenching withdrawals, but also why the onset of withdrawal symptoms was delayed the first time she checked into Lexington: Dolophine, also known as methadone, is a relatively long-lasting narcotic. That is one reason why it is widely used in maintenance programs.

on. You know, young people are very loud, very boisterous, and their voices would knock off them walls. That's why I think I worked all them hours in the hospital, so I wouldn't have to get in this line to go to breakfast and lunch and listen to that horrible screaming. If somebody said "hello" to me I couldn't hear them. That changed when they had a Dr. [Emil] Trellis come in there, I think around '57. He seemed to command a great deal of respect from them girls. I never knew why until I heard him speak one day. Then I began to see: they knew what he said, he meant. I think that was what they needed from the beginning and didn't have.

This time I saw a shift in the population. There was an enormous amount of blacks. They came mostly from Chicago and New York, the big cities. They used to say, "Well, here comes a bunch on the chain from D.C."—there were a lot of blacks from D.C. If you were arrested and brought there you were hooked up and chained, handcuffed to one another.

There were quite a few whites, but not as many as I had seen earlier. The whites were from more rural areas. Some of them were paregoric users: they became addicted to huge amounts of paregoric. This surprised me, how anyone could drink that. To take a pint of that, to get it all down in one day . . . you see, they would have awful stomach trouble behind all that.

I had seen a young woman when I went there in '53. She was a security aide, or psychiatric aide, in Population. Most of the psychiatric aides were from Lexington, or in around that area. This young lady came to work, she was about twenty-eight years old, very nice and very sociable. Seemed like a very kind person. When I came back in '56 she had changed so I couldn't believe it was the same person. She had toughened, and hardened, and wouldn't smile. Some of the nurses had changed too, but not that drastically.

The hospital itself, the prison population, was well kept. There was inspection with white gloves—this was run by the Coast Guard. Security would come around and check the rooms. Everything would be taken out of the rooms by the girls, the beds scrubbed, the windows, everything. Patients would clean them rooms and have them looking spotless. The withdrawal ward wasn't bad either; it was a clean hospital area.

There was music at Lexington. See, I loved music all my life. I took piano lessons when I was younger. I was interested in music in every way. Jazz—why I used to go to the Black and Tan Club on the South Side of Chicago. That's where I met Anita O'Day, Billie Holiday. That crowd impressed me with their music. When I was in Lexington, I began to see that black people—while they kicked the habit—had that jazz music going constantly. In the beginning, I didn't pay too much attention to it. I was too sick the first week. None of us could sleep, and we'd be laying on that cold bathroom floor when one of the girls would bring a record player in and plug it in. And I began to see the soothing effect that music had. No matter what kind of music it was, I had it on constantly after that.

At the end of six months, I went right back on Dilaudid. I couldn't wait to get out of there. The whole time I was there, that's all my mind was on. For one thing, that's all people ever talked about at Lexington. That was the topic of conversation: how much drugs this one used, that one used, where this one got them, how that one got them. I had an introduction to the good heroin, the poor heroin—before I ever got outside I knew all about heroin. [Laughs.] But I don't ever remember any being snuck into the hospital.

I went back one other time, in '67, on my own. By that time things were getting very bad: drugs were hard to get. The government and the states began to toughen up on narcotics, both from druggists and from doctors. A lot of doctors that had written, stopped. My husband and I were in Savannah, Georgia. We couldn't get a prescription, so we forged one for Dilaudid. I was in a motel. My husband said, "I'm going to try one more drugstore and see if I can get this filled." He went into the druggist and the druggist told him, "Well, I don't have it right now. If you want to leave the prescription you can come back tomorrow." My husband told him, "No, I'll just take the prescription. If I get a chance, if I'm still in the area, I'll pick it up tomorrow."

The pharmacist got his license plate. That night, when I was walking the dog, I saw a patrol car pull into the motel, swing around, and start looking at all the license plates on the cars. I walked by the patrol car— they said "Hi" and I said "Hi"—then I immediately went into my room and said to my husband, "We're getting arrested." He said, "Why?" I said, "It can't be nobody but us." "Why are you saying that?" "I just instinctively know: the way they're checking license plates, it's us." He said, "Go take a walk, get a cup of coffee or something across the street, see if they're still out there." I said, "I'm telling you, you better get rid of whatever we have here."

All we had in the hotel was liquid opium. It was a prescription for hemorrhoids: two ounces of deodorized opium, two ounces of olive oil, and ten drops of phenol, which is carbolic acid. Doesn't do a damn bit of good when applied to hemorrhoids [laughs], but years ago I guess someone's imagination told them it did. You pour the oil off the top, put the remaining black opium in a little pan, put a match to the top of it, and the alcohol will burn off. Then you let it boil and pop. When the popping stops you've burned off the phenol. What you have left is the opium. We had this as a safeguard in case we couldn't get anything else. But it was terrible to inject because, if you missed the vein, it burned the skin.

My husband got rid of this opium. He put it out the bathroom window which led into an alley, so he could get it later. While I was sitting in the restaurant, drinking a cup of coffee, I felt a tap on my shoulder. I told them, "All right, I already know." I got up and went back to the room. The policemen said, "You're under arrest." I said, "What for?" He said to my husband, "You were downtown last night trying to cash an illegal prescription. The pharmacist called the druggist [*sic*] where the prescription came from, and it's all illegal."

If you've ever seen a man be railroaded, my husband was, there in Savannah. He went before a court where he didn't even stand up to be sentenced, and the next thing you know they carted him off with a year in jail. They had absolutely nothing on him but a drugstore man saying that he had brought an illegal prescription in there; they didn't even have the prescription. It was a kangaroo court.

We didn't have any money by this time. He said to me, "Listen, I want you to go back to Memphis and ask Mama to lend you enough money." I went to his mother and asked her. She refused. But after a few days she said, "I'll think about it." I told her, "He's in there and it's not legal." So she sent a lawyer down there, and the lawyer got him out.

By this time, I'm telling you I was disgusted with everything. I told my husband, "Look, I'm gonna go back to Lexington and give it one more try. Do you want to go with me?" He said, "No, I've had enough of that place." I said, "Well, I'm going to try." This time I stayed there about four months. And when I came out, I really thought I was going to stay off drugs this time. I had convinced myself, *this is it,* I am not going to go through that no more. I'd give myself all the pep talks necessary.

But one thing complicated it: they had been giving me Librium every day after I came to Population. My nerves were very bad at that time. I would take two pills in the morning and two at four o'clock. But I thought they were nothing. I figured, "They're just tranquilizers. Anybody can stop taking tranquilizers"—never mind the fact that the Librium kept me functioning easier than all the other times I had been there.

When I left I didn't have any Librium to take with me—I just left. It wasn't the Librium by itself; it was stopping that and being off of the narcotics too. I was empty of everything, and everything seemed to fall apart for me. I looked around me and said, "I just give up. I don't know which direction to take now."

My husband was in Chicago, but I didn't go back there. I thought, "Maybe if I don't go back there I'll never get back on drugs again." On top of that I wanted to see my children, so I came to New York. I was here in New York a couple of months. I went to a doctor in Brooklyn—I was very sick, physically sick. I told him I had gone to Lexington and how long I'd been using drugs and everything. He said I had a myocardial infarction. It was like telling me I had an abscess: it meant absolutely nothing. I just knew I was sick, and something told me narcotics was the only thing that was going to make me feel right. This doctor gave me Dolophine pills, and I was right back where I started.

MARIE NYSWANDER

Addicts were not the only people we interviewed who had vivid memories of Lexington. Marie Nyswander, who later became well known as the co-developer of methadone maintenance, began her career there. Nyswander was born in Reno, Nevada, in 1919. When she was fifteen she was diagnosed as suffering tuberculosis and spent a year in a sanatorium; while recuperating she became concerned with the plight of poor TB patients and began reading widely in Marx and other anticapitalist writers. Nyswander joined the Young Communist League during the Depression but became disillusioned and left the organization. She retained, however, a lifelong concern for social issues. After graduating from the Cornell University Medical College and serving a surgical internship, she joined the U.S. Health Service in 1945 and, "by pure chance," was posted to Lexington.

I wasn't taught very much about addiction in medical school—maybe it was good not to get a prejudiced opinion. I knew about tolerance from pharmacology, but I never saw an addict: they weren't admitted to the hospital emergency room for treatment. Addicts were supposed to go to Lexington, Kentucky.

The year at Lexington was the hardest in my life. Prison is a terrible thing. If you have any kind of a personality that cares about your fellow man, working in a prison will simply blow you up with rage and frustration. What precipitates out in prison is a kind of bureaucratic personality that thrives on having prisoners work for them, on carrying a collection of keys, on speaking to people harshly, on being autocratic and self-centered. They indulged themselves: some of the medical staff used prisoners as servants in their homes.

I stayed in the Nurses' Home. That was a disaster. The nurses had worked in that prison for God knows how many years. I remember when Roosevelt died they all cheered. They referred to Negro patients as "niggers" and would order them around as such. That was pretty rough for a little girl just out of her internship, one who had no idea that people like this existed.

It was thoroughly indoctrinated that addicts were the lowest form of creature. There seemed to be an impression that they had some kind of wild, maniacal pleasure that the rest of us didn't know about, and for which they should be punished. It wasn't simply that addicts were minorities—back then the ethnic ratio was about the same as in society, except for an increase in Chinese patients. Some of the Chinese were bank presidents, very fine men who were arrested for smoking their opium pipe on Saturday night. Occasionally you'd hear a doctor say, "It's a shame these men were arrested for a cultural thing like this," but they never went to bat for them. The Chinese patients weren't treated any better; the nurses mocked them too—and these patients were far more cultured than the staff could ever be. [Laughs.] We had guards who had trouble making the required I.Q. of one hundred.

The patients were hardly anything to be desired either. People in prison—including myself—are transformed. That may not seem profound to you, but it was a profound discovery to me. The same patients I saw on the outside behaved so differently from those on the inside.

But I also had some very nice things happen with patients on the inside. There were several black addicts who worked in the kitchen of the Nurses' Home: they must have seen how miserable I was. I would just go in my room and cry at night—the whole thing was terrible. One night I heard a tapping outside my window. There were two black guys who worked in the kitchen with a milkshake and a sandwich. They just put them through the window and left. Every night that happened. Then I was invited to see a famous tap dancer who happened to be a patient at the time. He would tap dance in the laundry. They never treated me as less than a doctor, or called me by my first name, or did anything demeaning or inappropriate. They just wanted me to have a few minutes of pleasure. Well, I never forgot that.

These experiences caused me to begin to question the psychiatric approach to addiction. In Lexington, every time you diagnosed a drug addict you had to put "psychopath," because that's what it said in the psychiatric diagnostic manual. But you can't tell me that anybody who would be as considerate and observant as that could be a sociopath.

Did you ever meet Anslinger?

Oh-ho, my yes! I should say so. I wouldn't say I knew him personally: he'd walk out every time I would meet him someplace. His appearance was like a movie character of a despot [laughs]: he was baldish with a very thick neck and ruddy complexion. He didn't smile very much, at least not to me. He was very critical, and he would show his displeasure by getting up and walking out. There were several men, I assume his aides, who would get up and walk out with him.

He was the most powerful man, perhaps, in Washington. I think it was finally Kennedy who managed to retire him. I believe he was married to Mellon's granddaughter,[7] and he had his own P.R. system, which no one

7. Anslinger's wife, Martha Denniston, was in fact only a distant relative of Andrew Mellon, who served as secretary of the treasury during the Harding, Coolidge, and Hoover administrations.

else had there. I suppose it would be fair to characterize him as a man who quit listening; he certainly became very rigid, and dogmatic in his views. And very omnipotent, because he told me once, "When the doctors clean their own house, then I'll let you treat addicts—as long as they're doctor addicts." According to his own statement, he had a congressman whom he maintained on narcotics; I don't know who that was.[8] He was a law unto himself. He could do these things, yet if we gave even as much as one shot to a sick drug addict, we were liable.

Anslinger gave a speech to Congress once, I think it was around 1964 or 1965, after I'd started working on methadone maintenance. Anslinger sent me a little reprint of the speech, which I threw away, though I wish now I hadn't. He was describing this "so-called research woman" up in New York "who says she likes addicts." He said, "Can you imagine anyone of such a low moral character as to say that she likes addicts?" My feeling is that it was the Narcotics Bureau that turned the doctors against addicts, that scared them out of their treatment.

WILLIAM B. O'BRIEN

Marie Nyswander's dissatisfaction with the Lexington approach was shared by others. But some of the critics who rejected institutional detoxification also deplored indefinite maintenance and continued to cast about for other techniques that would enable their patients to achieve the traditional goal of abstinence. They found one possible alternative in Synanon, a therapeutic community that evolved in Ocean Park, California, in the late 1950s under the direction of Charles Dederich, an ex-alcoholic. Dederich made no bones about the authoritarian nature of Synanon; he consciously recreated an autocratic family environment to keep people in line. He also relied heavily on group encounters, led by a "Synanist," or experienced former addict. These encounters were intended to make the participants come to terms with their feelings, to assume responsibility for their own lives, and to learn to deal with their problems without recourse to drugs or alcohol.

Synanon was a relatively small-scale operation. Its real significance was that it inspired several physicians, clergymen, and social workers to establish "second-generation" therapeutic communities throughout the country. These were patterned after Synanon but incorporated significant individual variations. Several of the most important of these programs had their inception at the very end of the

---

8. It was, remarkably, Senator Joseph R. McCarthy. McCarthy's addiction and demand for access to morphine put Anslinger in a terrible bind: he hated the idea of maintaining anyone, but he hated even more the prospect of losing a powerful congressional ally, particularly one who shared his views on Communism. The McCarthy episode is recounted in John Caldwell McWilliams, "The Protectors: Harry J. Anslinger and the Federal Bureau of Narcotics, 1930–1962" (Ph.D. diss., Pennsylvania State University, 1986), 177–79.

classic era, in the middle 1960s. They did not rapidly expand, however, until the later 1960s and early 1970s, when the Lexington approach was officially discredited, the country was in the midst of a youthful drug epidemic, and private and public funding for community drug treatment programs of all sorts was readily available.

One of the leaders of the second-generation movement was Monsignor William B. O'Brien. Born in Yonkers, New York, in 1924, he decided in the fourth grade that he wanted to be a priest, and was ordained in 1951. He was also interested in psychology, which he studied in the seminary and at the University of Illinois with the help of a Lilly Foundation Fellowship in 1966. In 1963 he co-founded Daytop Village, Inc., and since 1972 he has served as its chairman and chief executive officer.[9]

I was interested in this field because, when I was stationed at St. Patrick's Cathedral, I became deeply involved in a major youth-gang murder case. The scene in New York at that time was very negative: youth-gang activity and neighborhoods which were all broken down into gang turfs, and there was a lot of violence. It all came to a head on July 30, 1957, in the infamous Michael Farmer murder case.[10] I thought the church should have been involved, and I got involved. Following that heralded murder trial, hundreds of kids were referred to me, and 90 percent of them were using drugs. I discovered that drug addiction was the underlying problem of this acting-out disorder. I began to look around for someone who knew something about drug abuse. I went to professionals, governmental experts, everyone. No one knew anything. Everyone said it was irreversible. There was no hope for the drug addict!

I didn't accept that, so I kept looking. It wasn't until 1959 that I found a house in Westport, Connecticut, called Synanon. I couldn't believe it. I went up there for a half-hour visit and I ended up staying all night. I discovered for the first time that drug abuse is only a symptom of the problem; it retreats when you deal with the deeply human pain and crises of the person behind the problem.

9. Prior to publication, Monsignor O'Brien requested that certain changes be made to enhance the accuracy of the narrative. We have incorporated the suggested alterations, most of which are quite minor.

10. Michael Farmer, a fifteen-year-old polio victim, was beaten and stabbed to death in a city park by members of the Egyptian Kings and Dragons gang. The murder, one of several involving gangs that summer, was widely publicized and focused attention on juvenile violence. (So did *West Side Story*, which opened two months later.) The ensuing trial, then the longest in New York City's history, resulted in the convictions of Louis Alvarez and Charles Horton for second-degree murder, and of two others for manslaughter. Alvarez and other gang members had been drinking cheap wine and whiskey the evening of the killing (*New York Times*, August 21, 1957, pp. 1, 18; April 16, 1958, pp. 1, 28; Lewis Yablonsky, *The Violent Gang* [Baltimore: Penguin Books, 1967 reprint ed.], 1–24).

Synanon was very good for the first five years after its founding in 1958. It was a godsend. But when they began going insane with power in 1963, Dr. Dan Casriel, a New York psychiatrist, and I expressed alarm. This occasioned a grave confrontation with them. Chuck Dederich, the founder of Synanon and "grand guru," was scheduled to come East to meet with us, but instead he sent his adjutant, Reid Kimball. We confronted him on five issues we felt were crucial. Firstly, there was the sudden shift in direction. Young people were no longer going to be returned to their neighborhoods, families, and loved ones on the premise that Synanon was the pristine, antiseptic, utopian society and that the world outside was irredeemably corrupt. Dederich wiped out reentry with a stroke of the pen. Secondly, we felt that Synanon had found the formula for the recovery of life, vis-à-vis the acting-out disorder, but we felt that they should permit research to find out *why* they were successful. Thirdly, we felt that, if the drug problem in America was going to be turned back, that Synanon had to enter into a partnership with health service professionals, so that there could be a coordinated response to drug abuse. Fourthly, we felt that some of the extremely harsh practices in Synanon—"pull-ups" we call them in the therapeutic community—were unnecessary and counterproductive: lowering people into cesspools, and like humiliations. Fifthly, the number-one drug impact area was New York. We wanted Synanon to open commensurately in New York.

We were turned down on all five counts. I left the meeting immediately, after ten or fifteen minutes, when I could see that they were rejecting our complaints. Casriel talked to them for another hour or so, without success. Shortly thereafter, we went and met with Mayor Wagner; within twenty-four hours we had established Daytop Village, the first of a second generation of therapeutic communities with all of our caveats built in. The acronym stood for: *Drug Addicts Yield to Persuasion*. David Deitch, an ex-addict and former director of the Westport House, left Synanon with us and became our new director.[11] Dr. Casriel was the supervising psychiatrist, and I set up a not-for-profit board of directors. And Daytop was born.

There are three different levels of mental illness: psychoses, neuroses, and character disorders—with corresponding symptoms of fantasy, anxiety, and irresponsibility. It is the last, the character disorder, that the therapeutic community has been uniquely successful in treating. This is generally a pure condition, but research tells us that about 3.6 to 4 percent

11. Deitch and O'Brien subsequently had a parting of the ways in 1968. Deitch was forced out because he was felt to be turning Daytop into a New Left cult, more interested in addressing society's problems than those of individual clients. Daniel Casriel's role is described in more detail in his book, *A Scream Away from Happiness* (New York: Grosset and Dunlap, 1972), 45–58.

of character disorders show signs, in addition, of neuroses or psychoses. We have to refer these people to our psychiatric division, and probably refer them out of Daytop for more traditional treatment.

The basic factor in the character disorder is the emotional infant. Its roots are in society. Parents in their role of pedagogues (teachers) must have operative a process called "maturation." In the simplest terms, maturation concerns the successful transference from parental-imposed controls to self-imposed controls, so that the youngster is the captain of his or her own ship by the age of seventeen, eighteen, nineteen, or twenty. Maturation is achieved through the instrument of challenge. But the parents of today were children of the Depression. Many have decided that their children are going to have the things they were deprived of. So they give rather than demand. Instead of getting a daughter to take increasing responsibility for her own room, the parent reasons: "I'll clean it myself!" Instead of a son going out and earning, perhaps via a newspaper route, the money for a car, the parent reasons: "I'll buy it for him as a gift when he graduates from high school."

The net effect of this is the physiologically mature child who has stopped growing emotionally some years earlier. It's a seductive process, because parents fail to discern what is actually happening. With the best of intentions, they are convinced that they're helping their children, but they're actually harming them. They think that they're acting out of genuine love, but fail to realize that it is self-love, expiating their own guilt. So now they have a nineteen-year-old daughter, who emotionally is at age eight. An eight-year-old cannot accept the stress surrounding an adult world. That stress becomes a huge and ever-present threat.

If you analyze threats, there are only four available ways to respond. The first springs from the emotion of anger, and the instrument is *violence*—like the chap in Atlanta, Georgia, who some weeks ago drove his car through the plate glass window of the telephone company. He was out of work, and they kept sending him phone bills. Violence was the option, trying to destroy the threat or reduce its influence over him—that's the character disorder. We have people in Daytop who only use violence as their tool to deal with the threat of stress.

The second way to respond to stress, instead of anger, is *fear*, with the instrument of *flight*. We simply take off. The extremities of America, interestingly, are filled with a lot of men who ran away from their marriage obligations. They've fled the threat.

The third way to deal with stress, long overlooked, is similar to the turtle pulling its head under the shell: *withdrawal*, with the instrument of chemicals. It's most readily available and widely used: alcohol and other drugs. That's the alcoholic and drug addict, withdrawing.

The fourth way to deal with stress is to do the maturation process over again, to grow up emotionally, to be nineteen years of age emotionally while locked into a nineteen-year-old's body. Then one doesn't need to react in an irresponsible way.

Now, in Daytop, in a therapeutic community, we close off the first avenue. We prohibit violence, or even a threat of violence. The second avenue . . . well, though we don't lock anybody in, we charge the addict: "That's the route you've been following while you've been on the streets. You've had all the freedom you've wanted and you've been constantly running away. If you want to continue taking that route, you don't belong in Daytop. But think seriously about flight, deal with your fears." That's tantamount to closing route number two. And route number three is as strongly blocked as route number one: no chemicals are permitted anywhere or anytime.

So we encourage the addict to travel the fourth road. We create, in the therapeutic community, in Daytop, the ambiance of the natural family, recreating the nutrients of that family environment. But we replace the element of consuming, destructive love, well intentioned as it might have been, with demanding love. We put in place parental-imposed controls. The resident often asks: "Why?" We respond that the addict is essentially "the baby" whose mother wouldn't let them near the street when they were small, or play with matches, because they could hurt themselves. "But who would shoot a needle into their arm, or pop pills into their mouth? That could destroy you, could be lethal and, in any event, it's upsetting the chemistry of your body. Who would do this? Only a B-A-B-Y. You don't have a drug problem, you have a B-A-B-Y problem. You had all the freedom you wanted, and you couldn't handle it. Do what you're told." That's what they do for the first five months. The orders are coming from ex-addicts who are role models for them. It's much easier to obey them because they were there on that same floor some months earlier.

Then, after the fifth month, we begin thrusting responsibility upon them. Thus begins the transference to self-imposed controls. That's why you can have 165 people at Daytop Swan Lake right now and have only 8 on staff; the responsibilities are assumed by the members of the house.

By the time ten or twelve months have gone by, the residents find themselves governing their own lives and they're taking responsibility for others. Soon, it is decided that they are ready to come into the reentry house, which is the stress-house. We deliberately introduce stress into their lives. For example, recently I came across a young fellow looking very dejected. I knew he had a date with his girlfriend over the approaching weekend. He explained: "I just called my girl to cancel the date. I've been pulled in." I inquired: "Why?" His answer: "I don't know why, but it must be for my good, because the staff said that they were withdrawing my permission."

Now on Monday in a group he's going to find out that life is like that, that one must expect setbacks and rejection. "We wanted to see how you would handle this." He'll be told that his being "pulled" was a clinical decision. Most of these experiences in reentry are bona fide, life-created, stress situations. However, if a youngster is doing so extremely well that we have to artificially manufacture stress, we do it to test them.

Even though you were artificially introducing stress to an innocent third party, namely, the girlfriend?

The girlfriend in most cases is involved already in one of our Wednesday night groups. We encourage the spouses, the girlfriends of our residents to participate in specialized groups engendering emotional growth. In many cases, the woman responded to the young fellow before he entered Daytop with consuming destructive love. She thought love and sympathy were going to help him. She did all the wrong things, not realizing at that time she was prolonging his agony. She needs to grow emotionally, also, if she's going to be able to keep abreast of his growth and to establish a viable relationship when he graduates. So she would understand this particular situation.

As a Catholic priest, do you see an analogy between the therapeutic community process and the sacrament of penance?

A very real one. The first therapeutic community can be traced to the early Christians. Early Christianity was essentially a small group movement. In those times there were no churches or cathedrals and people had to meet in homes thus limiting the size of their gatherings. These groups or communities were closely knit and held together by love, a love of God and a strong love for each other. It was in these communities that we first see the practice of what is known in Greek as *exomologesis*. The practice of *exomologesis* consists of total honesty and openness about one's life and is followed by important personal change with the support of the other group members. In other words, when I messed up or in Catholic terms, when I sinned, I had to confess my failure publicly before God and my Christian family, and beg His forgiveness and theirs. The priest served as mediator. The process involved the demand of the community upon the individual for a change of behavior and the imposition of a public penance, because I have not only disturbed my relationship with God but I've damaged my relationship with the other members of the community. So there were no five Hail Marys, no cheap grace. There was bona fide restitution. In Daytop, a similar process takes place only we call it "clean-up"—where I had to repair the damage of my destructiveness! And from this kind of group experience came *koinonia*, a Greek term meaning a deep sense of fellowship as well as community support of my behavior to continue to change and grow, to learn from that experience and to improve my life. That basically is the therapeutic community, although we use different names for it.

There's one school of criticism that says that therapeutic communities are almost too successful for their own good, in that it is difficult for long-term residents to reenter society, they've become so attached to their therapeutic "family."

There was validity in that criticism for a long while, when therapeutic communities in the United States were aping Synanon in many ways. But, now, I think we've learned a lot, especially through our national association.[12] Our mandate is to accept the young person, to put him through the wringer and get him back to his family at the earliest possible time. That's the mandate of Daytop, Phoenix House, Odyssey—all these programs. The accent is on returning him to his family. Even those who come back as our staff, about 2 percent of the total, we shoot back to their families first, and leave them out in society for about two years.

Daytop is the biggest bargain in America. Eighty-eight percent of our people would be in a jail cell if they weren't here. They'd each cost twenty-six thousand a year; here they cost only eight thousand. And we score in recovery scales the exact reverse of the 8 to 9 percent in the criminal justice system. Ours is 90 to 91 percent. That's for graduates. But it's still the best bargain in drug treatment, even when you count the splittees. About seven or eight years ago, our research division was doing a follow-up on splittees and graduates. George De Leon of the Phoenix House research division was doing the same thing independently. The outcomes were congruent. Basically, of those who graduated, ninety-two out of a hundred were successful. (Success was measured on the basis of three variables: no further drug use, no further crime, and positive life-style, which means finishing secondary school or college, marriage, employment record and performance.) But these studies also showed that, the longer a client is exposed to therapy, the higher his level of success. If he's with us six months, there's a 68 percent improvement in performance; if twelve months, 87 percent, almost the same as graduation, which is roughly eighteen months. So you had a performance improvement, whether splittee or graduate, which was remarkable. Remember, when we started this program there was *zero* turnaround, whether at Lexington or Fort Worth.

12. Therapeutic Communities of America, Inc., established 1975. This organization was begun to heal divisions, collect and disseminate information, and provide a united front for the various therapeutic communities. O'Brien was co-founder and served a term as president.

14.

Methadone Maintenance

Although Daytop Village and other early therapeutic communities represented a *significant departure from the Lexington model, they were by no means the most* *radical treatment alternative to develop during the 1960s. That distinction would* *have to go to methadone maintenance. It was not that methadone was a new* *drug; it had in fact been used for years to gradually detoxify addicts in Lexington.* *It was the way in which Drs. Vincent Dole and Marie Nyswander proposed* *using it, as part of a regimen of indefinite treatment, that was so revolutionary.* *This, of course, violated the Bureau of Narcotics' basic policy against maintenance* *and represented a standing challenge to all treatment programs, large or small,* *predicated on abstinence.*

The original premise behind methadone maintenance was that addicts had *undergone a permanent metabolic change, that they needed narcotics in a visceral* *way, the way a diabetic needs insulin. This explained relapse, and why abstinence* *was not a realistic goal. But methadone maintenance could satisfy the underlying* *craving and enable the addict to lead a normal and productive life. Methadone* *could be taken orally once a day, so addicts would not have to constantly in-* *ject themselves with possibly contaminated needles. At a sufficiently high dose* *methadone blocked the euphoric effects of a shot of heroin, so that addicts would* *not be tempted to continue using illegal narcotics. Nor would they need to, since* *methadone, itself a narcotic, prevented withdrawal sickness. Finally, methadone* *was cheap and legal, so that addicts could escape the grind of hustling and scoring,* *thereby improving their lives and reducing the amount of crime.*

There was, inevitably, a reaction, as both the premises and results of metha- *done maintenance were called into question. Critics said that the hypothesized* *metabolic change was mere speculation; that methadone was just a quick chemical* *fix, substituting one drug for another; and that it failed to significantly reduce* *criminal or antisocial behavior because it ignored the underlying problems of* *addicts—inferior or abnormal personalities, broken families, anomie, inebriety,* *ghetto squalor, deviant peers, or structural unemployment, and so on down the* list. *Others charged that methadone did too much, that it was an insidious form of social control aimed at turning restive inner-city minorities into harmless zombies; or that it was dangerous, because large amounts of methadone were diverted into the black market and consumed by those who might not otherwise have used drugs. Probably the fairest and most accurate thing to say about these criticisms (and this is just a partial list) is that they arose from mixed motives: there were real and unresolved problems with methadone maintenance, but there were also vested interests to be defended, especially by those whose funding and prestige were tied to competing addiction theories and treatments. Medical controversies are seldom fought on purely scientific grounds, and methadone is a classic case.*

The addicts we interviewed were not much interested in the finer points of the controversy, but they were glad that methadone maintenance became available when it did. Thirty or forty years was a long time to survive as an addict in the Anslinger era—it amounted to perhaps three or four lifetimes of normal stress and danger—and by the 1960s the older survivors were starting to play out. Although they had some reservations about methadone, several interviewees remarked that it had been a lifesaver for them. "My worst enemy I wouldn't wish my heroin habit on," Amparo cried out. "The time I spent on heroin was hell. That's why I get emotional whenever anyone asks me about it. That's why I'm comfortable on methadone now." Others expressed no regrets whatsoever about heroin or opium use and, were they given a choice, would have continued using them. "I'd smoke opium for the rest of my life," was Al's comment. But even those who preferred the drugs of their youth allowed that methadone was a great convenience. Given the adulteration of street drugs, the dangers of scoring, and the difficulty of hustling, there was really no other choice open to them save detoxification, and they had failed so often to achieve and maintain abstinence that they were not very sanguine about the prospect. Dusty summed it up:

Methadone's a crutch, in a way. You feel safe. I've said so many times, "I wonder what I'd be doing if there wasn't any methadone program?" I wondered if I'd still be alive. Because, without methadone, it would have been heroin, or cocaine, or something else, and the way the quality of drugs has deteriorated, I guess I would have shot five times as much as I shot before to find any satisfaction in it.

The first part of this chapter relates the experiences of three survivors with methadone: how they found out about it, what effects they observed, what problems they encountered, and the like. The second part is devoted to the memories of Dr. Vincent Dole, who co-founded methadone maintenance and who, more than any other individual, was responsible for its legitimation during the 1960s.

SAM

I never did anything illegal. That is to say I never stole narcotics, bought them in the street. I never put anything into my body that wasn't either given to me by a physician or prescribed by a physician and given to me by a pharmacist.

I would elicit with two or three, maybe four, pharmacies a certain understanding. Certain monies would exchange hands in return for which they would honor my prescriptions, even though they knew they were being given with a regularity that was far in excess of any normal usage.

Three physicians were as many as I could juggle at one time. I used three to let them save face. I wouldn't go to a physician on a Monday and then go back for another prescription on the following Monday. But with three of them working at the same time I could wait a decent interval of a month. Then he could say to himself, "Well, what the hell, a month, that's not too bad. I'll give him another prescription." That way I got my drug.

Eventually, though, I had to quit. My mind had become such a maelstrom of emotions, I was so mixed up. Through desperation I tried to commit suicide. The hopelessness of it, the unending corridors of addiction—I could see no way out, nothing ahead but more addiction. I sat down in a little hotel in Florida, wrote my daughter a note, took a good handful of pills, about forty, put them in my mouth, and knocked it all back with about half a pint of paraldehyde. Now, you take a three-hundred-pound truck driver who is obstreperous and give him a tablespoon of paraldehyde—in thirty seconds he's on the floor. And I took half a pint of it, and swallowed the pills.

By pure happenstance I was found and taken by ambulance to a hospital down there. I had my stomach pumped—just in time, I was given to understand. Another few hours would have done it. I stayed in that hospital about two weeks, perhaps three, then was taken to the Institute of Living in Hartford,[1] where I stayed five months.

This was one of a number of private sanitaria and hospitals I was in and out of while I was taking all these things. The last one I went to—at the time, I was just addicted to barbiturates—was Gracie Square Hospital, on the East Side. My physician at Gracie Square was a society doctor

---

1. The Institute of Living (originally chartered in 1822 as the Hartford Retreat for the Insane; the name was changed in 1943, for obvious reasons) is a private asylum with a reputation for treating wealthy and famous patients.

who charged me fifty dollars a day. I don't know how long I spent at the hospital, but there were weeks when I didn't see him. Those days I did see him he would pass me in the hall, pat me on the head, ask me, "What did I eat for lunch that afternoon?" and that would be that day's session. I quote this literally. I'd be running after him, asking him, "When are you going to see me, when are you going . . . ?" "Oh, we'll fix that," he said. When I finally did get to his office, he'd be on the telephone, transacting huge real estate deals involving the purchase of buildings and half-acres of land in the financial district of New York. He was married to a society woman and was a very wealthy man, but he certainly had nothing to do with me. I don't think he even knew my name.

It was while I was in Gracie Square, about '67 or '68, that I first heard the word "methadone." This was a third-hand rumor from a patient. I didn't know what it was, but I learned that it was something that got you off everything, that it was a catchall for all addictions. When I left the hospital I went immediately to the Gracie Square methadone clinic, just up the street. I was clean, but I can tell you first hand that it would not have been long before I went back to the barbiturates or the Alvodine or the Demerol.

When I first went to the clinic a woman psychiatrist whose name I unfortunately forget—she was very kind to me and very good—made it clear to me that here was a possible avenue of escape from the nooses around my neck, that methadone was a possible key. I went into it willingly: anything to get me out of the mess my life was in at that point.

I know now that methadone is a narcotic, the worst of them all. God, I think it's the hardest to break away from. Here's how I know. I was transferred to another clinic in the South Bronx. You went there for your dosage—you just walked in and walked right out. The clientele was almost exclusively black and Hispanic. But then one day, about five years ago, another woman doctor asked me why I came up so far to the Bronx to get medication. I said, "Because I was told to come here." She said, "Well, I'll move you down to another clinic"—it was Ninetysomething and Park Avenue.

That's where I was given the placebo. It's unthinkable, but it happened. I went to the clinic, was interviewed by the doctor—a heavy-set man, very nice—and filled out the usual forms. It was the pharmacist who gave me the placebo. You'd line up, you know; he would give you your medication over the counter. The first day I went there I swallowed the preparation— the medication, supposedly—that he had given me. It was bitter, it tasted like methadone, but it didn't take much to figure out that it wasn't. I was very uncomfortable that day, very sick. I complained about it. He said something about my not being used to . . . it was some double talk. Again, he gave me medication. That night I was in terrible, terrible condition. I was vomiting, jerking; I couldn't stand still long enough to urinate, that's how badly I was jerking [mimics seizure]. I was j-jerking convulsively, y-you co-co-couldn't talk!

That was only the second day. The third day I went back there, I said, to this man, "Look at me! Something is very wrong here, I don't know what is happening." He said, "Don't worry about it." I assumed he was thinking, "New kid on the block. I'm going to take his methadone, stick it in my pocket, and I'll be ahead."

That night was cold, wet, raining. I remember crawling on my hands and knees into the apartment terrace at three o'clock in the morning, trying to urinate. My bladder was so full, but I couldn't urinate standing up—I couldn't sit, stand, lie down, talk, eat, do anything. I was convulsing violently every three or four minutes.

The next morning I was prepared to go over the terrace: I was going to kill myself. I could no longer stand it. I don't think anybody could, three days without methadone. But there was a girl here and a man, friends of mine, who withheld me physically. I remember about 5:30 that morning they took me out of a taxicab, supporting me under my arms, and dragged me into the clinic. There was a line of people there, but I forced my way ahead, just pushing them out of the way. I grabbed this young pharmacist by the lapels of his coat and smashed my way into the pharmacy. I said, "Now, either you give me my medication or I'm going to kill you." Somebody had a lead pipe and was ready to hit me over the head, because they didn't know what I was, or what I was doing. They thought I was robbing the clinic. But he gave me some medication, or something. I know that it takes from a half-hour to forty-five minutes for methadone orally to take effect. My friends, again supporting me under the arms, walked me up and down the block for over an hour and a half. Nothing was happening, and I knew again that nothing was going to happen.

Then this girl took me in a cab to the office of a doctor—I don't want to mention his name. He was known then as Dr. Feelgood. While in his office I had a convulsion, I threw myself from a table which came down out of a wall, eight feet across the room, and hit the wall on the other side. When I came to, I don't know how much later, he was standing over me. He had administered something, and there were tongue depressors in my mouth.

What else could it have been except a placebo? Nothing else could have produced that sort of reaction. I was on one hundred milligrams of methadone, but I hadn't been using barbiturates. I was clean.

This doctor whose hands I fell into has a charisma you cannot believe until you meet him. He's an elderly man, but his personality is such that a president of the United States became one of his patients and closest friends. The minute you meet this guy, you fall in love with him: he is the most charming, wonderful man in the world. You get so that you go to him every day. You have to wait two or three hours in his waiting room, and the levels of society you meet there you won't believe.

I went to him for over three months. When he sees you he sits opposite and injects you in the little veins and capillaries on the backs of your hands, so that he leaves no marks. He also injected me several times in the jugular, several times in the groin. I never knew what he injected me with, and he never told me. He would go to the end of the room, turn his back to me, mix up some damn thing, hold it up to the light, mix it again, then put it together. He used an enormous syringe with a tiny needle. There was a lot of liquid, I know that; it was colored pink, and the moment the injection began I could taste Vitamin B, so I know that one of the ingredients was vitamins. There must have been amphetamines there too, because you instantly felt better.

He was expensive. Early in the game, I would go to him four or five times a day, at fifty dollars a clip. That was two hundred dollars a day, sometimes two hundred and fifty. During the summer this doctor took a home in Oyster Bay.[2] I couldn't drive a car in my condition, and the trains wouldn't operate at the hours I had to go out there. He was an early riser, and I had to be at his Oyster Bay home at five o'clock. So I would have chauffeur-driven limousines in front of my door three and sometimes four times a day, making round trips. Now, that would be running four to five hundred dollars a day, between the cost of his treatments and the cost of these limousines. But I had to do it. I was hooked on this doctor. I wasn't hooked on drugs or narcotics, or barbiturates, or methadone: I was hooked on him.

I was also dependent on whatever was in the pink solution, but he slowly took me down from four times a day, to three, to two, to one. Then to three times a week, and then once or twice a week. Finally, he said, "I don't think you need me anymore." I said OK, and we said goodbye, although we continued to meet socially.

That was the only literally drug-free period I have had in the last thirty or more years. But I was so depressed that I thought constantly of suicide. I wasn't sick—and whenever I use the word "sick," you must understand that among narcotic addicts, among "junkies," the word sick has only one connotation: withdrawal sickness. I wasn't sick: I didn't have that snake in my stomach, or that terrible need for narcotics. I was just terribly depressed. I think I had become, over the years, so . . . how to put this?

2. On the northern shore of Long Island, about twenty-three miles from midtown Manhattan.

So drug-oriented, oriented to taking some artificial substance, be it drug or Maalox or two aspirin at night. That contributed to the depression.

After three months I went back to the woman psychiatrist who originally recommended methadone. I told her my experience with this doctor and I said, "Shall I go back on methadone?" She said, "It's not a question of shall you; it's a question of how quickly can we get you back onto methadone." I went to the clinic to which I am presently going. The depression disappeared instantly. It was as dramatic as that.

Looking back, I don't feel I was led to methadone under false pretenses. But I think that they're not being entirely fair with the patient, in that they don't give him warning that he's going into treatment that lasts a lifetime. It's a lifetime maintenance program, although I have reason to hope that I can get away from methadone sometime before I die. I know they're still experimenting with it, but until the time comes when they find other drugs to get you off methadone, once you start it, you're on it for life.

Methadone is much better than Alvodine or Demerol though. Infinitely. It's better for the very simple reason that I lead a normal life. I don't have to scheme to get drugs. I no longer need a drug so long as I drink my medication every morning with a little bit of orange juice. There is no euphoria, or very little euphoria, involved. And taking it only once a day is an enormous advantage. My life has stabilized one hundred percent. If you weigh assets and liabilities, methadone has been a good thing for me. Not only a good thing, but the only thing.

Then why do I want to be off methadone someday? Because I'm on a leash. I'm retired, I have no financial worries, there are no roots keeping me in my apartment, and I plan to travel. Say I wanted to go to Kansas City, or Indianapolis, or Baton Rouge. I would first have to get an OK from my clinic doctor. That would be readily given, but he is restricted to giving me medication only for a certain number of days—I don't think it exceeds two weeks. If I wanted to be a gypsy and get into a mobile home and bum around the States, I couldn't do it. I can't go abroad. If there's no clinic in Lido, Venice or Naples, Italy, or Paris, France, I can't go there. Because where am I going to obtain medication? That's what I meant by the leash. It's always there.

RED

The traditional police approach and methadone maintenance seem, at first glance, to be at odds. One attempts to suppress the narcotic traffic, the other to provide addicts with a regular supply. But a useful, unanticipated relationship evolved between the two. The greater the police pressure, the more the expense and adul-

teration of heroin; the worse the heroin, the better cheap and unadulterated methadone looks to a prospective patient. "I'm sure that bad dope was one of the things that turned my mind around about heroin," said Red. "I'd thrown so much money away on junk, absolute horse junk. I said, 'I'm not going to spend any more. I'm going to quit this thing.'"

All of my life I've been a working man. I've come to know a lot of addicts through meetings, all kinds of addicts. Some people get their money to buy their dope by killing somebody that day, or they may have stolen it, or held somebody up. They'll steal goods, articles, *anything* that's salable. But I wasn't in that position. I was a musician. Most of the money I earned went for dope. Not all of it—I have a certain amount of intelligence, and there's a couple of things I always maintain. I like to stay clean. I've never been dirty, like the average addict leaning out on the street. He's filthy, hasn't had a bath. I never endured that kind of stuff. I don't want to smell myself, or anybody else to smell me.

But about 1962 I started suffering, because I wasn't that much on call. The popularity, working, recording with bands, staying on call, plenty of money—all of that was behind me. I was a married man now, and the work just wasn't coming in. It was a scuffle to get money together. But I never did enter the other life, you know, the ripping and running.

One night, somewhere up near the end of the year, I gathered together a few dollars—incidentally, this was some of our rent money, saved mostly through my wife's efforts—and I went out into the street to cop. I found somebody that had some, and I purchased it. When I came home it was snowing to beat the band. It was a night in New York City! Hardly any traffic could move, the snow and the ice were so heavy. At that time I lived in upper Manhattan, and I had quite a little way to go. I had to take the subway and go through all those dues: waiting in the late hours for a train, and all that. When I got home my wife was fast asleep, because she was going to work the next day, like I should've been doing. I sat down to do my thing, but somebody had put pure quinine in this ten-dollar bag. Not even a trace of heroin. They had beat me. Boy, I sat there on the edge of the bed and cried like a baby. I was so sick and miserable. My wife tried to comfort me—she started talking to me then. She started to make the same suggestion I had heard from others in the street: "I hear there are programs now. There are people out there who will try to help you. Now, honey, why don't you try to get behind one of those things?" She had said this to me before, but I had deaf ears. Up to that time I didn't care what I had to go through or how far I had to go, I would find that heroin. But now my ears were open. I listened to her, and I was sincere.

I didn't sleep all night. I couldn't. That very next morning I was up bright and early, dressed, and I left with her when she went to work—in fact, I got on the same subway. I went downtown to a hospital on

Eighteenth Street, seeking help. I applied for the methadone program. I even met the main doctor and his wife: Drs. Dole and Nyswander. This was around 1964, '65. They weren't accepting too many people at that time, and there was a long waiting list.

For a time I was able to buy the methadone. Someone had told me, "There are different guys in the street who sell their medication. You know, they have enough to go over, and they can do without for a day or so. You can get some that way, so you can stop hurting." You see, when I was sick, when I didn't have the heroin, I felt it in one place: my tummy. My abdomen gave me hell—and still does right now if I don't have the methadone. So, after I was told about the street methadone, I bought my first bottle from this fellow. I paid ten dollars for it. [Laughs.] Later on I found out the going price was eight, so he beat me for two dollars. But when I drank it I noticed, in a short time, that I evened off. I wasn't high, but I wasn't sick. I had a slight euphoria, but I wasn't nodding all over the place. My next aim then was to get on a program, although I had to continue buying heroin when I couldn't find the street methadone. Eventually, a couple of years later, I happened on an introduction to Dr. Lowinson. She believed in me right away. She wanted someone who was well motivated, who had it together in their head. So I went into Bronx State Hospital, where I was stabilized on methadone. They had a special floor for methadone patients—in fact, it was almost like jail. You just couldn't walk in and out; all the doors were locked and maintained. I think the minimum amount of time you could stay there was a month. But then, after I was discharged, I became an outpatient.

I think this program's been wonderful for me. It's actually almost a miracle. I find only one fault: the fact that it just won't absolutely cure me, so I can just say, "Make that forty milligrams I'm taking zero." I still have to hang on. It's the only thing that I know of that will keep me hurting as little as I am now.

Although the program's worked for me, I've seen it not work for a lot of people. I see one thing in particular that's very foolish: people who ask to be detoxed, then detox themselves so fast that, when they're down to just about zero, they can't let it go. Then they have to reclaim higher doses, until they're almost back to where they started.[3] I've also seen people

---

3. Depending on the philosophy of a particular program, patients are permitted, encouraged, or required to detoxify completely. Whether detoxification or even reduction to a lower dosage (say, from a hundred to thirty milligrams per day) should be a goal of methadone programs is an issue that has provoked controversy (Leon Brill, "High Versus Low-Dose Maintenance Therapy: A Review of Program Experiences," in Carl D. Chambers and Leon Brill, eds., *Methadone: Experiences and Issues* [New York: Behavioral Publications, 1973], 149–62; cf. Vincent P. Dole, "Addictive Behavior," *Scientific American* 243 [1980], 148, 150).

detox all the way, quit the program, and then come and beg to get back on the program, because they relapsed. And I've also seen people on the program cheating. They come in, get their dose, but then all through the week they're taking dope. It's very common: men and women, every day. Lots of them cheat. And most people who are not using heroin drink. There was a girl up here just last Tuesday—I remember her well because she was almost naked, with a little pair of short pants on, just bouncing herself all around. She was as drunk as she could be. She's coming to a maintenance program to get her dose, and she's drunk. Ossified.

But not everyone in the clinic cheats. There are those who don't. I don't cheat. I have never cheated. My mind is definitely made up. I've been clean all these years.

JERRY

Although it is not generally known, methadone maintenance was practiced infor-mally before Drs. Vincent Dole and Marie Nyswander began their pilot programs in the 1960s. Some addicts, unable to obtain opium for smoking, or disillu-sioned by the declining quality and rising price of heroin, switched to Dolophine (methadone hydrochloride) during the 1950s.

Jerry was among them. He was born into a middle-class Jewish family in Brooklyn in 1915. His father, a shohet, or ritual slaughterer, died when Jerry was twelve. Shortly thereafter he was caught burglarizing homes for money to buy toys and was sent to a Jewish military academy for delinquent children. He returned home when he was fifteen, worked at "some cockamamie jobs which didn't mean anything," and then drifted into a life of thievery.

I started robbing with a gun when I was about seventeen, eighteen. A lot of us kids, we wanted to be wise guys. We thought it was smart to be a hoodlum, and I fell into them things. Then I became involved with opium when I was about eighteen, nineteen. I learned through friends, so-called friends that I met and got acquainted with. They had them "lay-down joints," they called it. Somebody would run one of them pads. We used to buy hop two toy for five. They called it a "toy"—it was about as big as a cap from a soda bottle. And he would chef for you and you'd lay down and smoke it and it felt good.

At first I didn't smoke on a regular basis. Once a week, once every three weeks. And then came a time I started to smoke more often. To get hooked you have to smoke about, I imagine, two months, every day. If you let forty-eight hours go by, you're safe. But if you keep smoking every day, every other day, there's a good possibility that you'll get hooked after two months or so. It's up to what kind of system that you're made of, what kind of system you've got. Some of them were going through a kind of resistance their body had. I knew a guy who smoked for a month steady. Then he would stop, and drink, and stay away from it and he'd be all right. But, mainly, if you fooled around too often and too close, you got hooked.

I didn't consider myself a junkie even after I was hooked. The type of people that smoked were a different class. I started to get in with show people, smart-money people, you know, bookmakers. In fact, I wouldn't bother with anyone that used anything else. They were like low-life. We looked down on them.

"Smart-money people"? They made money with their wits. Con men had rackets, entertainers had good incomes where they didn't break their backs. The women I smoked with, there were some showgirls and there were some married women. They were all a better class. There weren't no low-lifes like that you'd be ashamed to be seen with or anything like that. There were some of them that came from wealthy homes; wealthy incomes they had. But the women I smoked with, not one that I knew of was hooked.

I was with the same woman for years. We were living common-law. When I went away and when I came back, we took up again. She wasn't an addict. Once in a while she would smoke. I used to marvel at her and say, "How the hell do you do it?" I remember, when she went to California on a visit, she asked me to give her a double toy in case she wanted to smoke. She was gone about a month. When she came back, she gave me back the double. She didn't even use it.

We didn't have any children. That had to do with the opium. My wife had about four abortions—she didn't want to have a baby, figured maybe the kid wouldn't be right, being I was hooked.

I started to buy larger amounts: a half a pound, a quarter of a pound of crude opium. I would cook it up myself and convert it into opium. It was the shape of a brick. It was like dried leaves, very dried leaves; it was packed and [claps hands] compressed. You boiled a big pot of water, put it in there, and let it cook for about two hours. Then I would strain it off and recook it. Then I'd give it another strain and recook again to make sure it's clean. Otherwise it would clog up. And I would boil it down until —did you ever see what opium looks like? Like a black sauce. I would boil it down until I got the water out of it and it was the thickness I wanted to get.

You had to have your own place, your own pad, to smoke. When you're involved with a layout, you know, it wasn't something that you could go in a hallway and smoke. You had to have an apartment with gas, electric, and a bed. Then you were able to smoke. Mainly I smoked alone, but I had a lot of fair-weather friends that would come over. They'd look to use you. I could chef and it made you, like, the king of the walk. You were the main guy. Especially me: I had money, I had stuff. They'd call and they were glad if I said, "You can come over." They didn't pay me no money or anything. But when I got in the jackpot, they all disappeared.

I smoked for about four years and then I got busted. I got caught on a stickup, end of '36. I went away for a six-to-twenty-five. I done four years out of it. Naturally I was clean, I was off. Then, when I came home, I started chippying around and got hooked again. Because once you're hooked, you can't chippy around. Somehow it seems to catch you fast. Try to smoke twice a week, three times a week, then try to stay away a few days—it don't work that way. Even though I was away four years, in a month's time I was hooked again.

When I got out of prison in '41 I went into the business of selling. But I didn't sell to users, I sold to dealers. I made quite a bundle of money. I was dealing opium and I was selling H too. Kilo, half a kilo. You make friends when you do time; you meet people in there. You pick out certain people that you think you can trust—or they think they can trust you. When you get out, if they're out, you get together. Like, for instance, if we both done time, and I thought you was OK, and you thought I was, and we hit the street and, maybe a period of six months went by and I would say to you, "Look, do you know anything about this? Could you connect me?" Maybe you could. If you did, you connected me with a dealer or something, and that's how it got started. You can't just go up to anybody and say, "Hey, you want to sell me some stuff?" They'll look at you like you're crazy. It's all through connections. You meet people and get involved.

But then I got busted again—in '47, I think it was. I got picked up by the feds. They couldn't get nothing on me—all they found was a jar of hop that I claimed was my personal stuff. They had information, but they couldn't prove nothing. They couldn't prove that I was dealing. They were mad and all that shit. So I was sent back. I got two years for violation. And then when I came out, that's when I got a job and that was the end of my fooling around. This is when I started using dollies. I had heard another fellow say they were supposed to be pretty good. Being I couldn't get opium, and I was hooked, I got dollies. I didn't get loaded, but I didn't get sick.

I started my job in '56, somewhere around in there. I learned a trade and I went to work as a presser—in a factory, not in a tailor shop. In ladies' sports wear. I worked for about twenty-five years. I never smoked opium again. I didn't smoke it because I couldn't get it. About '54, '55, it started to dribble out. If I'd have been able to get it, I would have smoked it. But it was always in my mind that I've got to have something so that I can go to work.

You say, "Well, why didn't you kick it?" To break the habit—to me, anyway—the rougher part is after you've cleaned yourself out. It would take about eight months till I would actually feel the way, you know, you have to feel: normal. I always worried that I would blow my job if I looked to break it. See, in my trade, if you get a steady shop, which means that you work steady there, that's it. If you blow that job, you can't get another shop so fast. It may take a year, two years, three years. Meantime, you'll be shaken up, work a day here, two days there—the union sends you, you know. The reason is that there's more pressers than jobs. So if you have a steady shop, you don't want to lose it. If you lose it, you don't know if you'll be able to get a steady shop again, especially if it's a good shop where you make a good dollar.

So it was rough. But I'd get the dollies. I didn't take much. It was ten grains, each tablet. I would take two and a half a day. At first I probably went to somebody and was dealing or something and I asked them, "Could you get me opium?" "No." "Could you get me dollies?" He said yes, and he got me dollies. Then, later on, in the late sixties into the seventies, I copped from a doctor that I was going to for years, a family doctor. He would only give me a scrip once a month for about forty dollies. Not every druggist would accept the scrip. I would go mainly to the druggist that was in his office, so they knew. But there were some druggists that I went to, they'd look at the scrip and say they didn't want to fill it. Eventually I was getting it from somebody else—another druggist—who sold it on the street.

I entered the methadone program April 25, 1973. It was hard to get it at that particular time. In fact, I think there was a rumor around that they were going to stop making it altogether. And, besides, I felt that, if I can get it legitimately, why do I have to run late at night to get it?

With methadone, like I get up and I take the drink. I feel, after about fifteen, twenty minutes, a half-hour, and I have coffee—I start to feel that I'm coming to life. I feel normal. I get up, I go to work, I do whatever I have to do. But if I had a choice of opium or methadone for maintenance, I'd take the opium, because it's a great time killer. I like the way it makes you feel. Dollies don't make you feel that good. But I'll tell you this, though: I don't have no cravings or fantasizing for opium. I don't get the feeling that I want to party anymore.

VINCENT DOLE

Vincent Dole was born in Chicago in 1913 and received his early education there. A mathematics major at Stanford, he decided to switch to medicine because mathematics seemed too much "a game of the mind, rather than the real world." He did his preclinical training at the University of Wisconsin, then, since his primary interest lay in research, transferred to Harvard in 1936. After completing his internship and residency, he took a position at the Rockefeller Institute in 1941 and was married the following year. Although he did some research on infectious diseases for the Navy during World War II, he spent most of his time on metabolic processes and disorders, believing these to be among medical science's key unsolved problems.

Before becoming interested in addiction, Dole did important research in hypertension, lipid chemistry, and several other fields. In fact, if he had not already achieved a national reputation as a research scientist, his enterprise would almost certainly have met the same fate as that of Willis Butler. But Dole's prestige and prior accomplishments helped to protect him and his co-worker Marie Nyswander when they began their controversial experiments with narcotic maintenance. [4]

I'd been interested in the appetite control systems, and I had a feeling that there was absolutely open territory in the whole question of behavior, and to what extent metabolism had something to do with drive. That coupled with a social feeling that's likely to overcome people around the age of fifty, where you begin to feel some sense of responsibility. At the time I was commuting from Rye, New York, and would get off at the 125th Street Station in Harlem. Sometimes I'd walk to work or take the el down Third Avenue. I had the sense of moving between two highly privileged oases through a truly epidemic sea of misery. I began to realize that *nobody* in my community of scientists or people in Rye had any concept of that world. We were essentially living in the midst of an epidemic and ignoring it.

I was talking about this to Lew Thomas,[5] who had been one of the group of us here at Rockefeller during the navy days. Thomas was on the Board of Health of the City of New York, and he'd been chairman of the Health Research Council's Committee on Narcotics. This committee had been set up out of desperation, out of the feeling that there ought to be something the doctors should do about it. But nothing much had come out of it. I said what a shame it was that there was none of the scientific thought in the field of addiction that I had encountered in my other researches. It didn't have recognition as a scientific problem. Certainly there wasn't any research talent in it. Such talent as there was was limited to people who were in the main part pharmacologists and studied animals. They didn't have much concept of the problem of human epidemiology. I told this to Lew and he said, "Well, that's a great thing. I'm just going to go off on a sabbatical, and I haven't seen much come out of this committee. Why don't you become the chairman?" So, suddenly

4. Prior to publication, Dr. Dole requested that certain changes be made in the text of the narrative to enhance its accuracy and clarity. We have incorporated his suggested alterations, most of which involve minor changes in phraseology.

5. Lewis Thomas, the distinguished medical essayist, researcher, and administrator. Thomas's version of the following events may be found in his autobiography, *The Youngest Science: Notes of a Medicine Watcher* (New York: Viking, 1983), 147–48.

I found myself given the chairmanship of the Health Research Council's
Committee on Narcotics.

I read as much as I could, and made a point of meeting everybody in
the field who pretended any sort of expertise or who had been recognized
as an expert. Actually, the only person who made any sense to me, just as
a clinician, was Marie Nyswander. I had read her book,[6] and I had heard
about her from others. So I invited her to come and talk with me, to see
what advice she had. She impressed me as a very intense and intelligent
person who was working under absolutely hopeless disadvantages administratively. She was all alone, with a good heart and a lot of spirit, trying to
fight the establishment up and down the line. So I said, "If we're going to
move forward on this"—at that time I had already started some planning
to do some research at Rockefeller—"you come here and we'll get you an
appointment to the staff." That was in late '62 or early '63.

I had sort of a twofold job. One was the research side, which was pleasant and went in a relatively smooth motion. We were going into almost
uncharted fields, so almost anything could be discovered. The other side
was the rather strenuous business of fighting for our privilege to do so.
I had to fight, to a large extent, against the federal government and, to a
secondary extent, against the inertia or opposition of the research establishment in the field. The Federal Bureau of Narcotics had an absolutely
iron clamp on the field and had essentially driven out physicians for thirty
years or more. The general perception was that this was a problem to be
dealt with in a regulatory way by the enforcement authorities and, medically, only by sending people to locked institutions like the Public Health
Hospital in Lexington.

To be fair, the Bureau of Narcotics probably had a sincere belief that
the way to control the problem was to stamp it out—if it's not working,
then the punishment's not severe enough. This attitude of the Bureau
was surely not uniquely generated by them: they were articulating into
regulatory form a prejudice against addiction, a sort of Fu Manchu irrational terror about the whole thing. This still exists today, and I think
it has been and continues to be a limiting fact in dealing effectively with
what should not be that big a problem.

*Do you believe that the race and the class of the people addicted had anything to
do with this hard-line approach?*

Yes. Not strictly because of the race and class, but probably because of
their helplessness. When you have more influential, middle-class people
involved in a problem—as you do in, say, alcoholism—then you are forced

6. *The Drug Addict as a Patient* (New York: Grune and Stratton, 1956).

into a more benign approach. But a minority, and particularly a minority thirty years ago, was a relatively helpless group. There's a great smugness in a privileged majority when they congratulate themselves on not having *that* problem, so they're not really forced into any humility.

At the onset of our research Marie Nyswander and I had a rather simple plan. Narcotics are considerably different in the details of their pharmacology. With alcohol, you can talk about all sorts of different drinks, but the common drug is ethanol. That's not true with narcotics. There is an extraordinarily wide range of chemicals that have in common narcotic activity, which can be defined technically as a cross-reaction to morphine. They will relieve the symptoms of abstinence produced by the withdrawal of morphine in a morphine-dependent subject. They will also produce the same tolerance that morphine does, so that tolerance developed to drug A will exhibit itself as tolerance to morphine when the subject is challenged with morphine. These technical attributes of a drug sufficed to classify it with the morphine-like drugs, or the opiates.

In retrospect, it seems obvious how simplistic it was for doctors to think of "narcotic addiction" as a unitary condition, especially since it had been known for a long time that different narcotics have quite different effects in terms of their intensity of action, their potency, and even what organ systems they affect. It seemed open territory to explore on addicts the different effects of pharmacologically different drugs, all belonging to the opiate family. We also wanted to study the response of addicts to narcotic drugs. What kind of disablement does a drug produce? How much and for how long?

To be sure, if a person experiences a euphoric effect, that tends to remove him, for a period of time, from other types of normal functions. But that in itself is certainly not sufficient to condemn a drug in such violent terms. After all, if a person has a glass of wine, or for that matter a good meal, that may make them feel better; it may actually be something one would recommend. So the question I asked myself was, "What's so bad about narcotics?" Everybody starts off with the axiom, "Narcotics are obviously bad, and therefore we must wipe them out." I said, "Well, you're probably right. But let me just ask in a little more detail, specifically what are we fighting in narcotics?" If you were to ask me what was so bad about cigarettes, I would say that there was a strong statistical tendency toward lung cancer, to emphysema, and various other disabilities. What's so bad about alcohol is that it can disable a person in terms of day-to-day functions, and it can also produce damage to the liver and the brain. Translating this for narcotics, I wanted to study the health effects and to see what was so bad.

So we tried, without preconception, to observe the effect of reasonable doses of narcotics given to people with a long-standing history of narcotic addiction (after obtaining their informed consent, and after review of the protocol by hospital authorities). We didn't have rigid guidelines: we simply accepted addicts that Marie Nyswander or others knew about, half a dozen at first. They ranged in age from twenty-one up to forty or thereabouts. Naturally we limited the study to men, because I didn't want a woman to get pregnant and present a danger of damaging the fetus. And I didn't want to get into the hormonal variables of menstrual cycles. But those were our only restrictions: males in an adult group with several years' history of intractable heroin addiction.

We set up a schedule of different drugs and different doses, recording in a notebook how the addicts felt and looked, whether their voices and pupils changed, that sort of thing. It was really humdrum observational research. Most of these drugs were rather short-acting. In three or four hours the addict would be miserable and vomiting, needing another shot. The doses on which you could keep them comfortable kept going up and up; the addicts were never really satisfied or happy. It was not an encouraging experience. I was prepared, in the early stages of observing this process, to concede that there was a lot of wisdom in rejecting the maintenance approach. And I could see why Butler had a problem with morphine maintenance: he was using the wrong drug. His intentions were right, but you cannot succeed with morphine or heroin. These drugs have too short a period of action to provide stability of function. Undoubtedly there have been, and still are, some people who, in their own quiet way, can stabilize themselves on small frequent doses of morphine. But morphine couldn't do the job I was thinking of, which was to try to treat thousands of people who had become hopeless addicts. Administratively, one could *never* set up an apparatus whereby you could give each patient a shot every four hours, and have a hundred thousand people in treatment. All you have to do is take a paper and a pencil and look at the staffing and facilities you'd need. Or, if you think you're going to give bags full of heroin or morphine for addicts to take back to Bedford-Stuyvesant, you're being unrealistic. Commentators who have suddenly discovered, after all these years, that the answer to the addiction problem is, "Well, why not just give them the heroin?" don't know what they're talking about. In fact, that was one of the first questions I asked when I didn't know much about the problem. I said, "I don't see what's so bad about dispensing pure heroin when taking the junk on the street is killing them, and devastating society through the crime generated by high prices." But I learned what was wrong, just by watching these people on our metabolic ward: you cannot stabilize the dose with a short-acting drug like heroin or morphine.

In any case, the study hadn't gone too long, about two months, when it became obvious that the people who were being tested with methadone were not so demanding for increasing doses. They were content with a steady dose. Even more remarkable was the change in their conversation. I made a practice of spending two or three hours almost every day just sitting and talking with the addicts in a somewhat aimless way. I was just trying to get a sense of their way of thinking, their values, their experiences. They educated me about a world that was out of my reach, one that I had never been in and would never enter. I became so sensitive to their attitudes that I noticed the change when my conversations with the addicts on methadone began to diversify into topics like baseball or politics, rather than endlessly, endlessly recalling drug experiences.

One time, as part of a policy of trying to get others to support our work, I invited Harris Isbell, head of the Addiction Research Unit at Lexington, to visit our research ward. He talked with the methadone group, asking them all sorts of questions. They responded, telling him what they were doing—many of them were going back to school, taking correspondence or evening courses. A couple of them had jobs in the daytime, reporting back to the ward at night. When he got done with this rather long talk and we had left the ward, he said to me, in a nice, gentle way, "Well, Vincent, I'm sorry to tell you, but you're wasting your time. Those are not addicts." He left and I went back to the ward. Naturally these fellows were all particularly interested in this interview because they all knew him well from Lexington. When I told them what he had said, they all laughed and laughed. They said, "He sure didn't tell us that when we were at Lexington."

Episodes of this sort convinced me of methadone's potential for rehabilitation. What was new in our work was actually not the drug; that had been around since World War II. In fact, the drug had been used at Lexington for detoxification. But the Lexington group had always been thinking in terms of relatively acute pharmacology. They had given huge doses to people under the conditions of a prison ward. They had manipulated the dose and conducted various experiments, but they were not in the position to learn anything about rehabilitation or, for that matter, of establishing a cooperative relationship with a patient. There's something about a prison ward and a guinea-pig attitude toward a patient that leads to an adversary relationship. Since they never got to know their patients as human beings, how could they rehabilitate anybody?

From the beginning, the Bureau of Narcotics objected to our experiments because we were maintaining addicts. It was an intimidating atmosphere. Before I began the studies, I had asked Det Bronk, who was president of Rockefeller, whether it could cause him any problems if I got into such a politically controversial field. I said that this problem is too hot for any doctor or institution in this country to handle, as far as I knew. He said, "If that's so, then it's our job to do it." He didn't ever raise any questions about political pressures, and, I suppose, through his authority, he deflected them. Also, I talked to a number of my friends —and, fortunately, most of the people who were in leading positions in academic medicine in America were my friends. I said, "If I come under political pressure for undertaking these studies, then I'll call on you for help." They agreed to support me in such a case. Fortunately, I never needed to call on them. I also went to Don O'Brien, one of the attorneys representing Rockefeller University. His staff drew up a massive legal brief, and out of it came the interesting fact that there wasn't any substantive law that prohibited my doing what I was proposing to do, even though the Bureau of Narcotics had asserted otherwise for a long time. All this preliminary work took a year.

It wasn't long after starting work that the Bureau of Narcotics heard of our activities. They sent an agent who came in the most peremptory, arrogant way. He hammered the table and said, "You're breaking the law." I said, "I've been looking into that and, as far as I understand the situation, I'm not." He said, "You are, and if you don't stop, we'll put you out of business." I said, "Well, maybe that's the proper thing for you to do. Given the way that you understand the law, you ought to take me to court so we can have a determination on this point." This fellow's face suddenly changed. He abruptly ended the discussion and said he'd have to discuss it with his superiors.

This type of interaction was repeated in one form or another until they became persuaded that there was no easy way to force us out by threats. Then, oddly enough, the next thing I learned was that they had announced to various people that we were conducting a very limited set of research studies with their authorization and under their control. Nobody else would be permitted to do this, but because we were a special research institution, we would be allowed to continue. But there wasn't any cooperation in this. They assigned agents to monitor everything we did, and to come to us with threats like "You are not doing things that are bona fide" and "You'd better watch out." They infiltrated clinics and stole records, trying to get what they considered inside information. They spread false rumors and encouraged attacks on us.

In 1965 we published an article in the *Journal of the American Medical Association*,[7] a kind of progress report on methadone maintenance. The reaction was mixed. Some people criticized me for publishing so early; other people were critical of the fact that we had gone so far without prior publication. There was an enormous amount of skepticism because this went against the dogma in the field. The more gentle critics said that "the patients are so selected that they don't represent anything. They would have done well anyway." Or, "There's something very special about the climate at Rockefeller"—or about Marie, or me, or somebody that was inspiring them—"So it's not really a pharmacological result at all."

7. "A Medical Treatment for Diacetylmorphine (Heroin) Addiction: A Clinical Trial with Methadone Hydrochloride," vol. 193, pp. 646–50.

Or that we were just liars. That was the Bureau of Narcotics line, that we had fabricated the data. It was a rumor campaign—no public statements. They certainly wouldn't expose themselves to a lawsuit.

I think the *JAMA* article won a number of converts—that article, and a number of ones that were published during the next two or three years. I had promised many people that, as best I could, I'd keep my reports up to date so there'd be no big lag. But there was an unfortunate reaction to this: some people became overly converted. They felt, without reading our reports carefully, that all they had to do was give methadone and then there was no more problem with the addicts. As best I could, at meetings and in publications, I urged that physicians should see that the problem was one of rehabilitating people with a very complicated mixture of social problems on top of a specific medical problem, and that they ought to tailor their programs to the kinds of problems they were dealing with. The strength of the early programs as designed by Marie Nyswander was in their sensitivity to individual human problems. The stupidity of thinking that just giving methadone will solve a complicated social problem seems to me beyond comprehension, but it's still a limiting factor in people's thinking. Either they're against methadone, or they think that just because they're giving methadone they should solve everyone's problems—and if that doesn't happen, then methadone didn't work.

The golden age of antibiotics had preceded this, when people were looking for magic bullets and miracle drugs. Maybe methadone seemed to some people to be that, and they jumped to conclusions.

I think so. As a matter of fact, if you take the whole field of medicine, there has been a deterioration in the quality of relations to the patients. Antibiotics, perhaps, were part of the knell of human doctor-patient relationships. On the whole, today's doctors are quite abrupt in dealing with human problems. What some physicians expect is that you come to them, get the prescription, take your medicine, and you ought to be all right. If you're not, why, you're a crock. I've heard many patients in other areas and friends complain about that type of impersonal treatment. Insofar as I have had experience as a patient, I just hate to go to a medical facility. Whatever the technical quality of care now, compared to a generation ago, we've paid a price in human quality. And with addiction we're dealing, unfortunately, with a disease in which human relationships are integral to rehabilitation.

Even before I began research on narcotics, I assumed that chronic exposure to narcotics induced a metabolic change, manifested in the physical craving for opiates. In previous work I had become persuaded that the abnormal intake of food in obesity was a symptom of metabolic defect. Perhaps that theory influenced my view of addiction. In fact, I believe that all ingestive behavior is in some way responsive to the biochemical state of the body.

But we're no closer today to explaining the metabolic aspect of addictive behavior than we were twenty years ago. What we have gained, however, is a better climate of research and acceptance of the possibility —I should say now probability—that specific metabolic abnormalities will be discovered. The work during the last decade on endorphins has been most dramatic and interesting, and shows that there are important neuromodulators which must be significant in behavior. However, to date, efforts to find a specific abnormality in endorphin metabolism have failed in relation to narcotic addiction. I have every hope that this will unfold during the coming decade.

The interesting thing is that, today, the only principal attacks on the so-called metabolic theory of addictive behavior come from people with an ideological position, usually related to identification with drug-free programs, oriented toward abstinence. I would be delighted to have permanent abstinence as a goal, if it were an achievable one. But for chronic addicts a cure is very rarely achieved, although short-term abstinence is common. No therapeutic community has ever produced statistics to show that sustained abstinence could be achieved on a significant scale. They select a small minority who remit and advertise them as their typical product.

People oftentimes criticize methadone for being a "crutch." The image that comes to my mind is of a person using the crutches: if you come along and say, "We're going to take away these things, and it'd be better for you to hop on one leg," then you're not helping him. If some fellow comes up with a way to grow a new leg, why, I'd be very enthusiastic about it. But until it's done, what is evil about a crutch?

I would hate to see therapeutic communities abolished. Their essential service is in helping young delinquents in the early stages of experimenting with drugs. They can guide them to a better lifestyle and generally give them a sense of meaning through structured support. But for these agencies to advertise themselves as being the *only*, complete, and adequate treatment for the bulk of chronic narcotic addicts is not supportable.

What were some of the milestones in the spread of methadone maintenance? How did it go from being a relatively small, prototypical program to a national phenomenon?

The critical event was a discussion I had with Dr. Ray Trussell, Commissioner of Hospitals for the City of New York. We had been working for more than a year, and I felt the time had come to examine the potential of this type of treatment on a larger scale and in a more generally relevant environment. So, I made an appointment to see Dr. Trussell and brought with me graphs and statistics of our work. I talked to him for a few minutes and, to my surprise, he picked up the telephone, called up Beth Israel Medical Center, said that he was sending a doctor over, and he would like them to give me whatever I needed for my work. Then he said to me with a smile, "This may be what I've been looking for for ten years." Like Marie Nyswander, he had had a long history of frustration in dealing with the practical aspect of the problem.[8]

I went to Beth Israel and talked to the director, who had already had a long conversation with Ray Trussell while I was en route. He simply said that Commissioner Trussell had offered to subsidize whatever kind of research I wanted to do in the area, subject to the normal controls and clearances within the medical center. Within a short time—the next week, practically—Marie Nyswander and I went to an empty floor on the Manhattan General Hospital (which subsequently became the Bernstein Institute) and started a program. It became the model for the later methadone programs.

This is the period I like to remember: the results at Beth Israel, at Rockefeller, and at the two or three other clinics established in New York were so favorable, and the group of people involved was so enthusiastic, that it seemed that there was really hope in the field—substantial hope. With it went a great sense of pride on the part of the patients and the staff. This honeymoon stage lasted from 1965 to 1970. During this time the Bureau of Narcotics and other agencies carped, infiltrated, and attempted to discredit the program, but on the whole they were a peripheral nuisance. Some regulatory authorities even approached me and said they would cease their attacks and permit us to exist if only we would promise not to let the program grow. Of course, I couldn't accept a restriction that would deny treatment to people who needed it.

The regulatory counterattack really didn't come until about '73, after the program had grown and become more visible, and there was a sense that we were intruding into other people's areas of authority. During the 1960s there had been substantial growth, up to a thousand patients or so, but it really ballooned during the early 1970s, when there were

8. Trussell, whom we also interviewed, had been particularly disillusioned by the failure of the Riverside Hospital program for the treatment of adolescent addicts, located on North Brother Island in the East River. Opened in 1952, this operation was closed by Trussell in 1961, after it had become embarrassingly clear that nearly all of its detoxified patients quickly relapsed. Trussell recalled his first meeting with Dole as follows: "He said that he had been working with mainline heroin addicts at Rockefeller University; that he had discovered accidentally a technique for blockading the heroin effect or craving, by using escalating doses of methadone to a blocking level; and that he had at least one patient who had been maintained that way for a year. He had a total of, I think, six protocols with him. What impressed me, what made me give him some immediate attention, was the fact that all six protocols had exactly the same positive outcome."

political pressures from the Nixon White House to expand methadone maintenance, and overly enthusiastic or opportunistic people jumped into the field. That's when things became disorderly.

The difficulty was not that methadone expanded, or that it did so rapidly, but that it expanded faster than medical competence developed. Here in New York Dr. Robert Newman showed what could be achieved: he brought in twenty thousand new patients. This was done in a remarkably efficient way, with good data control, good statistics, and high spirits on the part of the staff. So rapid expansion was possible if medical competence and leadership were there. But across the country people who had very little understanding of the pharmacology of methadone, and no comprehension of the wider array of medical and social problems presented by addicts, jumped into the field, feeling that all they had to do was hand out the drug.

This invited the federal government to reenter the field in a vigorous way, to take command of the whole business and to set up regulations that, I think, have to a large extent damaged the programs today. It was an unprecedented entry into the practice of medicine. If treating people with methadone is a medical process—like treating people with congestive heart failure with digitalis, or diabetics with insulin, or Addisonians with steroid hormones—then it constitutes a new phenomenon in medical practice to have some federal agency, nonmedical at that, control medical decisions with detailed legislation. Rigid guidelines defined who could be treated, how long he could be treated, what dose he could be given, and what services, what reporting was needed, and what paperwork mandated. Anybody running a program became subject to unannounced inspections from the many agencies supervising it, putting physicians under the threat of criminal prosecution if they hadn't followed the strict regulatory guidelines.

Other seeds of trouble were present in the late sixties and early seventies. With the growth of the programs, there was an adoption of methadone by people who still fundamentally believed that this was a psychological problem. They were only using methadone as a means to engage somebody in treatment, with the idea that ultimately the cure would be through psychotherapy. So there entered into the field a kind of hybrid thinking, with methadone being considered only a limited expedient. This type of attitude was adopted and expanded into an official view by the federal government, and it was incorporated into their regulations by 1974. The goal of treatment was not rehabilitation but abstinence.

To treat patients effectively a therapist must be sensitive to their problems, not merely put them into a structure that forces them to take inappropriate services. I have in mind some dreadful programs out in California. We learned that one fellow there was forced to quit his job to attend counseling sessions. Their hypothesis was that, after all, addiction is a symptom of a weak personality, and if a person needs methadone he must have a weak personality, therefore, whether he has a job or not, what he needs is to come to their counseling sessions. This seems bizarre, but it's not unusual, unfortunately. We haven't succeeded in scotching the ghost of the personality theory; it's grown fatter and stronger than it was ten years ago.

It also seemed bizarre when we were criticized for treating narcotic addicts who had alcohol or pill problems, because they didn't do as well as others. I rejected this with all the vigor I could summon. My job as a doctor was to treat sick people, not to hunt among sick people for the ones that were easy to treat. In fact, the sicker or more complicated they are, the more they need treatment.

Methadone doesn't make other drug problems worse, although it does make them more visible. We found that people who were alcoholics or pill abusers on methadone were the same who had had these problems prior to coming into the program. There is an enormous amount of drug abuse in the community. But the usual middle-class person would rather keep these things hidden. Even when a clinic is very orderly and successful, but brings in black, Puerto Rican, or otherwise identifiably nonneighborhood types into a nice little cloistered neighborhood, there will be a tremendous amount of opposition to it. People would just like to have some big jail set up in some place remote, lock up the addicts, and get them out of sight.

In 1972 I was asked to set up a detoxification program for the New York City jails. The conditions there were extraordinarily primitive. Addicts were taken from the street and simply locked up in cells, with no specific treatment. If they complained of withdrawal symptoms, or nausea, or vomiting, they were simply ignored as "acting up," in the language of the prison doctors. At the same time, to keep the institutions quiet, assistants from the dispensary would circulate through the cell blocks once or twice a day, handing out all sorts of sedatives and tranquilizers, which were ineffective for relief of withdrawal symptoms. There was essentially no medical treatment, unless an inmate was sent to the prison ward of a hospital.

It would be hard to exaggerate the noise, overcrowding, heat, squalor, dirt, misery, tension, and hatred that seeped through the institution. These were the conditions that led to the riots that broke up the Tombs and caused a turnover in administration: Commissioner McGrath was discharged and a new commissioner, Ben Malcolm, was given the task.[9] Shortly after he was appointed, he consulted me about what he could see to be the major problem, namely, the agitated state of untreated addicts

9. Malcolm was appointed Correction Commissioner on January 19, 1972. He was the first black in the city's history to hold that office.

that had been abruptly removed from the streets. I told him that the first step was to develop a simple, medically standardized detoxification program to relieve their acute discomfort, and, secondly, to provide at least minimal care for their other medical conditions. I offered to set up the program with his backing.

He accepted this offer. I therefore began under the authority of the commissioner and reorganized the medical services for the Tombs. Since something like 50 percent of the inmates were addicts, it was not a question of setting up a small ward; we essentially converted half of the Tombs into a medical service. The key ingredient in this was having the dedicated volunteer services of my older patients, who knew the place intimately because they'd been in there themselves many times.

Within two weeks, the institution was so transformed and so quiet that I was able to take Mayor Lindsay on a tour of a place that shortly before even the guards refused to enter without crash helmets. When he left, I got on the public address system and said that the mayor had been so favorably impressed by the results of this treatment that he promised that, as far as his administration could influence it, there would always be a medical treatment for addicts in the New York City jails. For the first and only time in that dismal institution, the iron cages and the walls in the great vaulted rooms rang with cheers.

Epilogue to the 1989 Edition:
From Methadone to the Drug War

On August 4, 1986, President Ronald Reagan delivered a major speech on drug policy. His stated purpose was "not to announce another short-term government offensive but to call instead for a national crusade against drugs—a sustained, relentless effort to rid America of this scourge—by mobilizing every segment of society against drug abuse." He called for the elimination of all drugs from workplaces and schools; voluntary (or, for key government personnel, mandatory) drug testing; improved treatment and rehabilitation programs; greater public intolerance of drug abuse; and stepped-up enforcement against domestic and international traffickers. In remarks to Republican congressmen before the address, Reagan set as his overall goal a 50 percent reduction in drug use and promised that his escalating war would mean "Pearl Harbor for the drug traffickers."

A little more than a month later, on September 14, 1986, the president made a nationally televised address, accompanied by First Lady Nancy Reagan. Again Reagan relied on martial metaphors, drawn from World War II. Americans would have to swing into action, he explained, the way they did in the 1940s, when men and women rolled up their sleeves, built tanks and planes, and planted victory gardens. "We're in another war for our freedom, and it's time for all of us to pull together again," he said. The First Lady was equally adamant. This was a total war, a war in which there could be no middle ground. Do not use drugs, and do not tolerate those who do. Firm, private refusals would create an "outspoken intolerance for drug use" and would influence by example young people who might otherwise experiment with drugs.[1]

There is a sense of *déjà vu* about these speeches. Harry Anslinger might well have spoken the same words, and, had he been in the audience, he certainly would have applauded them. What the rhetorical continuity conceals, however, is the fact that Reagan and his successors must confront a much different, and in many ways a much worse, situation than

Anslinger faced in his time. It is not that there has been a fur change in philosophy; substances like heroin and marijuana are lawed[2] and their suppression remains a law-enforcement prior is different is the extent and especially the complexity of dr the country today versus twenty-five years ago. This is true in every respect. Legally, therapeutically, pharmacologically, and the problem has grown more complicated.

The situation has become more complex legally because methadone maintenance has been superimposed on laws aimed at prohibition and interdiction. Recall that, from the early 1920s until the middle 1960s, American narcotic policy had two key objectives: the quashing of legal maintenance and the suppression of illicit narcotic transactions through vigorous police enforcement. What has happened since then has been a qualified abandonment of the first goal, *but not of the second*. This was intentional: the liberal supporters of maintenance never espoused, nor could they have achieved, a libertarian resolution of the problem. The government was not about to get out of drug enforcement and proclaim *caveat emptor*. Most liberals were perfectly willing to see addicts, whom they regarded as victims, treated in clinics, and traffickers, whom they regarded as criminals, sent to jail. This arrangement is at best paradoxical; some critics have described it as confused and contradictory.[3] What about the addict who is also a dealer? Or the addict who is a predacious criminal, before, during, and after treatment? Or the addict who diverts methadone into the black market? Methadone programs have reduced the frequency with which their clients violated the law, but they certainly have not eliminated all of their legal or behavioral problems.[4]

These difficulties are not unique to narcotic policy. In virtually every area where liberals successfully challenged restrictive policies in the 1960s and 1970s, similar quandaries have arisen. Gambling is a good example. State-run lottery games and other forms of legal gambling are now freely available and widely advertised. But illegal gambling has not disappeared, as some liberals hoped or assumed; the police still have plenty of sports bookies and *bolita* operators with whom to contend. The public, meanwhile, gets a decidedly mixed message: some forms of gambling are acceptable, but others are not. The same is true of drug use. Classic-era narcotic policy, despite its faults, was at least consistent. Its message was unambiguous: drugs are bad for you. This is one reason why proponents of therapeutic communities remain deeply suspicious of methadone maintenance: it contradicts, both symbolically and actually, the traditional goal of abstinence. "It's just another political expediency," charged Dr. Judianne Densen-Gerber, founder of the Odyssey House therapeutic community. "There's no reason to change a heroin user to methadone, just as there's no reason to change a scotch drinker to cheap wine. . . . People should not have a dependency disease. They should be able to make decisions without being controlled by their need for a substance."[5]

Others have countered that the problem has nothing to do with methadone maintenance but with the regulations that have hamstrung the programs. The late Marie Nyswander, whom we interviewed in 1981, was amused to find herself "sounding like a Republican" on the issue of federal controls. "I don't think there's any question about it," she said. "If we had decent treatment, in *all* the ways people could be treated—clinics, hospitals, doctors—then we'd probably take in the majority of addicts. But right now methadone is operating at only 30 to 50 percent of its potential."[6] Why not, she urged, permit stable, long-term patients to simply receive a several months' supply from a private physician? For Nyswander, contemporary narcotic policy was insufficiently reactionary; that is to say, the clock should have been turned all the way back to 1914, when doctors still had wide latitude in maintaining addicts, rather than to 1919–23, when a handful of municipal programs struggled to treat patients in a hostile regulatory environment. Indeed, the 1970s and 1980s might be aptly described as the New Clinic Era, with methadone maintenance understood as the vehicle of a long-delayed, but ultimately limited, counterrevolution.

Not all of the limitations were due to bureaucratic meddling, however. Dr. Robert Newman, who presided over the expansion of methadone maintenance in New York City from 1970 to 1974, also emphasized the strength of community opposition. The first twenty clinics breezed through, he recalled, but "the next twenty were pretty darn tough. . . . Finally, it became an insurmountable problem when the neighborhoods were given almost veto power. Since 1975 I think there's been one clinic opened in the City of New York, and that over tremendous opposition." Newman was chagrined to discover that methadone, despite its popularity with the crime-conscious Nixon administration, still served as a political lightning rod:

I remember trying to open one clinic up in the Bronx, and speaking at a community meeting. I talked for forty-five minutes about methadone and I thought I did an absolutely great job. I was sure I had everybody convinced. When I asked for questions, the first one was from some lady in the back who said, "Why don't you pick up our garbage?" I said, "What do you mean, pick up garbage?" I thought that the woman was crazy, or that I was in the wrong meeting. I said, "This isn't the Sanitation Department; we're talking about opening up a methadone clinic." She said, "*You* know what I mean. You're the City of New York, and you haven't picked up my garbage in two weeks." I said, "Lady, that's another department." She said, "Yeah, I know, you're always passing the buck. Whoever we talk to, it's never their department, it's somebody else's. Well, by God, you haven't picked up my garbage and I'm not going to allow you to do what you want to do up here with this methadone clinic."

Then there was the hatred and the concern regarding addicts and addiction. It's a lot of things: it's race and class; it's fear, the realization that addicts have to commit crimes to support their habit; and it's a resentment that people are feeling that good three, four, five times a day. It's hard to express this hostility, because there's nothing to focus against. But a methadone clinic brought all these problems together. It was *a building*, in front of which you could picket, or wheel your baby carriages, or go to the press about. I think people really wanted to express their hostility against a problem that was so evanescent that they couldn't do it any other way.[7]

Finally there were the addicts themselves, many of whom balked at entering treatment programs. There were garbled fears about methadone, complaints that it would "get into the bones" or render patients dependent for life. "It's very, very hard to quit methadone," remarked Ivory. "When a guy gets to be my age, getting off methadone pret' near kills you. I think methadone's got me hooked until I die." He conceded, however, that methadone had its good points:

Like, I used to live in Harlem. I knew a whole lot of people that used to be tramps. They wouldn't clean up, or wouldn't try to do nothing for themselves, sleeping out there on the street. Since this methadone came out you see them nice and clean, with a tie on and shoes shined, and working every day.

This amounts to a summary of the original thinking behind methadone. The drug may be a powerful narcotic, and treatment may be indefinite, but what does it matter if the patients turn their lives around? The problem, however, was that not all addicts wanted to turn their lives around, nor were they necessarily enamored of shiny shoes and daily work. They regarded methadone, or for that matter any other treatment program, as a form of surrender. An addict who sought treatment had to admit to himself and his peers that he no longer "had enough spunk to stay on the street and support a habit," as Jack put it. Ethnographic studies of untreated addicts have shown that their self-image is often that of an accomplished hustler, street-wise and disciplined enough to keep themselves in money and drugs. The "righteous dope fiends" consider addicts in methadone programs ("methadonians," "zombies," "blimps," "meth-heads" or "murdocks") to be losers, while those who enter therapeutic communities are totally *infra dig*. One successful long-time user, much like the survivors interviewed for this book, started to have foot trouble as he approached his middle fifties. His hustling suffered, and in desperation he sought help at Synanon. He quickly left. "Synanon wasn't for *me*," he exclaimed. "I wouldn't stand being thrown down the shit bowl [degraded] by those foul garbage junkies, snitches, winos, and sissies."[8]

These attitudes have persisted, and help to explain why more users do not take advantage of treatment opportunities. They also explain why, once in treatment, many patients leave or fail, since they are constantly reminded of and tempted by their old self-image, the smooth operator leading a free and exciting life. There is more to becoming an ex-addict than detoxification.

For all of these reasons the treatment revolution of the late 1960s and early 1970s has proved to be something of a disappointment, despite its great utility for the particular group of aging addicts we interviewed. According to one estimate, only 7 percent of the approximately 2.5 million Americans who have a serious drug problem are currently in treatment. Many of those who remain untreated "are undergoing progressive and chronic physical deterioration, as well as committing crimes and being involved in accidents that lead to injuries to themselves and others." There is an economic cost associated with this, as well as a human one. It is far less expensive for an addict to be in a treatment program than in and out of hospitals and jails.[9]

That is, if the untreated addict survives at all. One recent, frightening development has been the spread of AIDS, a uniformly fatal disease. Caused by human immunodeficiency virus (HIV, formerly known as LAV or HTLV-III), AIDS is spread among intravenous drug users through the sharing of syringes and needles.[10] There is no evidence that the virus can be spread through casual contact or the use of noninjected drugs; however, it can be spread through both homosexual and heterosexual contact and to the fetus *in utero*.[11] The number of persons infected with HIV who will ultimately develop clinical AIDS is not yet known with certainty, but it is at least three in ten—possibly as many as ten in ten.

The period between initial exposure to HIV and development of full AIDS averages seven or eight years.[12] This long latency period has permitted the rapid, unknowing spread of the virus within groups of intravenous drug users. The situation is especially bad in New York City, where there are both large numbers of cases of AIDS and high seroprevalence rates (a high percentage already infected) among intravenous drug users. By mid-1987 a third of the city's ten thousand AIDS cases were drug addicts; in nearby New Jersey and Connecticut, more than half of all diagnosed AIDS cases were addicts, their sex partners, or children.[13] Nationwide, nearly a quarter million intravenous drug users may already be infected.

It is difficult to say what the long-term effect of AIDS on narcotic addiction will be, since developments in AIDS are occurring very rapidly, both in the spread of the epidemic and in research on ways of potentially controlling or treating it. Nevertheless, current studies on the reactions of intravenous drug users to AIDS show that the epidemic has had a profound effect, and hint at the possibility of reducing the practice of illicit drug injection, or at least of making it more circumspect. Death has always been common among intravenous drug users, but AIDS forces a radically different psychology of death in the group. Involving a protracted and painful death, often with stigmatization and social isolation, AIDS conjures up none of the escapist fantasies associated with overdose deaths. The virus may also develop long after a person has ceased injecting drugs; one cannot be certain that stopping drugs will prevent the development of AIDS. Finally, there is the possibility of infecting friends and family, through sexual or *in utero* transmissions of the virus. These considerations have apparently prompted changes in the behavior of intravenous drug users in the New York area: addicts are increasing their use of sterile needles and reducing the numbers of persons with whom they will share drug injection equipment.[14] They are, in other words, becoming more like the subjects of this book, more concerned with needle-transmitted infections. It is possible that "safer" needle use will become the norm for intravenous narcotic addiction in the future. Fear and natural selection are both operating in that direction.

Another great potential for change in narcotic addiction may be in the recruitment of new intravenous drug users. Novices usually learn to mainline through contact with experienced users whom they admire and depend upon for the equipment for their first injection.[15] Over time, the fear of AIDS is likely to reduce both the admiration felt for experienced intravenous users and the willingness to borrow or experiment with their needles and syringes. No one wants to borrow death, especially death by AIDS.

The threat of AIDS could reduce illicit drug injection to the point where not enough new persons are recruited to replace those intravenous users who die or quit. This would not necessarily eliminate narcotic addiction, however. It would still be possible to become addicted by sniffing or (more rarely) smoking heroin, or by the regular use of a synthetic opiate. Thus, even if AIDS should virtually eliminate intravenous drug addiction, there is no guarantee that other forms of addiction will disappear. They may even expand, as has recently happened with cocaine smoking.

One last point about AIDS. Although there is some evidence that intravenous drug users are motivated to seek treatment for fear of the disease, most addicts remain at large, as noted earlier.[16] The danger that they pose to themselves and to others underscores the fact that a large percentage of users remain outside of treatment programs. *Any* modality, whether geared toward maintenance, short-term detoxification, or long-term abstinence, is safer than street trafficking and use—especially if the patients do not cheat on the program.

Of course, patients could not cheat if street drugs were unavailable. That was a point Anslinger made repeatedly: get the addicts clean through institutional treatment and then keep them from temptation by drying up the illicit supply. Unfortunately, the strategy did not work particularly well for him, nor has it worked at all well during the 1980s. The country, in fact, is flooded with drugs. Retail (street-level) drug transactions probably exceed 100 billion dollars, up from an estimated 79 billion in 1980. Heroin imports, which generated 8 billion dollars in 1980, grew 50 percent by 1986, from four to six metric tons per annum. Heroin purity levels were low in the early 1980s, in the 3-to-5-percent range, but they have recently increased, due to an influx of "China White," Mexican "black tar," and other highly potent varieties. Much of the Mexican heroin is smuggled by illegal aliens, whose chances of being caught crossing the border are as low as one in five.[17]

Nor is Mexico the only source of the problem. Large amounts of heroin are also shipped from Southeast Asia, a region that became a major source of supply during the Vietnam era. "Transportation was very easy," Ralph Salerno pointed out,

You didn't need a passport to fly into Vietnam. A lot of people, including minorities who had joined the military looking for a decent job and a reasonable career, made contacts in Southeast Asia, where there has always been opium and heroin use. They found, "Gee, you know we can make a buy. What the hell, the CIA is paying the Montagnards with heroin to fight on our side. Let's grab some, let's buy some cheap." So you began to get a second source of supply building up.

A third source of supply, Southwest Asian heroin, emerged in the late 1970s and expanded rapidly during the early 1980s, in the wake of political and military turmoil in the region. (Whatever the defects of the Shah's police, they were more efficient at controlling the narcotic traffic than Khomeini's Revolutionary Guards.) The one signal law enforcement accomplishment, the disruption of the famous "French connection" in the early 1970s, proved to be a transitory victory. Turkish opium processed into heroin at Marseilles, the single most important illicit source for most of the classic era, became very scarce in the U.S. after 1973. This was of little strategic significance, however, since the combined Mexican, Southeast Asian, and Southwest Asian supplies have more than made up for the deficit.[18]

The failure to stop the heroin traffic was by no means the only or even the worst setback for law enforcement since 1965. Officials have also had to contend with the emergence of several new street drugs, such as LSD and PCP; the diversion and abuse of licit drugs, such as Methedrine and methaqualone; and the increased popularity of illicit nonopiate drugs, such as marijuana and cocaine. Simply stated, more people from more different backgrounds have begun using more drugs.

This became apparent during the 1960s and early 1970s, as marijuana smoking spread rapidly among those whom sociologist Erich Goode described as "the growing edge of American social life." These were the baby boomers, then entering their late teens and early twenties, the prime drug-experimenting years.[19] "Probably the most affluent, confident, indulged crop in human history," Timothy Leary called them. "[This] generation of young Americans threw caution to the winds and recklessly rejected the fear-imposed systems that have kept human society surviving —the work ethic, male domination, life-style conformity, inhibition of sensuality and self-indulgence, reliance on authority."[20] Leary's generalization is only half-correct: most of the pot-smoking students graduated, trimmed their hair, and went to work for hierarchical enterprises, motivated by "fear" of an empty checking account. Despite their economic assimilation, however, they retained many of the hedonic, antiauthoritarian values of their youth, including tolerance of marijuana and other drugs.

The speed with which marijuana use and trafficking expanded was remarkable. In one state, California, marijuana arrests rose from 7,560 in 1964 to 50,327 in 1968. Nationwide, federal seizures of marijuana increased more than tenfold between 1969 and 1973, hashish seizures more than twentyfold. By 1979 an estimated 50 million Americans had tried marijuana at least once, including two-thirds of all young adults. Marijuana use has declined somewhat during the 1980s, but it remains a popular illicit drug, and source of huge profits for both international traffickers and domestic cultivators.[21]

Equally remarkable was marijuana's popularity among high school and junior high school students. Peter Santangelo, a former undercover narcotic agent who worked in southern Connecticut in the early 1970s, was struck by the youth of those who bought and sold marijuana and other drugs. "Teens, early teens, seventeen, eighteen; dungarees; long hair, never brushed, dirty; parents well-to-do" was the way he characterized his quarry.[22] Nationwide, the number of twelve-to-seventeen-year-olds who had ever tried marijuana rose from virtually zero in 1960 to three out of ten in 1979.[23]

This was a portentous development, not only because the young marijuana smokers might "burn out" with daily use, but because they were also more likely to experiment with other illicit substances. Marijuana, like tobacco and alcohol, was a gateway drug. A pattern emerged: first beer or wine, then tobacco or hard liquor, then marijuana, then another illegal drug. Or several, as in the case of George, a blond, genial Californian who started smoking pot regularly when he was fourteen, dropped acid at fifteen, and shot speed at sixteen, losing twenty-eight pounds in the process. Another man, Johnny, started at fifteen and went on a binge that lasted thirteen years. "I was a garbage-can addict," he admitted. "I wasn't choosy. I took pills, drank like a fish, used hallucinogens, did cocaine." Like Sam, he carried around assorted pills in a box, and took them "according to how I wanted to feel." More astonishing still was the private pharmacopoeia of the late comedian John Belushi, who first sought treatment for drug dependency in 1976. His physician, Dr. Michael Rosenbluth, wrote the following in Belushi's file:

Smokes 3 packs a day.
Alcohol drinks socially.
Medications: Valium occasionally.
Marijuana 4 to 5 times a week.
Cocaine—snort daily, main habit.
Mescaline—regularly.
Acid—10 to 20 trips.
No heroin.
Amphetamines—four kinds.
Barbiturates (Quaalude habit.)

The sole negative on the list—"no heroin"—did not last for long. It was, in fact, an overdose of heroin and cocaine that killed Belushi in 1982.[24]

The older addicts did not have much sympathy for such behavior. They disapproved of indiscriminate polydrug use, particularly among teenagers, whose habits they considered shocking and unprecedented. "Dumb kids," "no finesse," and "pill heads" were among the many epithets we heard. Ann, describing her Bronx high school in the mid-1930s, said, "There were no drugs. None. Oh my God, 'drugs' was a word that meant something foreign—really, it was connected with hospitals. I didn't even know there were such things." Her biggest escapade was rendezvousing in a candy store to sneak a cigarette with two other girls. "There was nothing like the sixties or seventies."

There is, however, one limiting detail in the case histories of younger users given above: Belushi was the only one of the three to try heroin. Neither George nor Johnny reported using narcotics. Some of their peers did, thereby contributing to the heroin epidemic of the early 1970s, but they were exceptional. Most marijuana smokers, if they went on to other drugs, chose pills, hallucinogens, or stimulants.[25] It was in the ghetto that the ultimate graduation to heroin was still most likely to occur; epidemiologic studies continued to show that minorities, especially black and Hispanic males, were heavily overrepresented among narcotic users.[26] What happened after 1965, in short, was the superimposition of a new pattern of largely recreational, largely youthful, largely white, and largely nonopiate drug use upon the existing pattern of inner-city narcotic use and addiction.

A partial exception to this generalization is cocaine, a cross-over drug that has experienced a renaissance among both white and minority users. Popular around the turn of the century, cocaine fell into disuse during the classic era. "Cocaine addiction has disappeared," Anslinger flatly declared.[27] The drug still had a few devotees, mainly individuals who were privileged, or socially marginal, or both. Among them were jazz musicians, stage and screen stars, pimps, prostitutes, and bohemians. But if federal seizures were any indication, cocaine was a remote second to heroin and other opiates. As late as 1970, only 478 pounds of the drug were confiscated nationwide.[28]

Today cocaine seizures are measured by the ton. Virtually all indicators of use—admissions to treatment programs, overdose deaths, student surveys, and chemical analyses of urine samples—have shown a marked increase in its consumption. By 1985 an estimated 40 percent of graduating high school seniors had tried the drug at least once. Illicit sales are so vast that the transportation and processing of money has become as difficult for cocaine traffickers as that of the drug itself. One dealer went to the point of removing the play money from several Monopoly games, replacing it with real money, sealing the boxes back up, and then shipping them to Colombia. A portion of such fabulous profits is naturally plowed back into production; between 1982 and 1986 the world's supply of cocaine was roughly doubled by the planting of new coca bushes in South America.[29]

One of the many groups to become involved in the cocaine revival of the 1970s was, ironically, methadone patients. At a sufficiently high dosage, methadone blocked the euphoric effects of heroin; that was one of its selling points. Methadone did not, however, necessarily blot out the desire to get high, and many patients soon discovered that nonopiate drugs, including cocaine, would do the trick. "Methadone . . . takes care of my heroin problem," explained one forty-two-year-old addict. "But I still need something, so I'm using coke. I'm shooting it." He financed his purchases with his welfare check and, when that was insufficient, by breaking into cars.[30] Others raised money by selling part of their methadone on the street. Proponents of methadone maintenance were caught in a political bind: not only was methadone pharmacologically irrelevant to the growing number of nonopiate users, it appeared (erroneously) that the programs were responsible for financing their indulgence. "The television stations in particular never tired of arranging an arrest with a local police department," Robert Newman complained. "An undercover agent would go up to one of the patients in front of a clinic, offer usually twice the going rate for illicit methadone, get as many people as they wanted to sell, while all this was filmed by a clandestine TV camera."[31]

In reality, methadone patients made up only a fraction of the new cocaine users. Several other forces were also at work. One of them was the waning popularity and availability of the amphetamines. "*Contra speedamos ex cathedra,*" pronounced Allen Ginsberg, a warning seconded by various counterculture notables. Speed killed. It also incarcerated, with the advent of stricter production regulations. Fear and short supplies of amphetamines made cocaine attractive as a "safe" alternative stimulant —at least until 1986, when the death of college basketball star Len Bias made it abundantly clear that cocaine could also kill.[32]

The highly publicized troubles that black athletes and celebrities had with cocaine were, in one sense, misleading. Because the Willie Wilsons and Richard Pryors of the world had huge amounts of disposable income and worked in high-pressure occupations, their cocaine consumption fit into what might be thought of as the traditional show-business pattern. What was different about the 1970s and 1980s was the spread of cocaine beyond these rarefied circles to the middle and professional classes, notably among baby boomers who had gone to college, flirted with the counterculture, smoked marijuana, and learned to discount official warnings about drug abuse. They also had the money and the disposition to become users, albeit on a lesser scale than the superstars. After 1982, when a glut of South American cocaine dropped wholesale prices by a third or more, those of modest means could partake.[33] With vials of "crack" (potent, smokable cocaine) retailing for as low as five dollars, no one was priced out of the market. Indeed, crack now rivals heroin as the drug of choice in the nation's ghettos.

Cocaine has had more going for it than declining prices and favorable word of mouth. Its use was also initially reinforced by the mass media. Rock stars glamorized the drug; so did several popular motion pictures. Counterculture newspapers and magazines carried lengthy articles, as did mainstream periodicals. Retailers got on the bandwagon with cocaine handbooks and paraphernalia; gold spoons and razor blades were enshrined as risqué symbols of conspicuous consumption. Suddenly, cocaine was *au courant*.

Historically, these developments can be understood as the recasting of elite drug use around cocaine instead of opium. Cocaine sniffers, like the opium smokers of the 1920s and 1930s, tended to dress nattily and look down on slovenly street addicts. They also boasted of their sexual prowess and regarded the drug as an aphrodisiac.[34] The after-hours clubs they frequented were like the opium dens, secret places of organized sin governed by strict rules of etiquette: don't lick your spoon, don't sniff from your fingernails, and don't hoover other people's cocaine.[35] The crack houses that have recently supplanted the after-hours clubs also resemble the dens of yore in the narrow sense that patrons gather there to smoke a purified form of the drug. Crack houses are apt to be more dangerous than the old dens, however, since regular, heavy cocaine use can produce violence and paranoia. The effects of crack are also likely to wear off much more quickly, making it harder to enjoy the long, leisurely sojourns that so appealed to the opium smokers.

Despite its drawbacks, crack smoking has transformed the urban cocaine scene since 1983. Crack caught on because it was easy to smoke, requiring no complicated preparations with dangerous chemicals, as had been the case with "free basing." Crack delivered the rush of intravenous injection without the risk of AIDS and other infections. A few users have experimented with smoking crack *and* black tar heroin, a combination likened to "firing both barrels at the brain's pleasure centers."[36] Two barrels or one, this method is likely to produce dependence, since the powerful doses soon disrupt the brain's chemistry, creating a depressed, anhedonic state that can only be overcome by more and more cocaine. Some users have also been drawn into a secondary dependency on tranquilizers and depressants, such as diazepam and barbiturates, which they take to combat the hyperstimulation and nervousness resulting from the cocaine.[37] Awareness of its addictive potential, together with concern over its relation to street crime, has hardened public attitudes toward the drug and altered the tone of press coverage.[38] Since 1965, cocaine has gone from complete obscurity to Public Enemy Number One.

Like many historical changes, the altered pattern of use has left linguistic traces. During the classic era, government officials, when describing their task, spoke unselfconsciously of combating the narcotic traffic. This was technically inaccurate, since cocaine and marijuana were not narcotics, but it made practical sense, because most of their arrests and the bulk of their seizures involved opiates. Since the 1960s, however, the word "narcotic" has been replaced by the more general term "drug," as in "drug problem," or the still more capacious adjective "substance," as in "substance abuse." This change was forced by the growing prominence of marijuana and cocaine, as well as the development of novel practices like glue sniffing or eating hallucinogenic plants and mushrooms. It made no sense, pharmacologically or otherwise, to lump these things together as "narcotic use," let alone "narcotic addiction." Some researchers sought to expand the concept of addiction itself when they saw that dependence could develop with nonopiate drugs. "We should define addiction in terms of the compulsion to take the drug rather than whether it causes withdrawal," Dr. Michael Bozarth explains. "In this sense, cocaine is at least as addictive as heroin."[39]

Or, one might say, as addictive as alcohol. Even as new patterns of nonopiate dependence were emerging, there was distressing evidence that the nation's oldest psychoactive nemesis was strengthening its grip on the population. Per capita consumption of alcohol rose steadily, from 2.1 gallons per capita in the early 1960s to 2.8 gallons in the late 1970s. One 1977 poll revealed that seven out of ten Americans drank, and that nearly one in five considered liquor the cause of trouble within their families. Although health concerns and adverse publicity have reduced alcohol consumption somewhat during the 1980s, it is still higher than at any time during the classic era.[40]

The pattern of American drinking has changed as well. In the 1940s and 1950s, the most numerous imbibers by far were the straight drinkers, people who regarded any substance other than alcohol (or tobacco) as beyond the pale. "Our national drug is alcohol," wrote William Burroughs in 1956. "We tend to regard the use of any other drug with special horror."[41] Ambivalence or outright hostility toward drug users persisted among straight drinkers after 1965. If the reader will indulge a personal anecdote: one of the authors was drinking beer with his friends on a warm summer night in 1970. We were sitting on a fence in the countryside, talking and laughing. A suspicious farmer called the police and a squad car was dispatched. The officer arrived, gathered our licenses, and radioed headquarters. When he discovered that we were all of age, that there were no warrants out against us, and that we had no drugs, he smiled. "Boys," he said, "We got a complaint, so y'all have to run along. If I was off duty, I'd get a six pack and join you." What we were doing was not only permissible, it was normal and expected—provided, of course, that no drugs were involved.

The reverse of this principle did not apply, however. Those who took drugs had no strong feelings against alcohol, tobacco, or other licit substances. Indeed, like John Belushi, they used them frequently. Some psychedelic enthusiasts of the 1960s preached that alcohol was a downer and that the faithful should renounce it, but they were disappointed by the response to their exhortations. The baby boomers were, so to speak, polypharmaceutically perverse: they cheerfully experimented with a range of illicit drugs while they drank alcohol and puffed cigarettes with their conventional elders. Linkages began to develop between their dependencies. Among recovering cocaine addicts, for example, drinking is one of the most common causes of relapse. Alcohol loosens their inhibitions; it also reminds them of their previous cocaine use, which often took place in a bar or other surroundings where drink was present. The memory triggers a sudden overwhelming longing, and they begin using again.[42]

The relationship of our classic-era addicts to alcohol was different, more a matter of either/or than both/and. Several interviewees, like Brenda or Low, drank before becoming addicts, but generally refrained while on narcotics. (If they had not, it is unlikely that they would have lived to tell their tales.) The same was true of cocaine. Occasionally they would speedball, mixing their heroin with cocaine. This was an infrequent pleasure, however, since the latter was very expensive, hard to find, relatively short-acting, and would not prevent withdrawal symptoms. They made it clear that they regarded cocaine as a luxury item and that, if forced to choose, they would always go with an opiate. This preference, as much as anything, dated them; it was incongruous to hear them speak so dismissingly of cocaine while the rest of the country was seemingly in the midst of an epidemic.

The foregoing raises some important questions. Why were law enforcement personnel, who remained individually opposed to cocaine and other drugs, collectively unable to contain their importation and use after 1965? Why did substances once comparatively rare become increasingly common? Why, despite larger budgets, expanded personnel, and more arrests, did the responsible agencies utterly fail to stop the influx of drugs?

The short answer is money. There was, in the first place, a great deal of money to be made from American users. It was not just that there were large numbers of adolescents in the 1960s and 1970s who were willing to experiment with drugs, it was that they had the wherewithal to do so. "I mean, these kids would say, 'Dad, I need fifty dollars so I can buy a tire,' or something," Agent Santagelo observed. "And Dad would give them fifty dollars." [43] Not all of the money went to the B.F. Goodrich Company. When these same youth graduated and became financially independent, they had more discretionary dollars at their disposal and could afford more expensive drugs in larger quantities. Gradually, a new stereotype, the white-collar professional squandering his salary on cocaine, emerged and joined that of the street addict who stole to support his habit. The traffickers were indifferent to whether American customers financed their use through work or theft; what mattered was that the money, or the fence-able merchandise, was there. The United States and, secondarily, Western Europe were the most logical targets for drug wholesalers because they were affluent, consumer societies, long on currency and short on moral strictures. [44] They were the perfect markets and drugs were the perfect products, since they could create and sustain their own demand.

The huge profits to be made in the United States not only provided incentives to drug wholesalers, they also bought protection for the traffickers through the familiar expedient of bribery. The sort of here's-two-thousand-dollars-now-let-me-sell-heroin-in-peace arrangement described by Arthur persisted after 1965, only on a much larger scale. Ralph Salerno was so alarmed by growing police corruption that it influenced his decision to take early retirement. "We're heading for one hell of a big scandal," he confided to a friend, "because the people in charge aren't all that knowledgeable [about the police force] or interested in its problems. And they'll explode." [45]

The explosion came in the early 1970s, when Detective Frank Serpico and Sargeant David Durk started talking to the *New York Times*. The articles led to the formation of an investigative commission headed by Whitman Knapp. The Knapp Commission's 1973 *Report on Police Corruption*, which highlighted problems with narcotic enforcement, made headlines for months. It also generated two books, *Serpico* (1973) and *Prince of the City* (1978), both of which were made into popular motion pictures. [46] Narcotic officers, who in Anslinger's time were cast in the *Untouchables* mold, were increasingly viewed with skepticism, as hero-villains who might be deep into the dirty business they were supposedly sorting out.

Domestic bribery, although a serious and demoralizing problem, seems minor when compared to the graft at the other end of the drug pipeline. Theoretically, it is much easier to choke off the commerce at its point of origin, before the drugs are concealed, shipped, and dispersed. Yet it is in those countries where drugs are grown and processed that corruption is most deeply entrenched. The bribes are actually calibrated: ten dollars a kilo for marijuana smuggled across the border at Tijuana, for example, with the local police commander earning upwards of $150,000 a week. Not only do Mexican authorities look the other way, they provide armed escort service for major shipments. They have also been known to torture, possibly to kill, interloping American narcotic agents. Some trafficking organizations, like the Shan United Army which operates along the Burma-Thailand border, are so large and well armed that they do not need to infiltrate governments; they are themselves autonomous political entities, lacking only a representative in the U.N. (The Palestine Liberation Organization, which has been suspected of dealing on the side, even has that.) Worldwide, the illicit narcotic industry has revenues estimated by some at a half-trillion dollars a year; it is easy and expedient to divert a fraction of the cash flow to protecting exports. Anyone who can stock Monopoly games with real money can afford a few strategically placed government officials. It is simply a matter of rationalizing risk.[47]

The problems of enforcement in the drug-producing countries are compounded by the global economic and political situation. Many of these nations are poor and, like Mexico, burdened by international debts. Drugs are a vital source of revenue, not only for their governments, but for the peasants who can earn more by cultivating poppies, coca, or marijuana than by producing licit commodities. In Bolivia, for example, lawful exports now produce only a fraction of the revenue brought in by cocaine, which is responsible for half of the country's gross national product.[48]

Despite their dependence on drug trafficking, Bolivia and other Latin American countries are widely supposed by U.S. officials to be targets of Communist subversion. They are withal our Cold War allies. This creates a conflict of interest: the State Department and the CIA may wish to protect, for their own geopolitical reasons, the same governments that the Drug Enforcement Administration suspects of complicity in smuggling. The 1988 attempt to oust Panama's General Manuel Antonio Noriega is the exception that proves the rule; information implicating Noriega in drug trafficking has been available since 1972. For years this information was simply ignored. The CIA has gone so far as to treat major traffickers as national security "assets," using their organizations for gun-running and counterinsurgency operations.[49] Foreign policy and antinarcotic efforts were occasionally at cross purposes during the classic era,[50] but on the whole Anslinger was successful at keeping the two in alignment. This is no longer the case. Domestic demand, unreal profits, systematic corruption, economic dependency, inconsistent diplomacy—for all of these reasons the interdiction strategy is in disarray. The borders are porous, price is declining, purity increasing, and new smuggling groups are continually surfacing. Even Jewish traffickers, whom our informants said left or were driven out during the 1930s, have reentered the picture.

The sense that the illicit drug market is out of control has provoked a debate over priorities. Some commentators have argued that, rather than worry about supply, we should concentrate on demand. "What is needed is broad societal *disapproval* of illicit drug use," emphasizes Dr. Mitchell S. Rosenthal, one of the pioneers of the therapeutic communities. "Active disapproval and the use of informal social sanctions might . . . make more aggressive law enforcement irrelevant." [51] Or, as Nancy Reagan put it, Americans would not have a problem if they learned to turn a cold shoulder to those who used or offered drugs.

There is some truth in this insight. Peer disapproval is more powerful than remote, impersonal laws; the host or hostess who says no is more effective than the prosecutor downtown. The difficulty lies in engineering such a massive change of attitudes and behavior, particularly among young adults accustomed to and tolerant of drug use. Many legislators, while willing to fund educational programs toward that end, have also resurrected the Anslingerian tactic of stiffer penalties for dealers, up to and including execution. The death penalty was, in fact, the most widely discussed aspect of the 1986 omnibus antidrug bill. Although capital punishment for major traffickers convicted of murder (a transparently political provision favored by House members up for reelection) was blocked by the Senate, the bill that did pass nevertheless specified longer prison sentences for those who recruited juveniles to sell drugs, or those who sold drugs near schools. The law also authorized $1.7 billion in additional expenditures, with most of the money to go for law enforcement and drug education. [52] Two years later, just before the 1988 general election, Congress passed a second omnibus bill. This time a capital punishment provision was included, as well as substantial new civil penalties for personal use and possession. Legislatively, the pendulum seems to be swinging back to the 1950s; we may be on the verge of a "neoclassic" era.

Is this a wise departure? Or, to put it another way, was the medicalization of the narcotic problem, the legitimatization of a hybrid approach in the 1960s and 1970s, a bad idea? Would the country have been better off if Anslinger had not retired, if he and his successors had been permitted to maintain an unwavering hard line?

The answer is almost certainly no. While it may be true that superimposing a clinical treatment model on a criminal justice base signaled official ambivalence to the public, it is doubtful that this produced many new users. There is one school that argues just the opposite, that criminalization inevitably glamorizes a drug.[53] The use of LSD, for example, peaked five years after it was made illegal: a few thousand users in 1966 swelled to an estimated five million by 1971.[54] This does not prove that criminalization caused increased use—that would be *post hoc, ergo propter hoc* reasoning—but it does suggest that the laws made little concrete difference.

The point can be generalized. Drug policy is best understood as a congeries of a society's history, values, and prejudices; it is not, in and of itself, the key variable governing the extent of drug use at a given point in time. Prevalence is more likely to be determined by outside events. These include wars, epidemics, population shifts, new technologies and pharmaceutical discoveries, physician behavior, economic conditions, media coverage, and changes in moral attitudes and religious beliefs. It should be remembered that Anslinger was head of the Bureau of Narcotics at a time when Americans were firmly opposed to narcotic use, when the press acted as his claque, smugglers lacked high-powered racing boats and Lear jets, and LSD, DMT, PCP, and other acronymic drugs were as yet unfamiliar to the public. These were far greater advantages than the Boggs Act. When circumstances changed, when the antinarcotic consensus eroded, the underclass grew and festered, new drugs became fashionable on campus, and hundreds of thousands of American troops were sent to fight in opium-rich Southeast Asia, then the scope of the problem was bound to widen. One factor alone, the coming of age of the nearly 80 million Americans born between 1946 and 1965, insured an upsurge in drug use; in epidemiologic terms, there was an unusually large number of susceptibles in the population immediately after the classic era.

If, as we have argued, government policy bears little on the prevalence of drug use, it does not follow that it is unrelated to the health and behavior of the users themselves. Quite the contrary. The real impact of punitive drug laws is on consumers, especially those who are addicts. It is hard to read the narratives in this book without seeing how practically every aspect of the addicts' lives was affected. Their hustling activities, patterns of association, routes of administration, risks of illness, prison histories, and the like were all shaped by the antimaintenance policy and its corollary, the black market. Mainlining, for example, was unknown before 1915, when addicts did not have to purchase adulterated narcotics. It is true that the preaddiction characteristics of users took a turn for the worse during the early twentieth century, and that numerous addicts, including many of our interviewees, would have led difficult, unhealthful, and crime-filled lives with or without the assistance of Harry Anslinger. The point is that their troubles, and those of the people they victimized, were exacerbated by legal strictures. Policy analyst Mark Kleiman has called this exacerbating tendency the paradox of vice control:

We make something illegal because it's a vice—bad for its devotees and bad for people around them. But for those who indulge anyway, prohibition and enforcement make the vice *more* dangerous; they also make these people more dangerous to the rest of us. Think of wood alcohol during Prohibition, the violence and disease associated with prostitution, the gambling debts collected by muscle rather than collection agencies.

That this paradox exists does not mean we should legalize everything—it seems to me that society is better off with 400,000 very dangerous heroin addicts obtaining the drug illegally than with 5 million addicts obtaining the drug from their doctors, even though each of them would be a little better off and a little less dangerous. It does mean that we don't get a free shot at drug dealing.[55]

Anslinger understood that his shot (or, more accurately, cannonade) at all types of drug dealing ultimately had to be based on some sort of least-misery-for-the-least-number rationale. That was why he continued to rail at the narcotic clinics and "dope doctors" long after they had been suppressed; they were the floodgates that must remain closed lest the country become awash with narcotics. For three decades he managed to convince the government and the public of the correctness of his utilitarian calculation, thereby maintaining "a policy of narcotics control unlike that of almost every nation in the world."[56] It was, nevertheless, a case built on bluff and intimidation. There is no objective evidence to support the idea that disallowal of maintenance saved the country from a series of mid-century narcotic epidemics.[57] While there were (and are) badly run, diversion-prone programs like the original New York City clinic described in chapter 12, there were also exemplary clinics like the one in Shreveport. Willis Butler's Shreveport narcotic clinic was, in a sense, the road not chosen. If Butler had gotten his way, if medical discretion and supervision had been permitted within the context of detoxification-or-maintenance programs, and if this approach had been widely emulated, then incalculable suffering, crime, and death could have been averted. Those who contemplate a purely preventative strategy for the future, who trust only in education and legal pressure, would do well to contemplate the implications of this. The combined medical-police approach, with all its contradictions and weaknesses, is by default the best policy available. The tragedy is that the country did not recognize this forty years sooner.

NOTES

1. "Reagan Urges Crusade Against Drug Scourge," *Hartford Courant* [from combined wire services], August 5, 1986, pp. A1, A8; Bernard Weinraub, "Reagan Seeks Drug Tests for Key U.S. Employees," *New York Times*, August 5, 1986, p. A24; videotape of President and Mrs. Reagan's televised address of September 15, 1986.

2. Under the Controlled Substances Act of 1970, rather than the Harrison Act and related federal laws of the 1910s and 1920s, which have been superseded. For an overview of the statutory and regulatory changes that occurred during the 1970s, see Edward Lewis, Jr., and William M. Lenck, "Role of Law and State," in Sachindra N. Pradhan and Samarendra N. Dutta, eds., *Drug Abuse: Clinical and Basic Aspects* (St. Louis: Mosby, 1977), 515–34.

3. Two very good articles on this subject are Mark Peyrot, "Cycles of Social Problem Development: The Case of Drug Abuse," *Sociological Quarterly* 25 (1984), 83–96, and Ronald Bayer, "Heroin Addiction, Criminal Culpability, and the Penal Sanction: The Liberal Response to Repressive Social Policy," in James C. Weissman and Robert L. DuPont, eds., *Criminal Justice and Drugs: The Unresolved Connection* (Port Washington, N.Y.: Kennikat, 1982), 94–103.

   "The current institutional system for dealing with drug abuse is a conglomeration of two contradictory approaches," Peyrot summarizes, "the newer, clinical approach has been 'tacked onto' the earlier criminal adjustment approach, rather than supplanting it" (91). Ch. 5 of Peter Conrad and Joseph W. Schneider, *Deviance and Medicalization: From Badness to Sickness* (St. Louis: Mosby, 1980), is also of interest. David F. Musto shows, in ch. 12 of the expanded edition of *The American Disease* (New York: Oxford University Press, 1987), that the hybrid police-medical policy was most in evidence during the 1970s; during the 1980s enforcement efforts received relatively higher priority.

4. John Kaplan, *The Hardest Drug: Heroin and Public Policy* (Chicago: University of Chicago Press, 1983), 169, 182.

5. Interview with Densen-Gerber, August 5, 1981.

6. Interview with Nyswander, June 22, 1981.

7. Interview with Newman, July 24, 1981.

8. Alan G. Sutter, "The World of the Righteous Dope Fiend," *Issues in Criminology* 2 (1966), 171–222, quotation at 200; see also Bill Hanson et al., *Life with Heroin: Voices from the Inner City* (Lexington, Mass.: Lexington Books, 1985), especially 126, 135–73.

9. Paul J. Goldstein et al., "Drug Dependence and Abuse," in Robert W. Amler and H. Bruce Dull, eds., *Closing the Gap: The Burden of Unnecessary Illness* (New York: Oxford University Press, 1987), 89–101; quotation at 97.

10. H.W. Cohen et al., "Behavioral Risk Factors for HTLV-III/LAV Seropositivity among Intravenous Drug Abusers," paper presented at the International Conference on the Acquired Immunodeficiency Syndrome (AIDS), Atlanta, April 14–17, 1985.

11. Robert R. Redfield et al., "Heterosexually Acquired HTLV-III/LAV Disease (AIDS-Related Complex and AIDS) . . . ," *Journal of the American Medical Association* 254 (1985), 2094–96; Normand Lapoint et al., "Transplacental Transmission of HTLV-III Virus," *New England Journal of Medicine* 312 (1985), 1325–26.

12. Kung-Jong Lui et al., "A Model-Based Estimate of the Mean Incubation Period for AIDS in Homosexual Men," *Science* 240 (1988), 1333–35.

13. Cf. Thomas J. Spira et al., "Prevalence of Antibody to Lymphadenopathy-Associated Virus among Drug-Detoxification Patients in New York," *New*

England Journal of Medicine 311 (1984), 467–68; Jörg Schüpbach et al., "Antibodies to HTLV-III in AIDS and Pre-AIDS and in Groups at Risk for AIDS," *New England Journal of Medicine* 312 (1985), 265–70; Giacchino Angarano et al., "Rapid Spread of HTLV-III Infection among Drug Addicts in Italy," *Lancet* (1985, Part 2), 1302; and J. R. Robertson et al., "Epidemic of AIDS-Related Virus (HTLV-III/LAV) Infection among Intravenous Drug Users," *British Medical Journal* 292 (1986), 527–29. See also Lawrence K. Altman, "New Fear on Drug Use and AIDS," *New York Times*, April 6, 1986, pp. 1, 30; Ronald Sullivan, "New York State Rejects Plan to Give Drug Users Needles," *New York Times*, May 18, 1987, Sec. 1, p. 38; Lionel C. Bascom, "AIDS Shift Seen from Gay Men to Drug Users," *New York Times*, July 19, 1987, Sec. 11, pp. 1, 19; and Philip M. Boffey, "Spread of AIDS Abating, but Deaths Will Still Soar," *New York Times*, February 14, 1988, Sec. 1, pp. 1, 36.

14. S. R. Friedman et al., "AIDS and Self-Organization among Intravenous Drug Users," forthcoming in the *International Journal of the Addictions* 22 (1987), 201–19; Don C. Des Jarlais et al., "Risk Reduction for the Acquired Immunodeficiency Syndrome Among Intravenous Drug Users," *Annals of Internal Medicine* 103 (1985), 755–59.

15. Don C. Des Jarlais et al., "AIDS and Needle-Sharing within the IV-Drug Use Subculture," in Douglas A. Feldman and Thomas M. Johnson, eds., *The Social Dimensions of AIDS: Method and Theory* (New York: Praeger, 1986), 111–25.

16. J. Jackson and S. Neshin, "New Jersey Community Health Education Project: Impact of Using Ex-Addict Educators to Disseminate Information on AIDS to Intravenous Drug Users," paper presented at the International Conference on AIDS, Paris, June 23–25, 1986; Jeffrey Schmalz, "Addicts to Get Needles in Plan to Curb AIDS," *New York Times*, January 31, 1988, Sec. 1, p. 1.

17. William French Smith, "Drug Traffic Today—Challenge and Response: Excerpts from a report [*sic*] to the President's Cabinet Council on Legal Policy, March 24, 1982," *Drug Enforcement* 9 (Summer 1982), 2–6; Michael Hanchard, "New Varieties of Heroin Showing Up More In State," *Hartford Courant*, June 9, 1986, p. C1; "Special Report: Black Tar Heroin in the United States" (typescript from Strategic Intelligence Section, Drug Enforcement Administration, March 10, 1986), i–ii; Peter Applebone, "On Border Patrol: Arrests and Futility," *New York Times*, August 3, 1986, Sec. 1, pp. 1, 22; and Peter Kerr, "Chinese Now Dominate New York Heroin Trade," *New York Times*, August 9, 1987, Sec. 1, pp. 1, 30.

18. John P. Lyle, "Southwest Asian Heroin: Pakistan, Afghanistan, and Iran," Miguel D. Walsh, "Impact of the Iraqi-Iranian Conflict," and John Bacon, "Is the French Connection Really Dead?" all in *Drug Enforcement* 8 (Summer 1981), 2–6, 7–12, and 19–21, respectively; Alfred W. McCoy et al., *The Politics of Heroin in Southeast Asia* (New York: Harper and Row, 1973), 53–54, 244–46.

19. Erich Goode, *The Marijuana Smokers* (New York: Basic Books, 1970), 3.

20. Timothy Leary, "Some Superficial Thoughts on the Sociology of LSD," in Lester Grinspoon and James B. Bakalar, eds., *Psychedelic Reflections* (New York: Human Sciences Press, 1983), 32, 36. Ch. 2 of Goode, cited above,

presents sampling data to the effect that marijuana smokers were more likely
to reject traditional values than nonsmokers.

21. Edward M. Brecher et al., *Licit and Illicit Drugs* (Boston: Little, Brown,
    1972), 422; U.S. Senate, *Marijuana-Hashish Epidemic and Its Impact on United
    States Security: Hearings Before the Subcommittee to Investigate the Administration
    of the Internal Security Act and Other Internal Security Laws of the Committee on
    the Judiciary* (Washington, D.C.: G.P.O., 1974), 7–8; Institute of Medicine,
    Marijuana and Health (Washington, D.C.: National Academy Press, 1982),
    36; Glenn Collins, "U.S. Social Tolerance of Drugs Found on Rise," *New
    York Times*, March 21, 1983, pp. A1, B5; James Mills, *The Underground Em-
    pire: Where Crime and Governments Embrace* (New York: Doubleday, 1986),
    passim; Christine Russell, "One-Third of College Students Try Cocaine . . .
    Use of Marijuana and Other Drugs Appears to Have Declined," *Washington
    Post*, July 8, 1986, p. A3.
22. Interview with Peter Santangelo, August 23, 1982.
23. *Marijuana and Health*, 37.
24. Richard H. Blum and associates, *The Dream Sellers: Perspectives on Drug
    Dealers* (San Francisco: Jossey-Bass, 1972), 91; Charles Leerhsen with
    Sandra Gary, "Getting Straight," *Newsweek* 103 (June 4, 1984), 63; Bob
    Woodward, *Wired: The Short Life and Fast Times of John Belushi* (New York:
    Simon and Schuster, 1984), 104–105. See also Denise Kandel, "Stages
    in Adolescent Involvement in Drug Use," *Science* 190 (1975), 912–14, and
    Bruce D. Johnson et al., *Taking Care of Business: The Economics of Crime by
    Heroin Abusers* (Lexington, Mass.: Lexington Books, 1985), 182, 226–29.
25. Table 1 in Kandel, above; 1982 National Household Survey on Drug Abuse
    data reproduced in Collins, "U. S. Social Tolerance," B5. It is also of interest
    that, among those who did progress to heroin, many apparently took precau-
    tions to avoid full-blown dependence. Heroin's reputation as an addicting
    drug preceded it. See Norman E. Zinberg, "Nonaddictive Opiate Use," in
    Criminal Justice and Drugs, especially 15.
26. Carl D. Chambers and Leon G. Hunt, "Epidemiology of Drug Abuse," in
    Sachindra N. Pradhan and Samarendra N. Dutta, eds., *Drug Abuse*, table
    2-2, p. 13; Irving Faber Lukoff, "Consequences of Use: Heroin and Other
    Narcotics," in Joan Dunne Rittenhouse, ed., *Report of the Task Force on the Epi-
    demiology of Heroin and Other Narcotics* (Menlo Park, Calif.: Stanford Research
    Institute, 1976), 124–26; Leon Gibson Hunt, "Prevalence of Active Heroin
    Use in the United States," and S.B. Sells, "Reflections on the Epidemiology
    of Heroin and Narcotic Addiction from the Perspective of Treatment Data,"
    both in Joan Dunne Rittenhouse, *The Epidemiology of Heroin and Other Nar-
    cotics*, NIDA Research Monograph 16 (Rockville, Md.: Alcohol, Drug Abuse,
    and Mental Health Administration, National Institute on Drug Abuse, Divi-
    sion of Research, 1977), 63–78 and 161–63, respectively; John C. Ball et al.,
    "Characteristics of 633 Patients in Methadone Maintenance Treatment in
    Three United States Cities: 45 Preliminary Tables" (Report of the Metha-
    done Research Project, 1986), table 602. Sells remarks, "A polarity can be
    observed between *low socioeconomic level street heroin users*, at one extreme,
    and the *youthful, middle class, maladjusted, nonopioid users*, at the other" (163;
    italics in the original). Among minority groups, use by Hispanics has grown

most rapidly in recent years, at least in New York City. See Blanche Frank et al., "Current Drug Use Trends in New York City, June 1986" (NYDSAS Report), 1.

27. Harry Anslinger and Kenneth W. Chapman, "Narcotic Addiction," *Modern Medicine* 25 (1957), 176.

28. Harold M. Schmeck, Jr., "Cocaine is Re-emerging as a Major Problem, While Marijuana Remains Popular," *New York Times*, November 15, 1971, p. 82. In 1937, by comparison, federal officials seized over 118 kilograms of heroin, as against only 827 *grams* of cocaine.

29. Thomas L. Dezelsky et al., "A Ten-Year Analysis of Non-Medical Drug Use Behavior at Five American Universities," *Journal of School Health* 51 (January 1981), 52–53; "The Growth of Cocaine Abuse: A Report by the Strategic Cocaine Unit of the DEA Office of Intelligence," *Drug Enforcement* 9 (Fall 1982), 18–20; Charles Blau, "Role of the Narcotic and Dangerous Drug Section in the Federal Government's Fight Against Drug Trafficking," *Drug Enforcement* 11 (Summer 1984), 17; Peter Kerr, "Rising Concern on Drugs Stirs Public to Activism," *New York Times*, August 10, 1986, Sec. 1, p. 28; Joel Brinkley, "Experts See U. S. Cocaine Problem as Continuing Despite Big Raids," *New York Times*, August 24, 1986, Sec. 1, p. 1; Louis L. Cregler and Herbert Mark, "Medical Complications of Cocaine Abuse," *New England Journal of Medicine* 315 (1986), 1495–1500; and Elaine Sciolino with Stephen Engelberg, "Drive Against Narcotics Foiled by Security Fears," *New York Times*, April 10, 1988, Sec. 1, p. 1.

30. Selwyn Raab, "Drug Flood Altering Patterns of Use," *New York Times*, May 20, 1984, p. 50. Statistical information on the use of cocaine and other drugs by methadone patients may be found in Ball et al., "Characteristics," tables 621–26.

31. Newman interview, cited above. See also Barry Spunt et al., "Methadone Diversion: A New Look," *Journal of Drug Issues* 16 (1986), 569–83, and James V. Spotts and Franklin C. Shontz, *The Life Styles of Nine American Cocaine Users: Trips to the Land of Cockaigne* (Washington, D.C.: G.P.O., 1976), 14. A good, if somewhat exaggerated, example of the criticism generated by diversion and "cheating" is Edward Jay Epstein, *Agency of Fear: Opiates and Political Power in America* (New York: Putnam, 1977), 246–50.

32. The idea that increased cocaine consumption was partly a substitute for the amphetamines is developed in Brecher, 267–303. Brecher published his study in 1972; since then amphetamine use has continued to decline as cocaine use has risen. See Robert D. Budd, "Drug Use Trends among Los Angeles County Probationers over the Last Five Years," *American Journal of Drug and Alcohol Abuse* 7 (1980), 59; Goldstein et al., "Drug Dependence and Abuse," 94.

33. Wholesale price data are in "Nation's No. 1 Concern, but Politics Blurs Facts," *New York Times*, September 9, 1984, p. 12; for retail prices see Thomas E. Ricks, "The Cocaine Business: Big Risks and Profits, High Labor Turnover," *Wall Street Journal*, June 30, 1986, p. 1.

34. Cocaine, because of its ability to generate more powerful sensations during orgasm; opium, because of its ability to delay male orgasm, and thus provide more satisfaction for the female partner. See also George R. Gay et al.,

"Love and Haight: The Sensuous Hippie Revisited. Drug/Sex Practices in San Francisco, 1980–81," *Journal of Psychoactive Drugs* 14 (1982), 115–16.

35. Jerry Williams, "Cocaine Culture in New York City," Columbia University Faculty Seminar on Drugs and Society, December 5, 1985.

36. "Special Report: Black Tar Heroin in the United States," 19; the shotgun analogy is from Dr. Frank Gawin, remarks made at "The Cocaine Epidemic: A Symposium on Assessment and Treatment Approaches," University of Hartford, June 13, 1986.

37. Robert D. Budd, "The Use of Diazepam and of Cocaine in Combination with Other Drugs by Los Angeles County Probationers," *American Journal of Drug and Alcohol Abuse* 8 (1981), 249–55. [William Hopkins] "A Study of Crack Smokers" (NYDSAS Report, June 6, 1986), 2, notes that a variety of drugs, including pills, alcohol, and marijuana, have been used to cope with the aftereffects of crack. For more on the spread of crack smoking and its consequences, see James N. Hall, "Cocaine Smoking Ignites America," *Street Pharmacologist* 9 (January 1986), 1.

38. *Newsweek* is representative of the change. In 1971 its coverage was balanced, matter-of-fact, and decidedly not alarmist; by 1986 crack was on the cover and held responsible for "an epidemic of urban lawlessness" and the destruction of "thousands of young lives" (cf. "It's the Real Thing," *Newsweek* 78 [September 27, 1971] and Tom Morganthau et al., "Crack and Crime," *Newsweek* 107 [June 16, 1986]).

39. Quoted in Erik Eckholm, "Cocaine's Vicious Spiral: Highs, Lows, Desperation," *New York Times*, August 17, 1986, Sec. 4, p. 24. See also the comments by Frank Gawin in Virginia Cowart, "National Concern About Drug Abuse Brings Athletes Under Unusual Scrutiny," *Journal of the American Medical Association* 256 (1986), 2459.

40. Sheila Blume, "National Patterns of Alcohol Use and Abuse," in Robert B. Millman et al., eds., *Research Developments in Drug and Alcohol Use* (New York: New York Academy of Sciences, 1981), 6; David E. Kyvig, *Repealing National Prohibition* (Chicago: University of Chicago Press, 1979), 202. On the recent decline in consumption, see U.S. Department of Commerce, Bureau of the Census, *Statistical Abstract of the United States, 1986* (Washington D.C.: G.P.O., 1985), 759.

41. "Letter from a Master Addict to Dangerous Drugs," *British Journal of Addiction* 53 (1957), 128. This article was written in Venice, Italy, in 1956, and published in January of 1957.

42. Gawin symposium remarks.

43. Santangelo interview.

44. On the European situation see Lee I. Dogoloff and Caroline M. Devine, "International Patterns of Drug Abuse and Control," in Millman et al., 17, and Laura M. Wicinski, "Europe Awash with Heroin," *Drug Enforcement* 8 (Summer 1981), 14–16.

45. Salerno interview.

46. The connection between drugs and corruption was emphasized in other films as well. Both *The Godfather* (Part 1, 1972) and *Scarface* (1983) featured grafting officers who misjudged the immunity conferred by their rank and who,

in a dramatic touch, were gunned down by the fictional gangsters Michael Corleone and Tony Montana. A similar fate, if different executioner, awaited the crooked cops in *Witness* (1985).

47. David L. Westrate, "Drug Trafficking and Terrorism," *Drug Enforcement* 12 (Summer 1985), 19–24; Alan Riding, "Colombians Grow Weary of Waging the War on Drugs," *New York Times*, February 1, 1988, pp. A1, A14; and Mills, *Underground Empire*, 3, 547, 561, 807, 1139–43, 1149–58, et passim. The DEA agents were Enrique Camarena, who was murdered in a way that suggests official collusion, and Victor Cortez, who was tortured by the Jalisco state police.

48. Mathea Falco, "The Big Business of Illicit Drugs," *New York Times Magazine*, December 11, 1983, p. 110; "Lucrative, Illegal and Corrupt," *World Development Forum* 5 (November 15, 1987), 2.

49. James Chace, "Getting to Sack the General," *New York Review of Books*, 35 (April 28, 1988), 52–53; Mills, *Underground Empire*, 218–23, 358–65, 383–85, 727, 731, 788–89, 1133, 1140–42; McCoy et al., *Politics of Heroin*, 218, 264–81, 309–13, 350.

50. Chiefly during World War II, which was otherwise such a boon to Anslinger's efforts to control the international traffic. The American branch of the Mafia collaborated with the Office of Naval Intelligence in providing waterfront security for New York City; the Sicilian branch helped the army with the reconquest and occupation of Mussolini's Italy. One result was that Luciano was released from prison, deported, and able to play a key role in reviving the postwar heroin trade (McCoy et al., 20–29).

51. "Time for a Real War on Drugs," *Newsweek* 106 (September 2, 1985), 13.

52. Although the Reagan administration subsequently reneged on some of the promised expenditures; cf. Linda Greenhouse, "Congress Approves Anti-Drug Bill as Senate Bars a Death Provision," *New York Times*, October 18, 1986, pp. 1, 33, and Bernard Weinraub, "In Reagan's Drug War, Congress Has the Big Guns," *New York Times*, March 15, 1987, Sec. 4, p. 5. The political logic of this bill, which President Reagan signed into law on October 27, 1986, is apparent when one considers poll data showing that Americans then ranked drug abuse as a national problem second only to the federal deficit (*Wall Street Journal*/NBC News Poll, p. 1 of the *Journal* for October 24, 1986). Politicians were not the only ones to jump on the antidrug bandwagon. Journalists and editorialists also scrabbled aboard, e.g., "It's time to take the gloves off. Time to act ruthlessly, without pity. Without remorse. Remove the scum that peddles this poison. What is so difficult? Arrest them. Lock them up and throw away the key" (full-page ad sponsored by *Hartford Courant*, November 19, 1986, p. E9). The same sort of rhetoric could have been found in virtually any Hearst newspaper in the 1920s and 1930s.

53. See Brecher et al., passim.

54. Grinspoon and Bakalar, eds., *Psychedelic Reflections*, 22.

55. Quoted in "What is Our Drug Problem?" *Harper's* 271 (December 1985), 51.

56. William Butler Eldridge, *Narcotics and the Law*, 2nd rev. ed. (Chicago: University of Chicago Press, 1967), 118.

57. For a review of the statistical information on this point, see ch. 4 of Alfred

Lindesmith, *The Addict and the Law*, and ch. 5 of Courtwright, *Dark Paradise*. There was a long-term decline in the total number of narcotic addicts between 1910 and 1940, but this was due primarily to a decline in *medical* addiction. Very few new medical addicts were being created and many old ones, left over from the nineteenth century, were dying off. The Bureau's efforts were targeted at nonmedical addicts, and their numbers did not appreciably diminish, except during World War II.

Epilogue to the 2012 Edition: America's Longest War

One day in 1980, as we were returning from an interview in Queens, a stranger approached us on the subway. He had the look of an out-of-town businessman: coat, tie, baffled expression. "Can you tell me," he asked, "what has happened to my city?" "What do you mean?" one of us replied warily. He didn't *look* like a crazy person. He wasn't. He had grown up in New York and moved away in the early 1960s. He had just made his first trip back to his old neighborhood, abandoned by manufacturers and blighted beyond recognition by drugs and crime.

The encounter came back to us when we wrote, in the original epilogue, of the extraordinary changes in the American drug scene after 1965. In 1980, when we began our interviews, rates of consumption for illicit drugs and alcohol had just reached their twentieth-century peaks in the United States. In the inner cities, where the rates were higher still, the consequences were obvious and devastating. By the time *Addicts Who Survived* appeared in print in 1989, the rates had begun declining, but the drug war had expanded beyond anything in Harry Anslinger's wildest dreams. Narcotic agents targeted not just heroin, but marijuana, cocaine, amphetamines, barbiturates, hallucinogens, and a host of other psychoactive drugs of minor concern before 1965. As we composed the narratives we realized that, like archaeologists scouting in a jungle, we had stumbled upon a lost world. Although drug use in the "classic era" was hardly innocent—our second interviewee was a convicted murderer—it was simpler and more contained than anything in 1980s America.

Now nearly another quarter century has passed. Despite many hopeful developments—new treatment and harm-reduction strategies, new therapies for HIV/AIDS patients, new scientific understanding of addiction—the American drug problem has become even more complex and politically fraught. The reissue of *Addicts Who Survived* has given us a chance to describe these developments and to revisit the question posed in the original epilogue: What have been the most important changes in drug use, policy, and treatment in the recent past?

Marijuana's comeback would have to rank at or near the top of the list. By virtually any measure—arrests, incidence, peer disapproval—adolescent marijuana use fell steadily during the 1980s. In 1979 about 3 million Americans tried marijuana for the first time; in 1990 only 1.5 million did so, a decline of 50 percent. Pot looked like the drug war's biggest victory. Unquestionably, it was the one most pleasing to suburban parents worried about their children drifting into a countercultural lifestyle.

Then, to the dismay of federal officials, the 1990s turned into the 1960s. Incidence began rising until, in 2000, there were as many new marijuana users (3 million) as there had been back in 1979. In 1986, when Ronald and Nancy Reagan declared war on drugs, just one in four Americans favored marijuana legalization. By 2000 one in three favored legalization; by 2011 one in two. The young and socially liberal were the most supportive, the old and socially conservative the most opposed—though Pat Robertson, the octogenarian televangelist, proved a notable exception. "If people can go into a liquor store and buy a bottle of alcohol and drink it at home legally," Robertson said in 2012, "then why do we say that the use of this other substance is somehow criminal?"[1]

The same logic applied to medicine. If patients could alleviate symptoms with other drugs, why not with marijuana? Medical marijuana advocates, as they came to be known, disputed the plant's legal classification as lacking any medicinal value. They presented case stories of sympathetic patients who benefited from using marijuana. And they pointed out that the denial of legal purchase for such patients produced no public health or safety benefit. These were plausible arguments, or plausible enough that, in 1996, voters in California and Arizona approved initiatives intended to let physicians authorize patients to smoke marijuana.

Critics called the medical marijuana movement a stalking horse for full legalization and a means of diversion to recreational users. Both charges contained an element of truth. No one supposed California's two hundred thousand physician-approved marijuana smokers were all chronically ill, or that all the state's lucrative marijuana crop was going to medically certified patients. Even so, thirteen more states and the District of Columbia enacted medical marijuana measures by the end of 2010. Marijuana turned out to be the weakest front in the drug war—not only in the United States but throughout the world, where cannabis remained the most commonly produced, trafficked, and consumed illicit drug.[2]

Stimulants other than cocaine made a similar comeback during the 1990s, although in a variety of guises. Illicit manufacturers cranked out methamphetamine; licit manufacturers produced Ritalin and Adderall and similar drugs used to treat attention deficit hyperactivity disorder (ADHD). In 2001 American pharmacists filled 369 percent more prescriptions for stimulant drugs than they had in 1992, primarily as a result of more frequent diagnoses of ADHD. Whatever the therapeutic intention, the pills did not always end up in the hands of those for whom they were prescribed. Some students took diverted pills to cram for exams and complete school work; others crushed and snorted them simply to get high. "I realized that taking drugs was fun so I wanted to experiment," explained a twenty-one-year-old prescription drug addict. "Before that I was against it but this [Adderall] was a pill from a doctor that helped you take tests better. . . . There couldn't be anything bad about it."[3]

Ecstasy, an amphetamine variant with weak psychedelic properties popular on the rave dance scene, attracted more than four times as many new users in 2000 as in 1995. Like the hepcats who dabbled in heroin or the baby boomers who embraced marijuana, Ecstasy users discovered an identity as well as a high. "Like you were either a skater or a prep, or, you know, a goth, or whatever," explained a nineteen-year-old named Natalie. "And like I didn't feel like I fit into any of those categories. And so then it was like, 'Oh, I'm a raver.' Like I finally figured out who I am."[4]

Cocaine, one of the few illicit drugs whose domestic stock fell during the 1990s, showed that identity could also work *against* recruitment. Teens, particularly black urban teens, were more inclined to taunt "thirsty crackheads" than to emulate them. They preferred pot, which was plentiful and seemingly benign—a misimpression, given that some users eventually became dependent. But there was no denying the generation gap. By 1992 arrestees in Washington, D.C., aged twenty and under tested positive for cannabis more often than cocaine. Those thirty-six and older still preferred cocaine. None of this deterred cocaine traffickers, who shifted more of their product to western and central Europe and Brazil to compensate for slackening demand in the United States.[5]

Researchers Andrew Golub and Bruce Johnson thought the marijuana boom of the 1990s illustrated an enduring truth about American drug epidemics. Teenagers liked drugs. But they shunned the ones that had messed up their elders, as heroin injection had done to the generation born in 1945–54 or cocaine and crack had done to the generation born in 1955–69. Yet older users—the ones who survived outside of institutions—continued to consume the hard drugs of their youth, which traffickers continued to supply. Like the markets for clothing or music or hairdos, the market for drugs was stratified by age.[6]

One thing that kept heroin from becoming completely *dépassé* was its rising quality. Colombian heroin, smuggled into the country by expendable couriers, was particularly potent. By 1994 street-heroin purity, which had averaged 3 to 10 percent in the 1970s and 1980s, had risen to 40 percent nationally, higher still in competitive markets like New York City. Heroin that pure could be sniffed or smoked, which reduced stigma and the risk of infection. Overdose remained a menace, as heroin-related deaths climbed from about two thousand annually in 1990 to nearly four thousand in 1996. Heroin dealers (many of whom also sold cocaine) served a mixed clientele: aging addicts from the Vietnam-era epidemic, cocaine and crack addicts who needed to come down, and a smattering of young bohemians. The last drew the wrath of newspaper editorialists, as did strung-out fashion models condemned for promoting "heroin chic."[7]

In hindsight, however, the late-1990s narcotic trend that had the most lasting impact was the growing misuse of narcotic pain medications. During the ten years after 1986, while the war on illicit drugs raged, specialists in pain medicine and palliative care mounted a quiet counterrevolution against the underutilization of prescription narcotics. A serious public health problem in the aggregate, untreated pain was an avoidable tragedy for individual patients. New research suggested that many patients with chronic, non-cancer pain could benefit from long-term opioid treatment. The dose could be "titrated to effect," or gradually increased while physicians monitored side effects.

A breakthrough of sorts occurred in December 1995, when the Food and Drug Administration (FDA) approved OxyContin for the treatment of moderate to severe pain. OxyContin contained oxycodone, a semisynthetic derivative of thebaine, an opium alkaloid chemically similar to morphine. But the pills had a time-release feature that reduced the risk of abuse, overdose, and addiction. Seizing (in fact, bankrolling) the new dispensation of liberalized narcotic prescription for chronic pain, Purdue Pharma aggressively promoted OxyContin to general practitioners. In theory, they could give pain patients their lives back. All they had to do was to establish and maintain the correct dose. In practice, that is what most physicians and patients did. OxyContin sales rose gratifyingly, from fifty-five million dollars in 1996 to well over a billion dollars in 2000.[8]

Other pharmaceutical boats rose on the same tide. Sales of all narcotic painkillers quadrupled between 1999 and 2010. American pharmacies dispensed sixty-nine tons of pure oxycodone in 2010 and forty-two tons of pure hydrocodone, a milder but nonetheless still potent narcotic. In 5 mg pills, that worked out to forty Percocets and twenty-four Vicodins for every man, woman, and child in the United States.[9]

The prescription narcotic boom had a dark side. A minority of patients—estimates ranged widely, from 3 to 40 percent—began manifesting addiction-like symptoms, such as seeking additional drugs. There was a limit to upping the prescribed dosage, as high-dose patients were more prone to falls, fractures, respiratory depression, overdose, and other life-threatening problems. "Risk goes up with dose, even if it's well done," explained psychiatrist Mark Sullivan. "We've never really exposed so many people to so much drug for so long. We don't really know what the long-term results are."[10]

Prescription narcotic users discovered that they could bypass the time-release feature by crushing the pills and then snorting or injecting the powder for a heroin-like high. Word spread among people who would have shunned heroin. "I don't have to go to the thug on the corner in the 'hood late at night to get my pills," said Ebony Davis, a social worker in Jacksonville, Florida. "I just go to a pharmacy. I can just smile, and the pharmacist looks at me, and it's all good, you know. . . . Even when you get to buyin' 'em off the street, or buyin' 'em from someone, they come in pill form, and we're taught as kids pills are OK if they're given to you." Paula, a blonde West Virginian, began experimenting with "oxys" at age twenty-one. "When you get that oxy buzz, you're happy," she said. "Your body don't hurt. Nothing can bring you down. It's a high where you don't have to think about nothing. All your troubles go away. You feel like everything is lifted off your shoulders." Lifted, that is, until addiction set in. "At first you do them to get high, and then after you're addicted, you don't do them to get high—you do them to survive."[11]

Mid-century heroin addicts described the addiction process with virtually identical words. What had changed, though, was the source of supply. Those who used oxycodone or other prescription narcotics like hydrocodone and methadone (also prescribed for chronic pain) ultimately got their drugs from pharmaceutical companies, not smugglers. They lifted pills from relatives' medicine cabinets, gave or sold them to friends, scored from middlemen and fly-by-night pain clinics, or wheedled prescriptions from doctors, much like Mike and Brenda (see pp. 135–41). The medical makeover of supply, which caught the Drug Enforcement Agency (DEA) off guard, occurred in just a few years during the late 1990s and early 2000s. By 2005 one in twenty Americans over the age of twelve admitted nonmedical use of prescription pain relievers during the previous year—more than any other scheduled drug save marijuana. Sheila Gordon, the nurse-manager of a Florida methadone clinic, watched as her patient population "flipped" from heroin to pills. "I'm actually a little surprised when someone comes in and says their primary opiate addiction is heroin, not oxycodone," she said in 2010. National studies confirmed the trend and showed that pill patients in methadone programs were both younger than the old-style heroin addicts and warier of injecting drugs.[12]

While needle-shyness reduced the risk of infection, the trend toward prescription drug abuse, aggravated by the common practice of mixing narcotics with benzodiazepines like Xanax or depressants like alcohol, triggered an overdose tsunami. In 2009, for the first time in memory, more people (37,485) died from drug overdoses than from motor vehicle accidents. That same year Michael Jackson became the John Belushi of prescription drug addicts, succumbing to benzodiazepines topped off by a lethal dose of propofol, his preferred nightcap to combat insomnia. Famous or obscure, the overdose fatalities were just the tip of a medical iceberg. For every prescription painkiller death, there were ten admissions for abuse to treatment programs and thirty-two visits to hospital emergency rooms for misuse or abuse.[13]

Equally striking was the change in the geography of overdose and addiction. During the classic era, most addicts used heroin and most heroin came into the country through New York City. Importers sold to wholesalers in big cities like Chicago, who resold to distributers in smaller industrial cities like Cleveland. Heroin seldom reached remote provincial cities, to which some jazz bookers refused to send bands, knowing that addicted musicians could not score. Urban, hierarchical distribution produced a pattern of urban, hierarchical use: addiction mapped onto availability. The increase in addiction among black urban migrants (see pp. 14–18) starkly demonstrated the importance of proximity to big-city heroin markets.[14]

Prescription narcotics required no proximity to street dealers. "I call a friend in Colorado and explain it to him," said an OxyContin addict from suburban Pittsburgh. "'Hey, I've got this crazy pill, an OC 80, an OC 40. You've got to go to the doctor and get it. Tell him your back hurts.'" When drugs were legally available, all that was needed was motivation and technique. This was true not only for prescription narcotics, but for domestic methamphetamine "cooked" from over-the-counter cold medications containing pseudoephedrine in ramshackle labs in remote, often depressed, rural areas. Drug abusers and traffickers began turning up in midwestern towns, Appalachian hollows, and white suburbs where nonmedical drug addiction had been vanishingly rare. As in the morphine boom of the nineteenth century, the new addicts were geographically diffuse and generally obtained their drugs through medical channels.[15]

This is not to say that illicit trafficking ceased. Colombians continued to ship cocaine and high-quality heroin. Mexican traffickers shipped cocaine, heroin, and lower-potency "commercial-grade" marijuana across (and sometimes via tunnels below) America's vast southwestern border, which supplanted Florida and other east coast states as the primary zone of entry. Mexican traffickers also stepped up their production of methamphetamine, taking advantage of their greater ability to obtain precursor chemicals and to set up industrial-scale processing labs. One 2012 army raid, on a ranch near Guadalajara, discovered fifteen tons of methamphetamine packed in rows of blue plastic barrels, like so much flour. Although the Colombian and Mexican governments sporadically cooperated with U.S. efforts at interdiction, neither controlled the large and remote drug-producing and transshipping regions under the sway of heavily armed militia and murderous criminal gangs. For the same reason Afghanistan, on the other side of the world, remained a global center of opium and heroin production.[16]

Most of the smuggled heroin and cocaine continued to find its way to cities, particularly inner cities abandoned by middle-class residents and employers. Sociologist Elijah Anderson liked to tell a story about his father, a black sharecropper from Arkansas who found work at the Studebaker plant in South Bend, Indiana. He supported a wife and five children and had enough money left over to buy a new 1950 Buick Dynaflow. "Today my father's counterpart works at McDonald's," Anderson said. A young black man from a tough neighborhood found it hard to get anything better. His zip code marked him as surely as a rap sheet. Even if he had bypassed hard drugs for marijuana, he would flunk a urine test. Employers did not want him. His mother could not support him. But he could deliver drugs, provided someone didn't rip him off. So he bought a 9 mm pistol and started packing.

Everyone else was packing too—if not guns, then their belongings to get out of the neighborhood. The problem fed on itself, nowhere more so than in Detroit, which became a city with more citizens under correctional supervision than in unionized auto-factory jobs. "Drug trafficking has become the free market's answer to deindustrialization," wrote historian Eric Schneider. "No drug policy will be successful without confronting the fact that the drug economy is a form of economic enterprise that has evolved over time and that has become increasingly prominent as other sources of employment have disappeared."[17]

Even as the drug economy grew, the penalties for becoming involved in it increased. New York's 1973 Rockefeller Drug Laws proved to be only the first of many state statutes that imposed stiffer mandatory minimum sentences for drug offenses or increased prison time for repeat offenders. The federal government followed suit in the mid-1980s, singling out crack dealers for the strictest punishments. The average sentence for federal drug offenders in 2004, seven years, was 17 percent higher than in 1988. Enforcement intensified at all levels. In 1980 police arrested about one in every four hundred Americans on drug charges. From 1988 through 2010 they arrested about one in two hundred, year in and year out. (Roughly half of these arrests involved marijuana.) Part of a larger story of mass imprisonment—by 2002 American prisons and jails housed two million prisoners, a quarter of the inmates on the planet—the drug war unquestionably had its greatest impact on black men, whose incapacitation and felony records kept them out of the job and marriage markets, further undermining the basic sources of community stability.[18]

Thus policy came full circle. After a period of experimentation under Richard Nixon, Ronald and Nancy Reagan launched a "neoclassical" revival that marked—indeed, that celebrated—a return to the stigmatization and strict punishment of the 1950s. This neoclassical phase proved to have sturdy legs, a surprise given the obvious failure to suppress trafficking, the blowback in minority communities, the turmoil in producer states like Mexico, the growing diversion and abuse of prescription narcotics, the rising dissent over marijuana prohibition, and the success of AIDS-conscious European governments in implementing innovative harm-reduction policies. It seems odd that these developments failed to prompt an official rethinking of policy such as occurred in Vietnam or Iraq, two other long wars of disappointing outcome.

The answer to the puzzle can be found in the political dynamics of yet another lengthy war, the one over moral and cultural issues that reshaped American politics after 1965. Following Nixon's lead, Republicans and New Right activists learned that they could tap popular anxieties over race riots, antiwar protests, the counterculture, welfare fraud, and rising crime to defeat Democrats and undermine liberal power. The strategy of accusing liberals of permissiveness worked well in the socially conservative South, a vote-rich region where the GOP became competitive and, by 1984, dominant among white voters. It also worked well in crime-plagued cities, where voters enraged by "dope addicts and welfare cheats" fired off angry letters to editors, mayors, and governors. One woman apologized for her failure to type, explaining that "my typewriter was stolen."[19]

The catch was that, once Republicans gained office, they could not deliver everything that the social conservatives demanded. Nor did Republicans necessarily want to, as they differed among themselves over questions like abortion. They therefore concentrated their fire on the safest of safe issues: street crime, welfare dependency, and drug abuse. Democrats learned that they had to compete with the Republicans on these same issues or be tarred with the brush of permissiveness. The ensuing who's-toughest competition produced the 1986 and 1988 federal antidrug legislation. Once in place, the new policies developed institutional and partisan inertia. Calls for reform invited charges of softness and appeasement. In that sense, the drug war became the political equivalent of the Cold War.

The same dynamic explains the checkered history of narcotic treatment and harm-reduction programs in the United States since the late 1980s. As our survivors pointed out, narcotics per se did not pose the greatest danger to users. Contaminated equipment and accidental overdose were the most lethal risks. That was why oral methadone appealed so strongly to public-health pragmatists: being alive had priority over being abstinent. Even so, methadone advocates continued to battle opposition from abstinence-oriented treatment providers, requirements for tapered withdrawal or low-dosage regimens (particularly ineffectual when rising heroin purity tempted less stable patients to "shoot over their dose"), and the usual not-in-my-backyard resistance.[20]

The problem was less methadone maintenance, whose efficacy study after study confirmed, than the stigma surrounding methadone programs and the reluctance to regard clients as normal patients. William White, a clinician and drug-treatment historian, located the core of the prejudice in the belief that recovery from narcotic addiction could not begin until the use of methadone and similar drugs ceased. Yet no one assumed the same for asthma, hypertension, diabetes, or other chronic diseases flexibly managed with or without medications. Attention to the needs of individual patients, providing drug-based treatments for some and non-drug-based treatments for others, was a hallmark of good medicine. But the methadone wars of the 1960s and 1970s, and the moralizing of the 1980s and 1990s, had produced good medicine's opposite: a treatment system in which patients were "siloed" in overregulated, stigmatized maintenance programs or in rigid, drug-free programs with high rates of relapse.

White and other advocates of medication-assisted treatment wanted to break down the silo walls, permitting clinicians to individualize treatment, upgrade and diversify services in methadone programs, and provide "pharmacotherapeutic support" (medically indicated drugs) for those in nominally drug-free programs. The goal for all patients should be recovery, which meant improved general health and reintegration into families and communities, as well as ceasing destructive behaviors like injecting illicit narcotics. In hindsight, many of our interviewees were pioneers of recovery-oriented methadone maintenance, as this idea came to be called. They found in methadone not only a drug that prevented withdrawal and craving, but a belated means of putting their lives back together.[21]

Others found hope in novel treatments. Beginning in 1992, new combinations of antiretroviral drugs greatly improved and prolonged the lives of HIV-positive patients, whether in methadone or other drug treatment programs. Then, in October 2002, the FDA approved buprenorphine as a treatment for narcotic addiction. A mixed opioid agonist-antagonist often administered with naloxone in pill form to discourage abuse, buprenorphine was, clinically speaking, methadone-lite. It offered the prospect of medication-assisted treatment that was safer, easier to manage, and more convenient, physicians being authorized to prescribe thirty-day take-home supplies. Between 2003 and 2010 buprenorphine took off. The number of grams distributed to retail outlets rose more than a hundredfold.

Unfortunately, the same problems associated with methadone—diversion, abuse, overdose, and relapse during or after gradual withdrawal—soon appeared. Suboxone, a commonly prescribed pill containing buprenorphine and naloxone, became a "standby drug" for heroin addicts "'til they get their true fix," explained an Ohio treatment provider. Novices got something more dangerous, a nice narcotic high. Even so, the medical evidence showed that stable, long-term buprenorphine patients had far better outcomes than untreated patients.[22]

Buprenorphine treatment reinforced the maintenance advocates' modest counteroffensive against the drug warriors. In 2009 the National Alliance of Methadone Advocates renamed itself the National Alliance for Medication Assisted Recovery, formally bringing buprenorphine patients and prescribers into the coalition. AIDS advocates were natural allies, as were health officials concerned with preventing the spread of HIV and other needle-transmitted infections. Medical literature reviews made it plain that maintenance treatment reduced HIV infection and risk behaviors among injection drug users (IDUs). Still, as of 2007, only 9 to 19 percent of American IDUs were receiving either methadone or buprenorphine.[23]

The continued exposure of untreated or undertreated IDUs to potentially lethal infections inspired other activists to establish needle and syringe programs (NSPs) designed to provide users with sterile injection equipment and other health- and addiction-related services. By 2009 three-quarters of American states had at least one NSP. Jonathan Gagnon was one patient. "I was at my friend's house and they were shooting up Dilaudid, and they said snorting it and popping it would give you nothing like the feeling of shooting it, so I said, 'OK, let's try it.' Once I did it I fell in love." He wound up at the Eastern Maine AIDS Network in Bangor for support services, counseling, and clean needles. Although he was already HIV positive, Gagnon wanted to avoid hepatitis C, another serious infection common among IDUs. (By 2007 more Americans were dying of hepatitis-C-related conditions than were dying of AIDS.) Every time Gagnon acquired a clean needle—one of four thousand the clinic distributed monthly—the odds of such an infection spreading further in the community diminished. From a clinical and public-health perspective, NSPs were win-win.[24]

As data accumulated that NSPs improved health and saved lives, advocates pushed for federal recognition and funding, much as had happened with methadone in the early 1970s. The issue came to a head in 1998, when a congressional ban on NSPs temporarily lapsed. The medical and scientific establishment and AIDS advocacy groups urged President Bill Clinton to approve federal funding to expand local and state programs. But Republican congressional leaders (who threatened to block any funding and hinted at retaliation by denying *all* federal money to AIDS groups that used private, state, or local dollars for NSPs) weighed in against the move, as did Office of National Drug Control Policy director Barry McCaffrey and dozens of antidrug groups. It made no sense to facilitate drug use, McCaffrey reminded the president, while spending $195 million for "educating kids that 'drugs are wrong, and they can kill you.'" Sheila Moloney, executive director of the conservative Eagle Forum, decried "taking American tax dollars and buying free needles for drug addicts." Clinton gave in, saying later "there's just no way we could have done it." The ban on federal funding remained in place until late 2009, when a Democratic Congress finally voted to remove it, only to have the Republican Congress reinstate it in late 2011. The Tea Party was as unenthusiastic about NSPs as the Eagle Forum. Like much else in the American political universe, drug policy remained hostage to cultural warfare and partisan maneuvering.[25]

Medical research highlighted the irony. In 1973 Nixon's research-friendly drug war gave birth to the National Institute on Drug Abuse (NIDA). Over the next three decades NIDA-funded experiments gave rise to a new scientific understanding of addiction. Addiction was, in the words of NIDA director Alan Leshner, "a brain disease." The disease, manifest in the loss of control over drug craving, seeking, and use despite adverse consequences, was chronic and relapsing in character. Although addiction had a social and genetic aspect, it also produced long-term changes in brain structure and function that researchers could see in reproducible imaging studies. Intriguingly, the images of drug addicts' brains resembled those of patients prone to compulsive gambling, sex, shopping, and eating. It turned out that drug and behavioral addictions activated the same neural pathways. Epidemiological and genetic studies described similar overlap, such as compulsive gamblers' greater propensity to abuse alcohol and drugs. Clinical studies revealed that narcotic antagonists could reduce compulsive gambling and pornography addiction, apparently by limiting these activities' capacity to augment dopamine, the key neurotransmitter in the brain's reward system. In the new dispensation, addiction was an acquired malfunctioning of the brain's reward center—a distinctive, organ-based disease that should be treated like other diseases.[26]

"That is the good news," Leshner wrote in 1997. "The bad news is the dramatic lag between these advances in science and their appreciation by the general public or their application in either practice or public policy settings." Most people continued to see drug abuse and addiction as social problems to be met with social solutions, principally the criminal justice system. However determinative social circumstances may have been in causing addiction, they still regarded addicts as blameworthy weaklings "unwilling to lead moral lives and to control their behavior and gratifications."[27]

That was a fair complaint if we add that addicts themselves often resisted medical approaches and labels. In fact, the most common reason they avoided treatment was that they were not ready to quit using drugs or alcohol, or that they thought they could manage their habits on their own. Financial worries over uninsured costs and lost work time kept others away. Even so, Leshner had put his finger on something important. The neuroscience revolution had neither halted the drug war nor eliminated stigma and resentment, present among wary clinicians as well as the burglarized public.[28]

None of this means that fundamental change is impossible. History is patient. It took more than four decades before the classic antimaintenance regime cracked in the mid-1960s. The neoclassical regime has shown similar signs of aging and strain, particularly on the state level. Legislators have retreated, however unevenly, from marijuana prohibition and long mandatory sentences for drug offenders. Even New York's Rockefeller Drug Laws, the harbinger of state drug-abuse reaction, were liberalized in 2009, permitting judges more discretion over sentencing. Drug courts, first established in 1989 and numbering over 2,300 two decades later, were another sign of tentative liberalization. Though they differed (and still differ) over the acceptability of medication-assisted treatment, drug courts identified and diverted non-violent offenders into various drug and alcohol treatment programs and then monitored compliance. They represented coercion, to be sure, but something less than "Go Directly to Jail."[29]

Recent history thus boils down to partial but contested revival of the public-health approach within a moribund but lingering drug war. Should researchers go beyond advances like methadone and buprenorphine, and develop new and more effective therapies for opioid and other addictions to curb craving and block drug euphoria, public-health advocates might finally break the policy logjam. Not even the most ardent social conservative wants to pay for prisons to control that which could be treated in examination rooms. Until then, however, the moral drawn in the 1989 epilogue still applies. Drug policy is neither a simple driver of drug abuse and addiction nor a straightforwardly rational response to it. It is instead a congeries of a society's history, values, and prejudices. The difference between then and now is that, despite the gains in scientific understanding, the congeries has become more tangled than ever.

NOTES

1. Substance Abuse and Mental Health Services Administration, *Results from the 2004 National Survey on Drug Use and Health: National Findings* (Rockville, Md.: Office of Applied Studies, 2005), fig. 5.1, http://oas.samhsa.gov/nsduh/2k4nsduh/2k4results/2k4results.htm; Jonathan P. Caulkins et al., *Marijuana Legalization: What Everyone Needs to Know* (New York: Oxford Univ. Press, 2012); Frank Newport, "Record-High 50% of Americans Favor Legalizing Marijuana Use," accessed November 12, 2011, http://www.gallup.com/poll/150149/record-high-americans-favor-legalizing-marijuana.aspx; Michael Felberbaum, "Pat Robertson: Pot Should Be Legal Like Alcohol," *Salon,* March 8, 2012, http://www.salon.com/2012/03/08/pat_robertson_pot_should_be_legal_like_alcohol_2_4.

2. David Samuels, "Dr. Kush," *New Yorker,* July 28, 2008, 49–61; United Nations Office on Drugs and Crime, *World Drug Report 2011,* accessed November 12, 2011, http://www.unodc.org/documents/data-and-analysis/WDR2011/WDR2011-ExSum.pdf.

3. Nicolas Rasmussen, *On Speed: The Many Lives of Amphetamine* (New York: New York Univ. Press, 2008), chap. 8; Sean Esteban McCabe, Christian J. Teter, and Carol J. Boyd, "Medical Use, Illicit Use and Diversion of Prescription Stimulant Medication," *Journal of Psychoactive Drugs* 38, no. 1 (March 2006): 43–56; The CASA National Advisory Commission on the Diversion and Abuse of Controlled Prescription Drugs, *Under the Counter: The Diversion and Abuse of Controlled Prescription Drugs in the U.S.* (New York: The National Center on Addiction and Substance Abuse at Columbia University, 2005). The quotation cited here appears on p. 16, while the percentage appears on p. 29.

4. Molly Moloney and Geoffrey Hunt, "Ecstasy, Gender, and Accountability in a Rave Culture," in *Drugs and Culture: Knowledge, Consumption and Policy,* ed. Geoffrey Hunt, Maitena Milhet, and Henri Bergeron (Farnham, U.K.: Ashgate, 2011), 171–94. The quotation cited here appears on p. 178.

5. Gina Kolata, "Old, Weak and a Loser: Crack User's Image Falls," *New York Times,* July 23, 1990; Mark A. R. Kleiman et al., *Drugs and Drug Policy: What Everyone Needs to Know* (New York: Oxford Univ. Press, 2011), 13, 86; Caulkins et al., *Marijuana Legalization;* "Younger Arrestees in U.S. Favor Marijuana; Older Arrestees Stay with Cocaine," *CESAR Fax* (hereafter cited as *CF*), 6, no. 26 (July 7, 1997) http://www.cesar.umd.edu/cesar/cesarfax/vol6/6-26.pdf; John Lyons, "Brazil's Emerging Market: Crack," *Wall Street Journal,* January 21, 2012, http://online.wsj.com/article/SB10001424052970203750404577172982033792126.html.

6. Andrew Golub and Bruce D. Johnson, "The Rise of Marijuana as the Drug of Choice among Youthful Arrestees," *Research in Brief* (Washington, D.C.: National Institute of Justice, June 2001), https://www.ncjrs.gov/pdffiles1/nij/187490.pdf.

7. David T. Courtwright, *Dark Paradise: A History of Opiate Addiction in America,* rev. ed. (Cambridge, Mass.: Harvard Univ. Press, 2001), 179–85; Blanche

Frank, "An Overview of Heroin Trends in New York City," *Mount Sinai Journal of Medicine* 67, nos. 5 and 6 (2000): 340–46.

8. John K. Jenkins, "OxyContin: Balancing Risks and Benefits," accessed November 14, 2012, http://www.fda.gov/NewsEvents/Testimony/ucm115180.htm; Tina Rosenberg, "When Is a Pain Doctor a Drug Pusher?," *New York Times Magazine*, June 17, 2007, http://www.nytimes.com/2007/06/17/magazine/17pain-t. html?pagewanted=all; Paul Tough, "Hillbilly Hell," *Observer*, April 6, 2002, http://www.guardian.co.uk/theobserver/2002/apr/07/life1.lifemagazine3.

9. Chris Hawley, "Painkiller Sales Soar around U.S. and Fuel Addiction," April 5, 2012, http://www.usatoday.com/news/health/story/2012-04-05/pain killer-addiction-fuel-common-addiction/54034032.

10. John Fauber, "Painkiller Boom Fueled by Networking," *JS Online*, February 18, 2012, http://m.jsonline.com/topstories/139609053.htm.

11. Kate Howard Perry, "Death by Prescription Drug Overdose Hard for Families to Swallow," *Florida Times-Union* video, 3:40, September 24, 2010, http://m. jacksonville.com/news/crime/2010-09-24/story/death-prescription-drug-overdose-hard-families-swallow; Tough, "Hillbilly Hell."

12. "Nonmedical Use of Prescription Drugs More Prevalent in U.S. than Use of Most Illicit Drugs," *CF* 15, no. 36 (September 11, 2006), http://www.cesar. umd.edu/cesar/cesarfax/vol15/15-36.pdf; Perry, "Death by Prescription Drug Overdose"; Andrew Rosenblum et al., "Prescription Opioid Abuse among Enrollees into Methadone Maintenance Treatment," *Drug and Alcohol Dependence* 90, no. 1 (September 6, 2007): 64–71.

13. Lisa Girion et al., "Drug Deaths Now Outnumber Traffic Fatalities in U.S., Data Show," *Los Angeles Times*, September 17, 2011; Centers for Disease Control and Prevention, *Policy Impact: Prescription Painkiller Overdoses*, accessed February 22, 2012, http://www.cdc.gov/homeandrecreationalsafety/rxbrief/.

14. Eric C. Schneider, *Smack: Heroin and the American City* (Philadelphia: Univ. of Pennsylvania Press, 2008), chap. 1; Courtwright, *Dark Paradise*, 149–52.

15. Tough, "Hillbilly Hell."

16. Mark Stevenson and Arturo Perez, "Mexico Meth Bust: Army Finds 15 Tons of Pure Methamphetamine," *Huffington Post*, February 9, 2012, http://www. huffingtonpost.com/2012/02/09/mexico-meth-bust_n_1266251.html.

17. Elijah Anderson, "Violence and the Inner-City Poor" (lecture, Univ. of North Florida, Jacksonville, Fla., March 13, 2006); Heather Ann Thompson, "Why Mass Incarceration Matters: Rethinking Crisis, Decline, and Transformation in Postwar American History," *Journal of American History* 97, no. 3 (December 2010): 708; Schneider, *Smack*, 203.

18. U.S. Department of Justice, Bureau of Justice Statistics, *Compendium of Federal Justice Statistics, 2004* (Washington, D.C.: Bureau of Justice Statistics, 2006), 2, http://bjs.ojp.usdoj.gov/content/pub/pdf/cfjs04.pdf, 2011; Marc Mauer and Ryan S. King, *A 25-Year Quagmire: The War on Drugs and Its Impact on American Society* (Washington, D.C.: The Sentencing Project, 2007), http://www. sentencingproject.org/doc/publications/dp_25yearquagmire.pdf; "Arrest Rate for Drug Abuse Violations Decreases for Fourth Year in a Row; Still Remains

Twice as High as Rates of Early 1980s," *CF* 20, no. 42 (November 7, 2011), http://www.cesar.umd.edu/cesar/cesarfax/vol20/20–42.pdf; "Marijuana Arrests Accounted for 52 % of All U.S. Drug Abuse Violation Arrests in 2010 While Heroin and Cocaine Arrests Decline," *CF* 20, no. 43 (November 14, 2011), http://www.cesar.umd.edu/cesar/cesarfax/vol20/20–43.pdf; David T. Courtwright, *No Right Turn: Conservative Politics in a Liberal America* (Cambridge, Mass.: Harvard Univ. Press, 2010), 156, 169.

19. Judy Kohler-Hausmann, "'The Attila the Hun Law': New York's Rockefeller Drug Laws and the Making of a Punitive State," *Journal of Social History* 44, no. 1 (Fall 2010): 77. The quotations cited here appear on this page.

20. Harold A. Pollack and Thomas D'Aunno, "Dosage Patterns in Methadone Treatment: Results from a National Survey, 1988–2005," *Health Services Research* 43, no. 6 (December 2008): 2143–46; Mary Jeanne Kreek, "Methadone-Related Opioid Agonist Pharmacotherapy for Heroin Addiction: History, Recent Molecular and Neurochemical Research and Future in Mainstream Medicine," *Annals of the New York Academy of Sciences* 909 (June 2000): 194.

21. William L. White, "Medication-Assisted Recovery from Opioid Addiction: Historical and Contemporary Perspectives," *Journal of Addictive Diseases* 31, no. 3 (July–Sept. 2012): 199–206; Shalini Shah and Sudhir Diwan, "Methadone: Does Stigma Play a Role as a Barrier to Treatment of Chronic Pain," *Pain Physician* 13, no. 3 (May/June 2010): 289–93. Another consequence of methadone's stigma was its underutilization in chronic pain cases for which it was otherwise well suited.

22. "Buprenorphine Availability, Diversion, and Misuse: A Summary of the CESAR FAX Series," *CF* 20, no. 34 (September 12, 2011), http://www.cesar.umd.edu/cesar/cesarfax/vol20/20–34.pdf; Ohio Department of Alcohol and Drug Addiction Services (ODADAS), *Ohio Substance Abuse Monitoring Network: Surveillance of Drug Abuse Trends in the State of Ohio: January–June 2011* (2011), 133, http://www.odadas.state.oh.us/public/ContentLinks.aspx?SectionID=16e8e052-c81f-4fae-9ebc-3cb5bedab3cd; Caroline Helwick, "For Prescription Opioid Dependence, Relapses Associated with Shorter Treatment Course," *Medscape*, May 24, 2010, http://www.medscape.com/viewarticle/722342.

23. James L. Sorensen and Amy L. Copeland, "Drug Abuse Treatment as an HIV Prevention Strategy: A Review," *Drug and Alcohol Dependence* 59, no. 1 (April 1, 2000): 17–31; Bradley M. Mathers et al., "HIV Prevention, Treatment, and Care Services for People Who Inject Drugs: A Systematic Review of Global, Regional, and National Coverage," *Lancet* 375, no. 9719 (March 20, 2010): 1014–28, esp. table 3.

24. Susan Sharon, "Ban Lifted on Federal Funding for Needle Exchange," *National Public Radio*, December 18, 2009, http://www.npr.org/templates/story/story.php?storyId=121511681; Kathleen N. Ly et al., "The Increasing Burden of Mortality From Viral Hepatitis in the United States Between 1999 and 2007," *Annals of Internal Medicine* 156, no. 4 (February 21, 2012): 271–78.

25. Courtwright, *No Right Turn*, 237–38. McCaffrey to Clinton, April 9, 1998, Moloney to McCaffrey, April 9, 1998, and other pertinent needle-exchange material, box 122, Domestic Policy Council: Bruce Reed Subject File, William J. Clinton Presidential Library, Little Rock, Ark.

26. David T. Courtwright, "The NIDA Brain Disease Paradigm: History, Resistance, and Spinoffs," *BioSocieties* 5, no. 1 (March 2010): 137–47.

27. Alan I. Leshner, "Addiction is a Brain Disease, and It Matters," *Science* 278, no. 5335 (October 3, 1997): 45.

28. "Lack of Motivation to Quit and Health Coverage Top Reasons for Not Receiving Needed Alcohol or Drug Treatment," *CF* 21, no. 7 (February 20, 2012), http://www.cesar.umd.edu/cesar/cesarfax/vol21/21-07.pdf.

29. Celinda Franco, *Drug Courts: Background, Effectiveness, and Policy Issues for Congress*, Congressional Research Service Report for Congress, October 12, 2010, http://www.fas.org/sgp/crs/misc/R41448.pdf.

Appendix: The Interviews

CORE QUESTIONS

Personal Background

When and where were you born?
What sort of family did you grow up in?
What was the occupation of your father? your mother?
How old were your parents when they died?
How far did you go in school?
What jobs have you held?
Why did you come to New York City (if not a native)?
Have you ever been married?
Have you had any children?

Onset of Addiction

When and where did you first use drugs?
Which drugs did you use?
Did you use other drugs before using opiates? alcohol? barbiturates?
cocaine? marijuana?
Why did you first use drugs? for medical reasons? curiosity? because
your friends were using?
When did you first notice that you were hooked on opiates?
What made you realize this?
Did the friends you were using with also become addicted?
How much did the drugs cost when you began using?
How pure were they?
How did you administer the drug? sniffing? smoking? skin popping?
intravenous?
What was your initial dose?

Addiction Career

Did you increase the dose?
If so, how rapidly?
What was the highest dosage you reached?
Which opiates were available when you became addicted?
When (if ever) did you first use heroin?
Did you change methods of administration? When and why?
Did you attempt to quit voluntarily?
How many times and under what circumstances?
Do you have any addict friends who managed to quit and remain
abstinent, without resorting to other drugs?
How did you obtain opiates?
How did your sources of supply change over time?
How did prices fluctuate over time?
When were opiates especially abundant? scarce?
Was there ever a time when you were forced to abstain because there
were simply no opiates to be found?
Were you able, during times of scarcity, to "make" doctors?
How did you do this?
Which opiates did the doctor provide?
How did you support yourself and pay for your habit?
Did you have to resort to hustling activities?
Were you ever arrested?
On what charges?
How many times?
Did you spend time in prison?
Were drugs available there?

Methadone

How long have you been on methadone maintenance?
Which program(s) have you been in?
How did you hear about methadone?
Did your addict friends advise you against it?
What made you decide to participate in the program?
How did it alter your style of life?
What is your opinion of methadone maintenance?

Present Circumstances

What are your present sources of income?
Are your needs being met?
How has your addiction affected your relationships with your family?
Do you regret having become addicted?

Given that addicts seldom reach old age, to what do you attribute your longevity?

EDITING PROCEDURES

In order to illustrate the way in which we assembled the narratives, here are two examples, one relatively simple, the other relatively complex. The way the tape would read in transcript is compared with the way it actually appears in the book. The first excerpt, with italics denoting the interviewers' questions and comments, is taken from an interview with Emily:

Could you describe what life was like on the Lower East Side at that time?
Well, I'll tell ya, life was all shooting and tough guys and, uh, they broke into my mother's house and put the lights out and steal the bulbs, and I had to fight with them. I took care of my brothers and my sisters— I was the tough one in the house.
Mm-hmm. [Nods head for her to continue.]
And, uh, my mother was a super; I had to help her out. My father worked as a presser. He made maybe nine dollars a week. So I had to get up in the morning and help them with the barrels to put out. And clean the toilets that they were in, you know, if the landlord was coming I had to wash the whole building, and the floor and the . . .
Were they—when you say "clean the toilets," you mean that people didn't have toilets in their homes, they . . .
No—all in the hall.
Mm-hmm.
And we had to clean them if they didn't clean 'em.
Mm-hmm.
So I wouldn't let my mother and father do it—I did it. I put on the rubber gloves and I cleaned 'em.
How many—about what size tenement was this?
Four.
Four stories?
Four stories.

This became:
Life was all shooting and tough guys. They'd break into my mother's house and put the lights out and steal the bulbs, and I had to fight with them. I took care of my brothers and sisters—I was the tough one in the house. My mother was a super; I had to help her out. My father worked as a presser. He made maybe nine dollars a week. So I had to get up in the morning and help them put out the barrels and clean the toilets. If

388 ADDICTS WHO SURVIVED

the landlord was coming I had to wash the whole building, and the floor. It was a four-story tenement. All the toilets were in the hall, and we had to clean them if the people didn't. I wouldn't let my mother and father do it—I did it. I put on the rubber gloves and I cleaned them.

The second illustration is drawn from the interview with Lotty. Although she had a knack for recalling anecdotes and characters, Lotty had trouble with chronology and her attention would sometimes wander. These problems, by no means uncommon, were related to old age and failing health. To cope with them we adopted a strategy of gently nudging her back on the track, of returning her attention to episodes not fully explained or satisfactorily dated. This was largely successful, but it meant that information about a particular person or event was often scattered throughout the interview, and had to be pieced together. For example, there are seven passages about her first husband and the circumstances in which she met him:

Excerpt 1: Tape 1, Side 2:
    . . . Then I got the shot of the H. So then I married this guy that had a liquor and a heroin . . .
    That was the same guy who gave you the shot?
    No.

Excerpt 2: Tape 1, Side 2:
    Now, earlier, you had mentioned that you had married your husband, and that he had both a heroin and an alcohol problem.
    He was very good to me, but I used to lose a lot of sleep. He was drunk all the time, and he'd shoot heroin.
    Was he addicted to heroin?
    Oh, yes.
    He was addicted and drinking at the same time?
    And, not only that, he'd take any kind of a pill he could get his hands on.
    When did you marry this man?
    Oh, God, I stayed with him . . .
    Well, just approximately. Like, was this after 1933?
    Oh, sure.
    Was it around . . .
    I stayed twenty years with him, so you know . . .
    Well, when did you break up with him, or when did he . . .
    Well, his—he met a girl. And this girl must have been—I don't know, one of those things.
    Well, OK—so he left for another girl. Do you remember when that was?
    And he took her to San Francisco.
    Do you remember when that was?

And then I met this man . . . [Continues with anecdote about how she met her second husband in the office of a physician who wrote prescriptions for Dilaudid.]

Excerpt 3: Tape 1, Side 2

We want to talk to you about the Dilaudid—that's very interesting, but . . .
Yeah.

But we want to—it would be simpler if we could sort of go in sequence. So do you remember if you married this man, your first husband, like in the mid-thirties? Say by 1935 were you married?

Well, to duck the army, he—oh, he did all sorts of things, you know, to get out of going in the war. He didn't want to go in the war, and so he didn't go. Then, when he didn't go . . .

[Reel ends. Excerpt continues Tape 2, Side 1]:

OK, now, we were talking about your first husband.

Well, he was a sort of a pain in the neck, because I always—I always had to sit up and watch him, that he didn't burn us up.

So how did you meet your first husband?

Well, to tell you the truth, I went on a . . . a heroin party. You know, like it was ten or twelve of us, and we bought a big . . . they were selling them in capsules then, for two dollars apiece. And three people could get fixed up with it, and it was only two dollars a cap. And, so, we, uh, went on a party, and that's how I met him. So right away he started making a play for me. And he was six-foot-four and very beautiful, very handsome.

What did he do for a living?

Nothing. He was a thief. He stole a forty-thousand-dollar necklace. And he was good to me, he gave me two—two emeralds, he'd give me stuff, you know, that he stole. But he'd tell me, "Don't wear it right away," you know. He'd be afraid they'd find it, you know.

This heroin party where you were getting these caps—had you been a heroin addict for long when you went to this party?

Oh, quite a while. But what made me stay with him at all was that he was so sweet. When—he was six-foot-four, and so handsome. He had blond-gold hair and . . .

So. And you say the reason he married you was to stay out of the army?
Yeah.

So, all right, this would date this party to about, uh, 1940, 1941 . . .
Uh-huh.

Because that's when they were drafting people, or even a little bit earlier, to go into the armed . . .

No, he died—he died after my second husband.

Oh, I see. So, OK, so you—all right, now, to back up just a little bit, around 1933, give or take a year, you started using heroin. And you were addicted to the white stuff during the thirties. And, toward the beginning of the Second World War, you met your first husband at a heroin party. So you'd actually been using heroin for some time.

Oh, yes.

Excerpt 4: Tape 2, Side 1:

This heroin party that you went to, were . . .

[Coughs.] Excuse me.

Were these rich people that were there, like the opium smokers, or were they poor people or . . .

No, they weren't rich. But they were thieves, most of them.

They were a different class of people.

[Nods agreement.] A class of people. And you had to understand them. Like, once my husband got a forty-thousand-dollar necklace . . .

That he stole?

Stole. And he couldn't sell it that way; he had to break it up—had the jeweler break it up. And he would sell . . .

A stone at a time?

Two or three stones at a time.

Did you—you say you were at a heroin party, this is very interesting to us, because several of the people we've spoken to said that they shot up their heroin alone, by themselves.

Nah.

During the thirties, did you usually shoot up with other people?

No—oh, if I was sick, I would shoot up alone.

But you preferred to party with other people?

I liked a big party, I liked to see something going on, you know.

What happened at these parties besides people shooting up?

Well, you know, some of them drank with it. I never drank with it; I never liked booze.

Now, did you have your own works at that time?

Oh, I always I carried my own, because . . .

In other words, in these parties, you'd use your own works?

Yeah, 'cause you never can tell what you can pick up, you know.

Did you let other people at the party use your works?

[Lotty shakes head.]

No?

No. I'd tell them, "Look, for all I know you might have leprosy." [Laughs.]

Excerpt 5: Tape 2, Side 1:

. . . Even when you were married to your first husband, you would act as a mistress to other men? And make—you had connections?

I had connections, but I didn't have to do it, because my husband made enough money. You know, when you're stealing jewelry, you're making a lot of money.

Oh, OK, I've got it now. From around 1931 until the time you married your, uh . . .

Second husband.

Well, wait a minute. From 1931 until the time you married your first husband, just right before the war, he was trying to avoid the draft . . .

Yeah.

You were in fact mistress to different men, you had several connections . . .

Yeah.

Excerpt 6: Tape 2, Side 1:

When were you married a second time?

Oh, the second time. My husband took a floosie to San Francisco. And that was my chance to get rid of him, because I had been trying to get rid of him for a long time.

Excerpt 7: Tape 3, Side 1:

Did you ever smoke opium again . . .

No.

After you started using the needle?

No.

Did you ever sniff heroin?

No.

So you went directly from the opium pipe to the needle?

Uh-huh.

What about pills, like the barbiturates?

Oh, I don't like them. Because—I guess because I saw my husband take so many of them. And the condition he'd get in, you know. He'd put his head down like this ["nods"], you know, and you'd have to watch him every minute. Otherwise, you could be burned to pieces or anything could happen, you know.

These seven excerpts were combined thus:

Just before the war I married this guy who had a liquor and a heroin problem. To tell you the truth, I met him at a heroin party—like it was ten or twelve of us. They were selling capsules then for two dollars apiece, and three people could get fixed up with it. I would shoot up alone if I was sick, but I liked a big party, I liked to see something going on. Some of them drank and shot heroin, but I never drank with it, I never liked booze. I carried my own works, because you never can tell what you can pick up. I didn't let other people at the party use my works. I'd tell them, "Look, for all I know you might have leprosy." [Laughs.]

They were a different class of people from the opium smokers. They weren't rich, but they were thieves, most of them. My husband was a thief. I went on a party and that's how I met him. Right away he started making a play for me. He was six-foot-four and very beautiful, very handsome, with blond-gold hair. He ducked the army—he did all sorts of things to get out of going in the war. That's the reason he married me.

I didn't have to act as a mistress to other men, because my husband made enough money. When you're stealing jewelry, you're making a lot of money. He once stole a forty-thousand-dollar necklace. He couldn't sell it that way; he had the jeweler break it up, and he would sell two or three stones at a time. He was good to me; he gave me two emeralds, he'd give me stuff that he stole. But he'd tell me, "Don't wear it right away." He'd be afraid they'd find it, you know.

He was very good to me, but I used to lose a lot of sleep. He was drunk all the time, and he'd shoot heroin—he was addicted to heroin. And, not only that, he'd take any kind of pill he could get his hands on. I don't like pills, I guess because I saw my husband take so many of them. The condition he'd get in. He'd put his head down and nod, and you'd have to watch him every minute. Otherwise you could be burned to pieces or anything could happen.

I stayed twenty years with him. Then he met a girl, a floosie. It was one of those things. He took her to San Francisco. And that was my chance to get rid of him, because I had been trying to get rid of him for a long time.

Glossary

What follows is a glossary, not a complete dictionary; no attempt has been made to give all possible definitions for the various drug and underworld terms. The only definitions given are those that correspond to the way in which the terms were actually used in the narratives. There are, for example, at least two subcultural meanings of "acid": 1. bad, adulterated narcotics, and 2. the hallucinogenic drug LSD. Since only the first usage appears in the narratives, only the first definition is given in the glossary. Readers interested in more comprehensive definitions should consult the following: Richard R. Lingeman, *Drugs from A to Z: A Dictionary*, second revised edition (New York: McGraw-Hill, 1974); "Glossary of Addict Argot," in Alfred R. Lindesmith, *Addiction and Opiates* (Chicago: Aldine, 1968), 249–66; and J. E. Schmidt, *Narcotics Lingo and Lore* (Chicago: Charles C. Thomas, 1959).

acid: bad, adulterated narcotics.
Alvodine: trade name for piminodine esylate, a narcotic analgesic.
bag: a portion of narcotics, usually heroin, sold in folded paper or a glassine envelope, e.g., a five-dollar *bag*.
beat: to rob or cheat, especially in a drug transaction.
behind: after, especially after using a drug, as in "I felt good *behind* the shot."
bit: a prison sentence.
bonita: milk sugar, commonly used to adulterate heroin.
bookie: one who organizes and serves as a liaison for illicit enterprises, particularly gambling or prostitution.
booking: arranging for others to gamble or have sex with prostitutes.
boost: to shoplift.
booster: shoplifter.
boot: a powerful, euphoric sensation.
break: 1. (v.) to quit using drugs; 2. (n.) a period during which drugs are not used.

bring-down: a depressing, annoying, or "square" person or circumstance.

broad: a woman, especially a prostitute.

bull: a policeman.

burned: cheated by the purchase of bad drugs.

bust: 1. (v.) to arrest a person, especially on a narcotic-related charge; 2. (n.) the arrest itself, as in "my third *bust.*"

caps: capsules of varying size that were once used to sell illicit heroin and, less frequently, cocaine.

cheat: to use illicit drugs while in a treatment program.

chef: 1. (v.) to prepare an opium pipe for smoking, usually by a group of people; 2. (n.) one who prepares same.

chemical: 1. bad narcotics; 2. an adulterant put in narcotics.

chippying, chippying around: to use narcotics occasionally.

clean: not using illicit drugs.

coke: cocaine.

cokie: a regular cocaine user.

cold turkey: abruptly and without any medical assistance, as in "I got busted and had to quite *cold turkey.*"

connection: source of supply of illicit drugs.

cook: 1. to *chef,* or prepare an opium pipe for smoking; 2. to refine raw opium so that is suitable for smoking; 3. to heat heroin and water until the heroin has dissolved and can be injected. Also referred to as *cooking up.*

cooker: a small container, such as a bent spoon, in which heroin and water are heated until the heroin has dissolved.

cop: to buy drugs.

cop out: to bargain for a lesser prison sentence.

cotton: piece of cotton or cloth used to filter impurities out of the heroin solution before it is injected.

croaker: a doctor, especially one who will write prescriptions for narcotics.

cut: 1. (v.) to adulterate drugs; 2. (n.) a substance used to adulterate drugs.

Darvon: a synthetic narcotic analgesic.

deck: a small amount of narcotics wrapped or folded in paper.

detox: 1. (v.) to detoxify, or eliminate narcotics and their effects from the system; 2. (n.) the process of detoxification, as in "I went through detox."

deuce: two dollars.

Dilaudid: a semisynthetic derivative of morphine.

dirty urine: a urine specimen that tests positive for the presence of illicit drugs.

do time: to serve a prison term.

dollies: Dolophine tablets.

Dolophine: methadone hydrochloride, a synthetic opiate.

dope: illicit drugs, particularly heroin.

dope fiend: 1. from the perspective of an opium smoker, a lower-class addict who resorts to the needle; 2. any narcotic addict, but especially one who consumes large amounts of drugs.

down: 1. hip, cool; 2. close, intimate.

drugstore junk: undiluted prescription narcotics.

dry: characterized by a scarcity of drugs, as a *dry* year.

eighth: an eighth of an ounce.

endorphins: peptides produced within the central nervous system that have effects similar to those of *opiates.*

fall out: to doze off after using a drug.

feds: federal law-enforcement authorities.

fish: a dupe or sucker.

garbage: bad, heavily adulterated narcotics. Similar to *acid* or *chemical.*

garbage junkie, garbage-can addict: an indiscriminate user who will take anything to get *high* and/or prevent withdrawal symptoms.

gee rag: a piece of cloth used to make the bowl of an opium pipe fit snugly into the stem.

get off: to use narcotics, especially by injection.

gob: a large amount.

good bag: relatively high-quality heroin.

green: inexperienced.

gun: a hypodermic syringe and needle.

H.: heroin.

habit: the condition of being addicted to narcotics, of having to use them continuously to avoid withdrawal symptoms.

hicks: shells, usually walnut shells, used in a sleight-of-hand game.

hide: a wallet.

high: a euphoric state, in a euphoric state.

hip: knowledgeable, particularly about drug use.

hit: 1. to inject with narcotics; 2. to adulterate narcotics.

hold: to prevent the onset of withdrawal symptoms, e.g., "One shot would *hold* me until I went to bed."

hooked, to get: 1. to become addicted; 2. to be arrested.

Hoosier: an addict who is not street-smart or experienced.

hoover: to snort greedily.

hop: opium prepared for smoking.

horse: heroin.

hot shot: an injection of poison, or of narcotics mixed with poison.

hustle: 1. (v.) to resort to illegal or quasi-legal activities to raise money; 2. (v.) more specifically, to engage in prostitution; 3. (n.) a particular criminal pursuit, as in "I never thought pimping was a good *hustle.*"

hype, hypo: hypodermic outfit.

jackpot: serious trouble, such as an arrest or prison term.

john: customer of a prostitute.

joint: 1. opium pipe and paraphernalia; 2. a place, such as a bar or brothel, where illegal enterprises are conducted.

Jones: same as *habit.*

junk: narcotics, especially heroin.

junkie: a narcotic addict, particularly one who is disreputable and/or uses a needle.

keep a habit up: to succeed in raising enough money and purchasing enough narcotics to use continuously, thereby avoiding withdrawal symptoms.

Kentucky: U.S. Public Health Service Narcotic Hospital at Lexington, Kentucky.

kick, kick it out: to endure withdrawal symptoms in order to quit using narcotics.

kilo: kilogram, the weight unit commonly used in higher-level narcotic transactions. One kilogram is about 2.2 pounds.

K.Y.: same as *Kentucky.*

lay-down joint: a place where opium is smoked, often a specially equipped hotel room.

layout: outfit for smoking opium.

lemon hustler: a con man who specializes in the *lemon game,* in which victims are enticed to meet beautiful women and, while waiting for them, are inveigled into a card, dice, or pool swindle.

Lex, Lexington: same as *Kentucky.*

Librium: a tranquilizer commonly used to treat anxiety and tension.

loaded: high on drugs.

lockup: jail.

LSD: a semisynthetic derivative of lysergic acid that acts as a powerful hallucinogen.

lush-worker: one who steals from drunks.

mainline: 1. (v.) to inject drugs intravenously; 2. (n.) a large vein, most often in the arm, into which narcotics are injected.

make a buy: to purchase drugs.

make a doctor: to get a prescription for narcotics by tricking, cajoling, or bribing a doctor.

manita: milk sugar used as an adulterant for heroin.

match players: con men who play the *match game,* which includes betting on and manipulating empty and full matchboxes.

max it out: serve a full prison term.

meet: an appointment to purchase drugs.

mess around: to use drugs.

methaqualone: a hypnotic and sedative drug best known in the United States under the name Quaalude.

Methedrine: trade name for methamphetamine, a central nervous system stimulant.

mill: a place where large amounts of heroin are processed.

mix: to adulterate.

monkey, monkey on my back: a narcotic *habit.*

morph: morphine.

mud: opium.

narcs: narcotic police.

Nembutal: pentobarbital sodium, a short-acting hypnotic and sedative.

Neosalvarsan: compound used to treat syphilis, somewhat less toxic than *Salvarsan.*

nod, nod out: to enter a dreamy, half-sleeping state after a shot of narcotics.

number: one's preferred drug.

O.D.: 1. (v.) to exhibit, or cause to exhibit, the symptoms of a narcotic overdose; 2. (n.) the overdose itself.

off: not using narcotics.

on: using narcotics.

opiate: a drug containing or derived from opium or its alkaloids.

out: a means of escape or release.

pad: a place where drugs are consumed, often an apartment.

panic: a period during which illicit narcotics are difficult or impossible to come by.

Pantopon: an opium preparation containing the alkaloids of opium, but with the inert gums and resins removed. Pantopon is one-half morphine.

paraldehyde: a hypnotic and sedative with a foul odor and taste.

paregoric: camphorated tincture of opium.

pat: to run one's hand gently over a victim's pockets in search of money or a wallet.

PCP: phencyclidine, an analgesic and anesthetic used by veterinarians that emerged as a black-market hallucinogen in the 1970s.

peel, peel off: to remove money, especially from a victim's wallet or purse.

P.G.: paregoric.

pickup: purchase of illicit drugs.

pill: 1. a pellet of opium placed in the bowl of an opium pipe; 2. a barbiturate or amphetamine drug, as in "These kids today are hooked on *pills.*"

pipie: an opium smoker.

pit: large vein in the arm leading to the heart.

Placidyl: a hypnotic and sedative prescribed for insomnia.

play around: to use narcotics irregularly and in small amounts.

pop: 1. (v.) to place in one's mouth and swallow; 2. (n.) an arrest; 3. (n.) a *skin pop.*

Population: see *Withdrawal.*

pot: marijuana.

punk out: to behave in a weak, juvenile, or inexperienced way.

pusher: the *square's* term for a drug dealer.

quarter: quarter of an ounce.

quinine: the antimalarial alkaloid of cinchona bark, sometimes used to adulterate heroin.

railroad: to convict after a hasty and/or unfair trial.

rainbow: a capsule of Tuinal.

rat: to inform the police.

red: a capsule of Seconal.

reefer: a marijuana cigarette.

Riker's, Riker's Island: New York City penitentiary in the East River, off the southeast Bronx shore.

ripping and running: stealing to raise money for narcotics.

roundup: coordinated arrests, as in a police *roundup.*

rush: an immediate and powerful sensation of pleasure associated with the injection of drugs.

Salvarsan: arsenical compound used to treat syphilis.

score: to purchase drugs.

scrip, script: a prescription, usually for narcotic drugs.

Seconal: a short-acting hypnotic and sedative.

sent away: imprisoned.

shake down: to extort money from someone engaged in an illegal enterprise, particularly when done by the police.

shit: 1. narcotics; 2. bad or inferior narcotics.

shoot up: to inject narcotics.

shooting gallery: a place, such as an abandoned building, where several addicts congregate to purchase and inject drugs, often using a common set of *works.*

short: lacking enough money to purchase drugs.

short count, to give a: to give short weight, i.e., to cheat by selling less of an amount than promised or expected.

shylocking: acting as a loan shark.

sick: experiencing withdrawal distress.

sixteenth: a sixteenth of an ounce.

skin pop: 1. (v.) to inject narcotics intramuscularly or subcutaneously, rather than in a vein. Cf. *mainline.* 2. (n.) an injection taken intramuscularly or subcutaneously, as in "She gave me a *skin pop.*"

snort: 1. (v.) to sniff heroin or cocaine up the nostrils; 2. (n.) the quantity of the drugs so consumed, as in "He took a *snort.*"

speedball: 1. (v.) to sniff or inject a combination of an opiate (most often heroin) and cocaine; 2. (n.) the combination itself, as in "She shot up a *speedball.*"

spike: 1. (v.) to *mainline;* 2. (n.) a hypodermic needle.

splittee: one who leaves—who "splits"—a therapeutic community before completing the program.

spoon: a small, variable quantity of narcotics used in lower-level transactions.

square: a conventional person who does not take drugs or *hustle.*

SSI: Supplemental Security Income provided by the Social Security Administration.

stash: 1. (v.) to conceal drugs; 2. (n.) place where drugs are concealed.

step on: to adulterate.

stick: stem of an opium pipe.

stool pigeon: police informer.

straight: the normal feeling that follows an addict's use of narcotics, the opposite of feeling or getting *sick.*

stuff: narcotics, sometimes also referred to as *hard stuff.*

take off: 1. to get *high* by injecting drugs; 2. to steal from; 3. to kill, as in "They *took* him *off.*"

tartrate: a small, collapsible tube with a hypodermic needle (Syrette) containing a single dose of morphine tartrate.

tea: marijuana.

tender: a tenderfoot or novice.

three-card monte: a game in which the dealer shows three cards, manipulates them by sleight of hand, places them face down on the table, and then invites bets on the location of a particular card. Three-card monte operators often employ a shill.

tie up: to use an improvised tourniquet such as a belt to distend the veins prior to an injection.

tight: close, intimate.

till-tapping: taking cash surreptitiously from a merchant's till.

tin: a small container of opium.

Tombs: New York City prison, so named because of the gloomy, Egyptian-style architecture of the original building on Center Street.

torn up: very *high.*

tracks: telltale marks of needle use, usually on the arm, caused by scarring and/or collapsed veins.

Tuinal: a hypnotic and sedative consisting of equal parts of Amytal and *Seconal.*

turn: to inform on or betray.

turn on: 1. to begin using drugs; 2. to get someone else to use drugs.

VDRL: acronym for Veneral Disease Research Laboratories.

vine: grapevine, or informal and clandestine information network.

Wassermann test: a medical test for the presence of syphilitic infection.

wasted: very *high* or intoxicated.

weight: relatively large quantities of drugs.

whack, whack up: adulterate.

white stuff: heroin.

Withdrawal: The place in Lexington Hospital where addicts were gradually withdrawn from narcotics before being sent to the general population area, known as Population.

works: apparatus for injecting heroin.

write: to write a prescription for drugs.

writer: a doctor who can be persuaded to *write*.

yellow sheet: record of arrests and convictions.

yen: craving for narcotics, especially during withdrawal distress.

yen-hok: needle used to hold and manipulate opium *pills*.

yen-pok: opium *pill*.

yen-shee: the residue, containing morphine, that accumulates in the bowl of an opium pipe.

yen-shee gow: instrument used for scraping *yen-shee* from the bowl of an opium pipe.

Select Bibliography

These works provide, from several different perspectives, detailed information on the social, legal, and medical aspects of American narcotic use during the classic era of narcotic control from the early 1920s to the mid-1960s:

Acker, Caroline Jean. *Creating the American Junkie: Addiction Research in the Classic Era of Narcotic Control.* Baltimore: Johns Hopkins University Press, 2008.

Anslinger, H. J., and William F. Tompkins. *The Traffic in Narcotics.* New York: Funk and Wagnalls, 1953.

Ball, John C., and Carl D. Chambers, eds. *The Epidemiology of Opiate Addiction in the United States.* Springfield, Ill.: Charles C. Thomas, 1970.

Belenko, Steven R., ed. *Drugs and Drug Policy in America: A Documentary History.* Westport, Conn.: Greenwood Press, 2000.

Bonnie, Richard J., and Charles H. Whitebread II. *The Marijuana Conviction: A History of Marijuana Prohibition in the United States.* Charlottesville: University Press of Virginia, 1974.

Brecher, Edward M., et al. *Licit and Illicit Drugs.* Boston: Little, Brown, 1972.

Burnham, John C. *Bad Habits: Drinking, Smoking, Taking Drugs, Gambling, Sexual Misbehavior, and Swearing in American History.* New York: New York University Press, 1993.

Burroughs, William S. *Junky: 50th Anniversary Definitive Edition,* edited and with an introduction by Oliver Harris. New York: Penguin Books, 2003.

Campbell, Nancy D. *Discovering Addiction: The Science and Politics of Substance Abuse Research.* Ann Arbor: University of Michigan Press, 2007.

Campbell, Nancy D., J. P. Olsen, and Luke Walden. *The Narcotic Farm: The Rise and Fall of America's First Prison for Drug Addicts.* New York: Abrams, 2008.

Chein, Isidor, et al. *The Road to H: Narcotics, Delinquency, and Social Policy.* New York: Basic Books, 1964.

Courtwright, David T. *Dark Paradise: A History of Opiate Addiction in America.* Cambridge, Mass.: Harvard University Press, 2001.

Eldridge, William Butler. *Narcotics and the Law: A Critique of the American Experiment in Narcotic Control.* Second rev. ed. Chicago: University of Chicago Press, 1967.

Erlen, Jonathon, and Joseph F. Spillane, eds. *Federal Drug Control: The Evolution of Policy and Practice.* New York: Pharmaceutical Products Press, 2004.

Joint Committee of the American Bar Association and the American Medical Association on Narcotic Drugs. *Drug Addiction: Crime or Disease? Interim and Final Reports.* Bloomington: Indiana University Press, 1961.

Jonnes, Jill. *Hep-Cats, Narcs, and Pipe Dreams: A History of America's Romance with Illegal Drugs.* New York: Scribner, 1996.

Kandall, Stephen R. *Substance and Shadow: Women and Addiction in the United States.* Cambridge, Mass.: Harvard University Press, 1996.

King, Rufus. *The Drug Hang-Up: America's Fifty-Year Folly.* Springfield, Ill.: Charles C. Thomas, 1972.

Kolb, Lawrence. *Drug Addiction: A Medical Problem.* Springfield, Ill.: Charles C. Thomas, 1962.

Larner, Jeremy, and Ralph Tefferteller. *The Addict in the Street.* New York: Grove Press, 1964.

Lindesmith, Alfred R. *Addiction and Opiates.* Rev. ed. Chicago: Aldine, 1968.

———. *The Addict and the Law.* Bloomington: Indiana University Press, 1965.

McWilliams, John C. *The Protectors: Harry J. Anslinger and the Federal Bureau of Narcotics, 1930–1962.* Newark: University of Delaware Press, 1990.

Morgan, H. Wayne. *Drugs in America, 1800–1980: A Social History.* Syracuse, N.Y.: Syracuse University Press, 1981.

Musto, David F. *The American Disease: Origins of Narcotic Control.* Third ed. New York: Oxford University Press, 1999.

Musto, David F., Pamela Korsmeyer, and Thomas W. Maulucci, eds. *One Hundred Years of Heroin.* Westport, Conn.: Auburn House, 2002.

Schneider, Eric D. *Smack: Heroin and the American City.* Philadelphia: University of Pennsylvania Press, 2008.

Terry, Charles E., and Mildred Pellens. *The Opium Problem.* New York: Bureau of Social Hygiene, 1928.

U.S. Senate. Permanent Subcommittee on Investigations of the Committee on Government Operations. *Organized Crime and Illicit Traffic in Narcotics: Hearings.* 5 volumes and index. Washington, D.C.: G.P.O., 1963–65.

White, William L. *Slaying the Dragon: The History of Addiction Treatment and Recovery in America.* Bloomington, Ill.: Chestnut Health Systems, 1998.

Index